Health

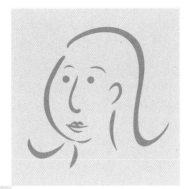

Gender Inequalities in Health

A Swedish Perspective

Edited by

Piroska Östlin,
Maria Danielsson,
Finn Diderichsen,
Annika Härenstam,
Gudrun Lindberg

Translated by Dorothy Duncan

Harvard Center for
Population and Development Studies

HSPH

Department of Population and
International Health
Harvard School of Public Health
Boston, Massachusetts, U.S.A.

Distributed by Harvard University Press

Library of Congress Cataloging in Publication Data

Könoch ohalsa. English
  Gender inequalities in health / volume editors, Piroska Östlin...[et al.].
    p. cm.
  Includes index.
  ISBN 0-674-00528-7 (pbk.)
  1. Health—Sex differences. 2. Medical care—Utilization—Sex differ-
  ences. 3. Sex discrimination in medicine. I. Östlin, Piroska, 1958
  II. Title

  RA564.85 .K6613 2001
  362.1´08—dc21

                                                              2001016628

Printed in the United States of America

HARVARD CENTER FOR POPULATION AND
DEVELOPMENT STUDIES
9 BOW STREET
CAMBRIDGE, MA 02138
USA

cpds@hsph.harvard.edu

Cover Design by Carol Maglitta Design

Contents

Preface to the English Translation

THIS PARTICULAR VOLUME IS the result of cooperation between various individuals from different disciplines and institutions on both sides of the Atlantic and was originally translated into English in response to interest from the Gender and Health Equity working group of the Global Health Equity Initiative (GHEI). This international network of researchers, funded by the Swedish International Development Agency and the Rockefeller Foundation, aims to support research and public debate on issues pertaining to the concept of fairness in health from the perspective of gender equity.

A first step towards this goal was to bring into the English domain a volume, showcasing Sweden's experience as a pioneer in the spheres of health achievement and gender equality. *Gender Inequalities in Health: A Swedish Perspective* provides a unique opportunity to review the lessons learned and the challenges remaining in addressing issues of social and health inequalities in a country, where unlike many other places, gender consciousness and social justice are prominently part of the public policy agenda. The volume documents how current health patterns in Sweden can be traced to historical social changes, and analyzes how the changing structure of Swedish employment and private life, create challenges in sustaining attempts to address gender and health inequalities in the future.

Apart from providing insights into the Swedish context, our hope is that *Gender Inequalities in Health: A Swedish Perspective* will be a valuable resource of comparative information on women's and men's health. In this volume prominent representatives of both social and medical sciences review previous research, basic concepts, explanatory models, possible hypotheses and new empirical data from Sweden and elsewhere, to understand more clearly how society over time shapes the different experiences of both men's and women's health. Apart from a general review of how gender analysis contributes to a better understanding of the biological and social patterns found in morbidity and mortality, this volume also details areas of health that characterize the complexity of some of these differences in specific areas. This includes areas that are traditionally associated with women, such as reproductive health, areas that are increasingly associated with women's higher health burdens like mental health, violence against women, and musculoskeletal disorders, and areas that are normally associated with men but that have important consequences for women, like cardiovascular disease.

Gender Inequalities in Health: A Swedish Perspective would remain unknown to the English speaking world, were it not for the encouragement provided by Lincoln Chen and Gita Sen in pursuing this project. In addition, we are grateful for the generous support provided by various donors, including the Swedish Council for Social Research, the Swedish National Institute of Public Health and the Swedish National Institute of Working Life. We would also like to express our gratitude to the Rockefeller Foundation for providing both financial and institutional support for the translation.

We were lucky to be able to enlist the excellent skills of Dorothy Duncan, our translator. We are indebted to the detailed attention paid and patience reserved by Dorothy and all the contributing authors over the two years it took to undertake numerous chapter revisions and updates. We would particularly like to acknowledge our debt and express our deepest gratitude to Asha George from the Harvard Center for Population and Development Studies for her never failing enthusiasm and hard work to complete this volume. Her review of all the chapters and insightful expert comments were extremely helpful for the authors. We owe much more to her than can be adequately expressed here.

Finally, this book could not have been transformed from a private, translated manuscript to a printed book in the public domain, without the commitment and coordinated hard work undertaken by Christopher Cahill and Winifred Fitzgerald at the Harvard Center for Population and Development Studies, Puritan Press, Ylva Strömberg at Studentlitteratur and Susan Seymour from Harvard University Press.

Piroska Östlin
Lead Editor

KAROLINSKA INSTITUTE

Foreword to the Swedish Original

THE PURPOSE OF THIS VOLUME is to provide a state-of-the-art understanding of gender inequalities in health by drawing on contributions from prominent Swedish experts in the fields of epidemiology, psychology, sociology, history and various medical specialties. The authors describe with empirical data from both Sweden and elsewhere the differences that prevail in men's and women's health and the reasons for them.

The volume advances the development of contemporary knowledge on gender inequalities in health. It presents current research findings on the health of women and men, along with insights into both the biological/genetic and social causes of the inequalities between them. Inequality in health between men and women, like inequality in the health of members of different social classes, is hardly new. Economic and social development processes perpetuate states of inequality. With this in mind, we argue that we all share responsibility for implementing appropriate public health policies to counteract these processes. This requires a steady stream of new insights and new solutions. Our hope is that this book will contribute to the public discussion of such solutions.

In addition to the authors, many people have contributed to this book. We would like to thank first all the members of the Network for Gender Studies on Health in Stockholm for their input during the planning stage. Special thanks go to Gunnel Boström, Maicen Ekman, Inga-lill Engkvist, Charli Eriksson, Margareta Falk, Maria Gerhardsson de Verdier, Malin Josephson, Eva Matell, Lennart Nordenfelt, Gudrun Persson, Claes-Göran Stefansson, Kerstin Tode and Denny Vågerö for valuable suggestions on the book as a whole as well as on individual sections. We would also like to express our appreciation to the National Institute of Public Health for its financial support. In addition, enabling resources were provided by the Centre for Epidemiology at the National Board of Health and Welfare, the Department of Occupational Medicine of Karolinska Hospital and the Department of Public Health Sciences at Karolinska Institute. Our sincere thanks to all of you.

STOCKHOLM, APRIL 1996

Piroska Östlin   Maria Danielsson   Finn Diderichsen
Annika Härenstam   Gudrun Lindberg

1

Gender and health: Concepts and explanatory models

Anne Hammarström, Annika Härenstam, Piroska Östlin

THIS ANTHOLOGY FOCUSES ON the concepts of gender inequalities in health, and examines various ways of explaining the links between them. The significance each of us attaches to these concepts has a great deal to do with individual factors (our own experience, education, philosophy of life, life circumstances, etc.), and is strongly affected by the cultural norms and values of society.

In a scientific context, a given concept can be defined in different ways, and thus its perceived significance depends on the discipline (medicine, psychology, sociology, economics, etc.) that forms the researcher's frame of reference. Moreover, even within a single discipline there can be different theoretical approaches and operational definitions of these concepts.

We do not seek to define the central concepts of this book using every scientific tradition or frame of reference. Nor is it possible for us to offer definitions or models on gender-related health differences that all of our contributing authors would wholeheartedly endorse. However, we would be remiss if we did not offer the reader some general discussion of the concepts with which we are dealing, and so we shall outline some of the most widely used and, in our view, most helpful concepts used in discussing gender perspectives on health.

In the following section we elaborate on the origin and significance of the concepts of gender and of health/illness. We also present some common explanations for differences in health between men and women.

The concept of sex and gender

The terms sex and gender are often used as synonyms in medicine, but in gender research the two concepts have fundamentally different meanings. "Sex" refers to the biologically given differences between men and women—a definition that at first glance appears to be relatively simple. Chromosomes, internal and external sex organs, hormonal makeup and secondary sex characteristics together determine an individual's sex.

The sex/gender distinction comes from the field of social psychology. During the 1970s, Gayle Rubin (1975) proposed a distinction between "sex" and "gender," the former being a biological, the latter a social concept. "Gender" generally

1

involves psychological, social and cultural aspects—the circumstances of a person's life, an individual's self-concept and behavior, how men and women are viewed in society, what they look like, how they think and feel, how they dress and how they perceive the world they live in (Puranen 1994). Thus, gender means the social, cultural and symbolic construction of femininity and masculinity in any given society.

From sex roles to the concept of gender

Sex roles became a central concept in research and discussion during the 1950s and 1960s. Women and men were seen as having been trained in stereotypical role behavior through their upbringing and other social influences. Role theories assumed a complementarity and a harmony between the sexes that played down social conflicts and differences.

However, the research into women's issues that emerged in the 1970s, particularly in the United States, dissociated itself from the concept of sex roles, believing that roles were being used as an explanation for gender constructions and discrimination against women. Criticism was heard from a variety of sources (Baude et al. 1987), which contended that role theories tended to end up simply describing a miserable situation, where women were passive objects of social norms. Moreover, the focus was frequently put on women's internal conflicts in such a way as to implicate women, rather than an imbalance of power, as the source of the problem. Critics felt that material conditions of society rather than forms of consciousness should form the starting point for analysis. Nonetheless, in Sweden research on sex roles had an important impact on policymaking and helped to promote equal opportunities for men and women.

Research on women's issues developed in Sweden in the 1970s in close cooperation with the international research community, and with close interaction with the new women's movement. Scientific objectivity as defined by the traditional male-dominated academy was called into question. Women's research showed how traditional theories and subjects, as well as methods, treatment and interpretation of results, failed to offer a true picture of the situation in society. Too little attention was given to women's lives, work and health, or the wrong conclusions were drawn. This led to the development of new questions, theories and methods. Women's knowledge and experience, which differed from men's, shed light on realities and connections that had previously been unrecognized. However, simply conducting research about women does not make it women's research (Harding 1986, Göransson 1989), as such research also involves examining conditions of inequality that have been shown to have a substantial effect on both women's and men's lives. Such conditions are found in the workplace, the private sphere and society as a whole (Carlstedt 1992, Koblinsky & Timyan 1993, Doyal 1995, Sabo & Gordon 1995, Hammarström 1994, Riska 1997).

Developments in theory have ushered in a change from women's research to gender research, in which the relationship between women and men is viewed as a socially mutable construction that is not predetermined by nature (Hammarström 1999). There is much discussion among gender researchers regarding concepts, theories and their applications. Maud Eduards (1995) points out the differences between women's research, equality research, gender research and feminist research by analyzing their political and theoretical implications. If research is aimed at increasing the influence of disadvantaged groups in society, it is essential that there should be a political link—in this case, to the women's movement. For this reason, Eduards sees a distinction with feminist research in the fact that it is based on both a theoretical and an activist political perspective.

The concept of gender

The fairly complicated question of the role of biological sex versus social aspects of being male or female was a focus of women's researchers in the 1970s. The term "gender" was employed to separate biological sex from the social, cultural and symbolic construction of femininity and masculinity. This represented a major departure from traditional male-dominated research, which used biological hypotheses to draw conclusions about women that had a devastating impact—including lower intelligence levels, passive sexuality and a genetic basis for maternal behavior and feelings (Lundgren 1993, Fausto-Sterling 1992, Hubbard 1992).

Before the term "gender" came into use, the word "sex" was applied to gender differences whether they were biological or socio-cultural in nature. Biological differences were regarded as the original and naturally occurring differences between men and women, and were considered to be of primary importance. Biology was, and still is, regarded by traditional medical research as unchangeable and deterministic. Biology was also seen to be the cause of a number of social and psychological differences between women and men.

The concept of gender was originally introduced in Sweden by Yvonne Hirdman (1988). She defines the gender system as the organizing principle underlying other systems. The gender system, based on two rules, organizes men and women into their respective gender. One rule is the distinct separation of almost all areas of life into male/female categories. The second rule is the male norm, that is a hierarchical system in which men are considered the standard for what is normal and valid. The system reproduces itself on three levels: the abstract level of cultural images, the institutionalized level and the interpersonal level.

It has become increasingly important to analyze the dichotomy between body and mind, nature and culture inherent in the two-fold concept of sex/gender. Gender researchers have criticized the stark distinction made between immutable biological sex, on the one hand, and socially-constructed gender on the other (Widerberg 1992, Lundgren 1993, Hägg 1993, Gunnarsson 1994, Hammarström

1999). Biological and social factors should be analyzed simultaneously; what is biological is also socially determined, and vice versa.

Gender research

Gender research is characterized by theoretical pluralism and grounded in multiple perspectives, where the use of one overarching theory can no longer be regarded as sufficient. Nevertheless, there is some common ground in the view of gender as a basic principle for how society is organized and in the impact of gender on all social relationships. Analyzing gender means investigating power relationships and the construction of the differences between men and women as well as the actual process that creates these differences. From a structural point of view, relationships between men and women can be characterized by male dominance, preferential right of interpretation and power. Although gender is a basic organizational principle in all societies, it is not a homogeneous category. Women, like men, are different principally in their age, social and ethnic background, religion, sexuality and geopolitical status (i.e., whether they live in developing or developed countries). These factors, along with gender, determine dominance in society. Lack of control and self-determination, in whatever form, contributes to the uneven distribution of health in society.

Our definition of gender research within the field of public health is:

> . . . research on health, where one basic question is the relationship between power and gender and its consequences for public health. The aim is to develop new and revised theories and methods and to seek systematic and comprehensive knowledge about the meaning of gender constructions, the importance of gender relations as well as the interplay between sex and gender in the uneven distribution of health in the population.

In public health, there is also a need for theoretical and empirical research on men. Like male gender researchers within men's studies,[1] we want to emphasize the importance of bringing a power and a profeminist perspective into research on men's health and illness.

Sandra Harding (1986) developed an overarching conceptual model of the gender system that can be helpful in understanding why this system is reproduced in an historical and cultural perspective. In her view, gendered social life is produced through three distinct processes:

1. Gender symbolism, which means that women and men are assigned different and opposing characteristics that cannot be attributed to actual biological differences, such as active/passive, rational/emotional, etc.;

2. Gender structure (or the division of labor by gender): Gendered social life is the consequence of organizing social activities in such a way as to fit in with the symbolic gender. The labor market, segregated along gender lines, is a clear example of this, with men and women on different hierarchical levels and within different occupational groups and branches;

3.   Individual gender as a process, where each individual is shaped by surrounding attitudes about what is appropriate for women and men, respectively.

The meaning of femininity and masculinity within these three forms of gender differs from culture to culture, although within any culture they act together. In Sweden, as in other countries characterized by a certain degree of equality between men and women, symbolic gender is a hidden but nevertheless important aspect in forming perceptions of masculinities and femininities.

How the basic gender system is to be viewed is one of the questions discussed among gender researchers and others who have examined the concepts used in research.[2] Hirdman (1988, 1994) uses gender as a sexual-power concept, describing the dominance of men and the subordination of women as one of the two underlying principles of the gender system. Harriet Holter brings up issues of male dominance, also pointing out that it is mistaken to believe that men have all the power and women none. Women should be viewed as active agents, even when they are oppressed by male structures. Nor should we lose sight of the fact that some men are powerless relative to other men, owing primarily to their class or ethnicity (Holter 1992).

Public-health research has used the class concept to study health differences among various population groups. This research has often turned a blind eye to gender. Gender research has criticized the scientific community for failing to study either women, their conditions or the power relationships between women and men. One example is a review of articles dealing with occupational epidemiology, which reveals that they seldom indicate whether the data for a given study refer to men or women (Ekenvall et al. 1993). Thus, it might be argued that established occupational research overlooks the gender aspect, which has resulted in insufficient knowledge of women's as well as men's work environment and health.

There are many different perspectives within current gender research. As a result, theoretical and conceptual developments continue in this field. Gender researchers today may hold different views and theories about how best to understand gender. It is therefore important to be aware of differences among researchers resulting from their gender, socio-economic status, cultural, ethnic and religious backgrounds as well as their home scientific disciplines. Whether we call ourselves researchers within women's studies, gender researchers or feminist researchers, it is critical that we define the theoretical and methodological bases of our work.

Additive research on women is not the same as gender research

The development of gender research is sometimes divided into different steps, where the first is to add knowledge about women to the already existing medical knowledge on men. It is relatively easy to argue that we need medical research not only on men, but also on women. Several of the chapters in this anthology are additive in nature, and this type of research can one day offer some insight into men's and women's health, ill health and life circumstances. But research on women per se is not the same as gender research. If it were, almost any research might be defined as gender studies, provided that the research were conducted on women or the results were divided by sex. Our experience as gender researchers within the field of public health has shown that when political priorities make grants and posts available, definitions and concepts may be applied opportunistically. Thus, any research on women (or men) might be defined as additive gender research, which would include, for example, all research in gynecology as well as any variable-oriented research.[3] In our view, the term gender research should not be applied to additive research on women. The concepts and theories used in gender research should always be defined accurately.

The concept of health

It is important to keep in mind the complexity and ambiguity of both general and scientific concepts of health and illness. The one-dimensional, biomedical view of health (sometimes referred to as the "engine trouble" model) that predominated for a very long time has been increasingly called into question in the last few decades. A broader view of what health means has emerged, with competition against the strictly biomedical view arising from humanistic and social-science perspectives on illness. This is only natural at a time when there is widespread agreement that findings such as health differences between men and women or different socio-economic and ethnic groups cannot be explained solely in terms of biology or genetics.

A holistic view of health and illness takes as its starting point an action-oriented perspective; central to this view is the individual's ability to act and to achieve essential goals (Nordenfelt 1987). In contrast, there is the analytic or bio-statistical theory represented by such researchers as Christopher Boorse (1977), whose point of departure is the function of an organ or a part of the body.

Analyzing gender and health requires using different concepts of health and describing health/sickness indicators of various kinds. Such a comprehensive view is essential, since the concept of health is many-faceted, and the distribution of poor health between men and women is not unaffected by the choice of health indicator. In discussing gender differentials in health, it is particularly helpful to address the distinction between disease, illness and sickness, as well as the links between these concepts. This is a distinction made most frequently in the fields of medical sociology, anthropology and philosophy. Andrew Twaddle, a proponent of such a trichotomy, proposed the following definitions (Twaddle 1994, pp. 22-6):

> Disease is a health problem that consists of a physiological malfunction that results in an actual or potential reduction in physical capacities and/or a reduced life expectancy. Diseases are events located at the organic level of organization. They are observable apart from subjective experience or social convention. They

are measurable with "objective" means. They fit the criteria of positivism. Diseases can be identified by measuring physiological changes. Disease is the all-but-exclusive concern of medicine as an occupation. The heart of medical practice is the ability to diagnose disease and to respond with appropriate treatment.

An illness is a subjectively interpreted undesirable state of health. It consists of subjective feeling states (e.g. pain, weakness), perceptions of the adequacy of their bodily functioning, and/or feelings of competence. Illnesses are events located at the personality level of organization. They consist of the internal experience of the individual. Whereas disease can be identified only through signs, illness can be identified only through symptoms. The statistical measurement of illness consists of self-reports of symptoms and/or self-ratings of health status.

Sickness is a social identity. It is the poor health or the health problem(s) of an individual as defined by others with reference to the social activity of that individual. Unlike disease, which is defined by organic functioning, or illness, which is defined by subjective feeling states, sickness is defined by participation in the social system. The most direct measures of sickness are made by either observing the social participation of the individual and his or her interaction with others or by interviews.

At the same time, however, the distinction between disease, illness and sickness should not be overdrawn. It is most common for them to coincide: Somatic changes (disease) and the experience of such changes (illness) generally bring about a social response (sickness). This is the case when the individual "feels unwell" because of changes in normal body functions, which are subject to diagnosis. When the person's level of performance does not meet a conventional social standard, he or she is certified as sick. There are, though, instances when disease, illness and sickness do not overlap: A person may suffer from high blood pressure (disease) without knowing it or feeling ill (illness). Moreover, people can experience pain, fatigue, etc. without any measurable deviation from normal bodily function.

The use of these concepts has a gendered meaning. For example, given the predominant positivistic view of knowledge within the field of medicine, a clash may easily occur between the patient (often a woman), who is expressing illness, and the physician (often a man), who is searching for disease. Women with diffuse symptoms and without disease find themselves at the bottom of the status hierarchy. A criticism of the prevailing view of knowledge is that medical diagnosis is neither objective nor a biological fact. Medical scrutiny is filtered through a layer of expectations and existing knowledge, which gives the physician the power to define diagnosis independently of the patient's experience (Hammarström 1997).

The significance of the concept of health has been discussed from various perspectives. The classical definition used by WHO might be described as taking a public-health perspective, in that it takes into account not only physical, but also psychological and social factors. Later on, the concept of health expanded to take in the health-field concept, which emphasized biological, environmental, lifestyle and health-care causes of good or poor health (Lalonde 1974). Even if the focus on lifestyle was questionable, this definition was an important one for preventive work, since it focused on the explanations underlying ill health. Starting with the 1978 Alma Ata declaration on primary health care, health has been viewed more and more as a resource rather than as a goal in life (Hallqvist & Janlert 1991).

In traditional research, state of health is almost always measured using the indirect method of studying the occurrence of sickness and poor health. Health is what remains when illnesses are factored out. This choice is motivated by practical considerations—there are relatively well-developed methods and concepts for studying illness, even if there is increasing awareness that these methods do not always apply to women's situations. However, the question of what health is and how it should be measured needs much more attention in future public health research.

Since we are dealing here with the central task of public health, which is to promote health, it is essential to have a positively formulated concept of health. The discussion of what is health has been beneficial in pointing out what may constitute health, what factors affect health and why we should try to improve public health (Hallqvist & Janlert 1991).

Various explanations for differences in health between men and women

There are two main types of models found in the scientific literature for explaining differences in health between men and women:

a. biological/genetic models, which emphasize sex differences in biological makeup in terms of genes, hormones and physiology, factors that lead to different risks of illness; and

b. socio-cultural models, which focus on gender differences in health-related behavior as well as on life circumstances such as work, family and other socially-determined factors that may pose a risk to health.

The biological/genetic model has developed within Western medicine, which is dominated by a positivistic, biologically-oriented discourse without being aware of social, cultural and historical context. In this discourse, the societal perspective has been neglected in favor of genetic and biomedical models. Biology stands out as unchangeable and deterministic. This model is also used by some researchers to indicate that biological differences between men and women are of primary importance, and subsequently cause social and psychological differences as well (Robert & Uvnäs Moberg 1994).

A great deal of criticism has been leveled against the sharp distinction made between biological/genetic and socio-cultural models (Hubbard 1990, Fausto-Sterling 1992, Lundgren 1993). Since cultural and social conditions are closely intertwined with biological factors, it is impossible to draw a clear distinction between the two. Socio-cultural circumstances also seem to affect factors that are clearly biological in nature, such as stress hormones, blood pressure, muscle mass, bones, the immune system, body shape and so on.

Criticism of the distinction between biological/genetic models and socio-cultural models can be particularly helpful when it leads to the integration of a gender perspective into more biologically-oriented research. Since there is currently a great deal of interest in biological research, it is particularly important to look at findings from this area from a gender-theory perspective and to show the links between men's and women's health and their life circumstances.

No single explanatory model can provide a complete framework for analyzing causes of gender inequalities in health. Research using a purely biological/genetic model can explain and describe biological and physiological gender differences, but that does not answer such questions as why women live longer but are sicker than men. Research based on a purely socio-cultural model can offer explanations for gender differences in risky behavior and in the inclination to seek medical care, and it can also give explanations of the links between health and life circumstances. But a socio-cultural model alone is equally inadequate to explain gender differences in health. The optimal research model for studying gender and health is one that takes into account relationships between men and women and the fact that there are reciprocal effects of biological sex and socio-cultural gender.

In the following sections we examine in more detail both biological/genetic and socio-cultural models and present examples of each.

Biological/genetic models

There are many examples of the close interaction between biological and social factors in gender-related health. Excess male mortality from cardiovascular disease before the age of 65 may have both biological and social explanations. Men not only lack the protection of estrogen, but their lives tend to be more performance-oriented and they are more likely to be alcohol abusers (National Public Health Commission 1998). Women, on the other hand, have a higher risk of osteoporosis and fractures, primarily of the hip, after menopause. Estrogen production is an important factor in this context, but other variables like smoking and physical inactivity are also significant (Medical Products Agency 1993).

Research on poor health among women has been conducted primarily from a medical perspective with a strong biological orientation, in which analysis of social influences has taken a back seat to genetic and biomedical models. Furthermore, genetic and biomedical factors have often been equated with each other, i.e., biological differences have been regarded as innate and immutable. Biological/genetic models, based on knowledge of the human body, seek to explain variations in health. A biological/genetic model looks for causation within the individual, in his or her genetic makeup and in factors (such as infections or physical deterioration) that cause harm to the human body.

The differences in the biological constitution of men and women can lead to different risks for a variety of illnesses and diseases. Workplaces, for example, are generally set up to accommodate the anatomy of a normal male, a fact that can pose health risks to women as well as to men with atypical body types. Since women have a higher proportion of fat tissue than men, their risk of harm from exposure to fat-soluble chemicals is greater. There are, then, sex differences in the absorption, metabolism and excretion of fat-soluble chemicals. Women also have thinner skin than men, so chemicals can more easily penetrate into their bodies and trigger allergies and eczema. Because women have a slower metabolism, chemicals remain in their bodies longer, resulting in higher concentrations of chemicals in the bloodstream. Studies to determine "safe" levels of exposure to chemicals in the workplace are performed on healthy volunteers, usually young men. Given the sex differences discussed above, there is some question as to how "safe" current exposure levels are for women and for men who do not fit the norm (Ekenvall et al. 1993).

The male norm is evident in clinical research, where results on men have been generalized to apply to women as well. Bias may be defined as the deviation of results from the truth, and bias in research related to sex/gender results from male dominance in almost all theorizing and decision-making in science. This androcentric bias means that white, middle-class men have defined the priorities of medical research (Rosser 1994). While women constitute the majority of patients, they hold few positions of power and continue to be a minority among medical researchers.

It has been noted in recent years that certain medical findings are based solely on research on men, with women excluded from the relevant studies (Hammarström 1991, Orth-Gomér & Schenk-Gustafsson 1992). Research on women may give different results, as in the case of risk factors, symptoms, diagnosis and treatment for cardiovascular disease (Kannel 1987, Khan et al. 1990, Dellborg & Swedberg 1993, Karlsson et al. 1993, Weaver et al. 1996).

Socio-cultural models

In addition to possible biological causes, explanations for differences in illness, disease and mortality between men and women have been proposed that involve gender differences in behavior patterns, living situations and life circumstances, particularly with respect to work and family. Verbrugge uses the term "acquired risks" (1989) rather than socio-cultural explanatory models to underscore the fact that these are risks that occur in the course of one's life. When distinguishing between acquired (social) and not acquired (biological) risks, she, like many others, seems to overlook the fact that biological differences, too, can be acquired.

Some scientific disciplines, like history, anthropology, demography, sociology, psychology and public health, are more likely than others to take as their starting point a socio-cultural model in studying gender and health. Common to all of them is a search for knowledge about cultural and social circumstances and the interactions between the individual and the structural framework that surrounds people. However, just as in medicine, gender is often left out as an analytic category.

Socio-cultural models include a number of different types of explanations, classified in various ways (Botten 1994, Verbrugge 1989, Hammarström 1999). There are also similarities to explanatory models of social genesis (Macintyre 1986), which can generally be applied to gender differences as well. Below we give an example of the thinking behind two different socio-cultural explanations, one focusing on life circumstances, the other on lifestyle and behavior.

Life circumstances

This model takes as its starting point the differing conditions of men's and women's lives and seeks to understand gender-related health differences by examining life circumstances. In recent years, more and more attention has been given to the different circumstances of men's and women's lives as an explanation for excess illness among women. Some of the most important factors in this context are structural aspects of society, with differing conditions for women and men in the workplace, in relationships between couples, in family life and in participation in social activities (Hall 1990, Lundberg 1990, Lundgren 1993, Schei et al. 1993, Hammarström 1996).

A labor market that is segregated by gender means substantially different working conditions for women and men. There are large gender differences, usually to the disadvantage of women, in such things as work compensation, whether in the form of status or money; career opportunities; and the presence of various ergonomic, physical and psychosocial risk factors in the workplace. Women have lower wages and a less favorable work environment than men, and this cannot be explained simply by pointing out that women are more likely to work part-time or perform different kinds of work. Wage differentials remain even when women and men are alike in all of these respects (Le Grand 1994, Karanta 1995). Furthermore, women clearly have less influence over their work and a lower degree of self-determination relative to men (Östlin 1996). In a variety of ways, all of these factors are reflected in different illness patterns for men and women (Joint Work Environment Council for the Government Sector 1994).

Domestic work is another sphere of great importance to gender-related health. In Sweden it has been calculated that overall, women perform two-thirds of all domestic work (Rydenstam 1992). This means that women spend 685 hours more per year on domestic work than men do, corresponding to 17 weeks of full-time employment. The health consequences of this have been shown in various studies, such as a Swedish study demonstrating that women's secretion of stress hormones increases significantly in the evening, while men's secretion of such hormones decreases (Frankenhaeuser 1991).

A serious and often hidden danger to women's health is posed by the violence and abuse to which more and more women are subjected, primarily at the hands of their partners or former partners (Kvinnofrid 1995). There is a real need to systematize and enlarge the body of knowledge in this field. More and more connections between abuse and ill health are suspected, as in the cases of anorexia and chronic pain. Other links have been verified, such as increased rates of depression, suicide, insomnia and fearfulness (Goodstein & Page 1981). There are also various somatic manifestations, like chronic abdominal pain and heart disease as well as direct injuries (burns, concussion, broken bones, damage to internal organs, etc.) and reproductive implications (STDs, miscarriage, small for date, gynecological trauma, etc.) (Schei 1990, Chez 1988, Harrop-Griffiths et al. 1988, Larsson & Andersson 1988).

Lifestyle and behavior

Differences in behavior and lifestyle can include general health-related habits, risk-taking with one's life and health, as well as illness-related behavior such as how one perceives and assesses symptoms, the inclination to take appropriate action in the case of illness or symptoms, etc. It has been reported that in the United States at least a third of the excess mortality of men relative to women is due to accidents, suicide, cirrhosis of the liver and diseases of the respiratory organs (Waldron 1976). Similar results have been obtained using Swedish data (Hammarström 1991). This type of mortality is largely caused by behavior that, in our cultures, is interwoven with conceptions of masculinity. This includes competitive behavior, an orientation toward performance, risk-taking (in traffic, on the job, etc.), violence and alcohol consumption.

Diseases of the respiratory system are increasing among women as a result of higher rates of smoking. Statistics show that the rate of lung cancer among women is increasing by four percent a year, while increases among men have come to a halt (Swedish National Board of Health and Welfare 1994). Over twenty years, the lung cancer rate for women has more than doubled. The gender gap is closing as more girls begin to smoke than boys, while many adult males are quitting smoking.

Men's alcohol consumption, behavioral patterns and care needs have been studied, but there is little corresponding information for women. Traditionally, women have been more cautious than men when it comes to alcohol. For fear of public disapproval, women are more likely to hide their abuse of alcohol and more reluctant to seek help. It is estimated that about four percent of women consume large quantities of alcohol, compared with ten percent of men. Alcohol-related illnesses and injuries are most common among young and middle-aged men (Swedish National Board of Health and Welfare 1994).

It is important to put human behavior in a larger perspective, in order to analyze behavior at the structural as well as at the group and individual level. Let us take, for example, the differences between men's and women's eating habits. Since women, generally speaking, are far more nutrition-conscious than men and have more knowledge and training in preparing food, they have better overall eating habits than men (National Public Health Commission, Swedish Government Official Reports 1998:43, p. 145). On the other hand, men earn more money and can afford to go out to lunch more frequently. Thus, they tend to eat a more nutritious midday meal than women, who are more apt to take along a light meal like a sandwich.

Interviews and questionnaires on health regularly show that women are more likely to report a variety of symptoms. Women seek medical care much more frequently than men. Women consume more medication than men. Women make use of the health insurance system more than men do; the difference between illness-related absences of men and women amounts to seven or eight days per year (Diderichsen et al. 1993). Furthermore, research shows that women do not seek medical care without cause; in the case of respiratory infections, for example, pathogenic bacteria are found with equal frequency among female and male patients (Söderström et al. 1991). Stenberg and Wall (1995) carried out a medical validation study to test the quality of information provided by male and female office workers regarding "sick building syndrome." Symptoms were reported by twelve percent of the women, but only four percent of the men. Clinical studies, however, showed that women had a higher rate of disease than men and that the actual gender differences may be even greater than the questionnaires indicated. This does not contradict the fact that women, owing to their reproductive role, menstruation, pregnancy, etc., may also be more observant and more conscious of their bodies than men are. Accordingly, women may find it easier than men do to report health problems and/or seek help when there seems to be a physical problem. Similarly, the traditional masculine ideal of remaining impervious to infirmities may also be an explanation for gender differences in self-reported illness (Hammarström 1991).

The need for research on gender and health

A public-health focus on gender issues is still quite new, and it is slowly being developed within a variety of disciplines. Two cornerstones are essential to this endeavor. First, it is crucial that work be interdisciplinary in nature.[4] New and exciting insights often arise in the interaction between traditional subject fields. Crossing borders that exist in research and education can lead to scientific breakthroughs at the interface between different disciplines. Both public health and gender research are interdisciplinary fields. Public health strives to enhance the health of the population by means of disease-preventing as well as health-promoting activities. This work requires collaboration between different disciplines, in which variation, breadth and depth are achieved by combining the perspectives of each discipline.

An interdisciplinary approach is necessary to develop a comprehensive gender-theoretical framework. Since gender research must be based on multiple perspectives, characterized by theoretical pluralism, no single discipline is sufficient. In the humanities and social sciences, the development of gender theories has continued over a long period, while in medicine it has only begun.

The second cornerstone is international involvement. This is another means of enhancing creativity and dynamism, as well as a prerequisite for guaranteeing high-quality research.

Internationalization would also mean an increased opportunity for multi-dimensional perspectives, i.e. looking at gender alongside race, class, sexual orientation, globalization, etc.

A gender perspective in health research raises many interesting research questions that urgently need to be addressed. Future priority should be given to our two main areas of research: The first is theoretical development, which has barely started within medicine and public health. Theoretical research is crucial to an understanding of the importance of power relationships and gender constructions in affecting people's health. A basic research program makes it possible to develop concepts, explanatory models and definitions in a variety of contexts. Such research might be focused on issues like the importance of the construction of gender for health and health behavior; the interplay between biological and social/cultural factors; and the significance of the body for health. Through the collaboration of researchers from different disciplines who are engaged in gender-oriented studies, the way can be paved for fruitful and creative cooperation to promote the development of gender theories in public health.

Our second main area of research is focused on developing more gender-sensitive methods. Here the need is perhaps most obvious in connection with sexualized violence. Past research has shown how difficult it is for the health-care system to identify sexualized violence as a cause of ill health (Rönnberg & Hammarström 2000), which points to the need to develop gender-sensitive methods in this area.

Research is being conducted at centers and forums for women's studies throughout Sweden, characterized by an interdisciplinary perspective and paradigm-critical gender-theory approach. Such research provides an opportunity to integrate various research traditions and models in the field of gender and health research; and this is, indeed, beginning to happen. We hope this positive trend will continue, and that research in public health and medicine will become more and more integrated in ongoing gender research.

The design of the book

This volume contains contributions from a number of research fields. Authors include physicians with a variety of specialties as well as epidemiologists, psychologists, sociologists and historians. Most chapters include both a biological and a socio-cultural explanatory model.

In Chapter 2, *Maria Danielsson and Gudrun Lindberg* describe Sweden's health situation today, dealing particularly with gender differences in health, but also touching on class differences. Using an epidemiological approach, they show gender differences in various age groups that represent particularly important phases in the life cycle. To put contemporary Swedish conditions into perspective, they offer international and historical comparisons of women's and men's health. A main aim of this chapter is to shed light on the gender paradox by scrutinizing what exactly ill health is, whether described as disease, illness or sickness.

Kajsa Sundström describes the reproductive health of women and men in individual and global terms in Chapter 3. On the individual level, this involves the biological ability to bring a child into the world and the social means of caring for and bringing up that child. Globally, there are substantial differences in reproductive health across different countries and among individuals within a single country. This chapter deals with forms and conditions of reproductive life, with a focus on the responsibilities of society, the health-care system and the individual from a historical and international perspective.

In Chapter 4, *Karin Johannisson* examines the health of women and men from a historical and cultural perspective. She presents gender-specific biological models from the medical world at the turn of the century that viewed biological gender as a critical factor in disease and ill health. Examples show how even today notions of male and female affect scientific theory and understanding of illness, the treatment of disease and the patient's own experience.

Chapters 5, 6, 7 and 9 discuss a variety of models that explain gender differences in the incidence of several common diseases. These chapters examine the interactions between biological and socio-cultural factors in the occurrence of such diseases. The authors define health in different ways. In Chapter 5, *Tore Hällström* discusses gender differences in both patient-experienced (e.g., nervousness, fearfulness) and diagnosed (e.g., schizophrenia, anorexia nervosa) mental illnesses from the perspective of various explanatory models. *Karen Leander* and *Maria Danielsson* describe in Chapter 6 the frequently hidden health problem of violence against women, with the harm it does to both body and mind. In addition to health consequences, they describe underlying factors, such as society's view and treatment of violence against women. *Eva Vingård* and *Åsa Kilbom* discuss in Chapter 7 what is known about the causes of a gender gap in the incidence of diseases of the musculoskeletal system. These diseases constitute a major public health problem, rarely causing death but placing a substantial financial burden on society and leading to a great deal of suffering on the part of afflicted individuals. A literature review makes clear the importance of understanding both the biological and the socio-cultural differences between the sexes so that progress can be made in preventing such diseases. In Chapter 8 *Töres Theorell* discusses gender differences in the incidence of cardiovascular disease, based on research conducted in recent decades on working life. There are obvious differences in the risk of becoming ill for women and men because of differences in exposure to environmental influences as well as in individual factors such as coping mechanisms and physiological response patterns.

In Chapter 9, *Örjan Hemström* discusses the gender differential in mortality, examining a variety of explanations posited by researchers from a number of disciplines. The chapter begins by presenting general explanatory factors; it is organized theoretically, discussing the significance of social factors at the macro level, followed by the level of the group and concluding with individual factors. Finally, the author describes various types of interactions of social and biological explanations for mortality differences between women and men.

The last three chapters describe how changes in the structure of society affect the living conditions and health of men and women. In Chapter 10, *Ann-Sofie Ohlander* takes a historical perspective in her discussion of how social changes have affected living conditions, focusing primarily on the situation of women. We follow women's struggles throughout history to cope with the demands of both production and reproduction, i.e. with making a living as well as fulfilling family responsibilities. In Chapter 11, *Rolf Å. Gustafsson* and *Marta Szebehely* show what changes in how the elderly are cared for today mean for the well-being and health of women and men. Shifting responsibility for caregiving means major adjustments for care recipients, care providers and relatives, adjustments that affect not only the groups themselves, but also relationships among these groups. Finally, in Chapter 12, *Annika Härenstam, Gunnar Aronsson* and *Anne Hammarström* discuss the effect of future social change on the health of women and men. Their predictions of future developments concern both public and private life.

Notes

1 E.g. the English sociologist Jeff Hearn as well as Sabo D and Gordon DF in their book *Men's health and illness. Power and the body.* London: Sage; 1995.

2 For an overview, see for example Baude et al. 1987, Acker et al. 1992, Hallberg 1992, Kvinnovetenskaplig tidskrift 1994 (3), Westberg-Wohlgemuth 1996, Widerberg 1992 and Holm 1993.

3 When gender differences are found within health-related research, the analysis often ends by concluding that there are such differences, instead of analyzing their meaning and consequences. This kind of research might be called variable-oriented research, and should be distinguished from gender research, which by and large starts with the differences (or similarities) between men and women.

4 "Interdisciplinary" needs to be distinguished from "multidisciplinary," which is additive, not integrative. Four interactions constitute an "interdisciplinary" effort: borrowing and solving problems, incorporating new subjects and methods as well as the emergence of an inter-discipline.

References

Alvesson M, Sköldberg K. *Tolkning och reflektion. Vetenskapsfilosofi och kvalitativ metod [Interpretation and reflection: Scientific philosophy and qualitative method]*. Lund: Studentlitteratur; 1994. (Available in Swedish only).

Askew S, Ross C. *Boys don't cry*. Milton Keynes; 1988.

Baelum J, Dossing M, Hansen SH, Lundqvist GR, Andersen NT. *Toluene metabolism during exposure to varying concentrations combined with exercise*. Int Arch Occup Environ Health 1987;9:281–94.

Baelum J. *Toluene in alveolar air during controlled exposure to constant and to varying concentrations*. Int Arch Occup Environ Health 1990;62:59–64.

Baude A et al. *Kvinnoforskningen igår och idag [Women's research yesterday and today]*. Chapter 2, Kvinnoarbetsliv, Arbetslivscentrum; 1987. (Available in Swedish only).

Bengtsson C. *Kolesterolvärdet ingen bra indikator på risken för hjärtinfarkt och tidig död hos kvinnan [Cholesterol level is not a good indicator of the risk of coronary infarct and early death among women]*. Läkartidningen 1989;86(11):945–9. (Available in Swedish only).

Boorse C. *Health as a Theoretical Concept*. Philosophy of Science 1977;44:542–73.

Botten G. *Könsskillnader i sjuklighet och dödlighet [Gender differences in morbidity and mortality]*. In: Schei B, Botten G, Sundby J, editors. Kvinnomedicin. Bonnier Utbildning AB and Ad Notam Gyldendal A/S; 1994. (Available in Swedish only).

Carlstedt G. *Kvinnors hälsa—en fråga om makt [Women's health: a question of power]*. Stockholm: Folksam/Tidens förlag; 1992. (Available in Swedish only).

Chez R. *Women battering*. Am J Obstet Gynecol 1988;158:1–4.

Dahlström E. *Debatten om kvinnor, män, samhälle: kvinnoforskning under trettio år [The debate on women, men, society: women's research for thirty years]*. In: Acker et al. Kvinnor och mäns liv och arbete. Stockholm: SNS Förlag; 1992. (Available in Swedish only)..

Dellborg M, Swedberg K. *Acute mycardial infarction: Difference in treatment between men and women*. Qual Assur Health Care 1993;5:261–265.

Diderichsen F, Kindlund H, Vogel J. *Kvinnans sjukfrånvaro. Arbetsmiljön orsak till kraftig ökning [Women's absences from work: Work environment causes substantial increase.]* Läkartidningen 1993;90:289–92. (English summary).

Doyal L. *What makes women sick*. Gender and the political economy of health. London: Macmillan; 1995.

Eduards M. *En allvarsam lek med ord [A serious game with words]*. In: Viljan att veta och viljan att förstå. Swedish Government Official Reports 1995:110. Stockholm: Ministry of Education and Cultural Affairs; 1995. (Available in Swedish only).

Edenvall L, Härenstam A, Karlqvist L, Nise G, Vingård E. *Kvinnan i den vetenskapliga studien—finns hon? [Women in scientific studies: Are they represented?]* Läkartidningen 1993;90:3773–6. (English summary).

Fausto-Sterling A. *The myths of gender. Biological theories about women and men*. New York: Basic Books; 1992.

Frankenhaeuser M, Lundberg U, Chesney M, editors. *Women, work and health: Stress and opportunities*. New York: Plenum Press; 1991.

Goodstein RK, Page AW. *Battered wife syndrome: Overview of dynamics and treatment*. Am J Psychiatry 1981;138:1036–44.

Gunnarsson E. Att våga väga jämnt. *Om kvalifikationer och kvinnliga förhållningssätt i ett tekniskt industriarbete [Daring to evaluate men and women equally: On qualifications and women's attitudes toward industrial technical jobs]*. 1994:157 D. Luleå: Luleå Institute of Technology; 1994. (English summary).

Göransson A. *Fältet, strategierna och framtiden. [The field, strategies and the future]*. Kvinnovetenskaplig tidskrift 1989;(3–4):4–18. (English summary).

Hall E. *Women's work: An inquiry into the health effects of invisible and visible labor*. Baltimore, Md: The Johns Hopkins University. School of Hygiene and Public Health. Health Policy and Management Department; 1990 [Thesis].

Hallberg M. *Kunskap om kön. En studie av feministisk vetenskapteori [Knowledge regarding sex: A study of feminist scientific theory]*. Gothenburg: Daidalos; 1992 [Thesis]. (English summary).

Hallqvist J, Janlert U. *Vad är folkhälsa? [What is public health?]* In: Folkhälsogruppen. Folkhälsans villkor. Stockholm: Allmänna förlaget; 1991, pp. 21–43. (Available in Swedish only).

Hammarström A. a) *Könsperspektiv på hälsan [A gender perspective on health]*. Socialmedicinisk tidskrift 68 (4) pp. 177–181, 1991. (Available in Swedish only).

Hammarström A. b) *Varför lever kvinnor längre än män, trots högre sjuklighet? [Why do women live longer than men, despite higher rates of illness?]* Allmänmedicin No. 2, pp. 67–71, 1991. (Available in Swedish only).

Hammarström A. *Health consequences of youth unemployment—review from a gender perspective*. Soc. Sci. Med. 1994;38(5):699–709.

Hammarström A. *Arbetslöshet och ohälsa—om ungdomars livsvillkor [Unemployment and health: The life circumstances of young people]*. Studentlitteratur 1996. (Available in Swedish only).

Hammarström A. *Det är bara psykiskt—om konstruktion av kön i mötet mellan läkare och patient [It's only the mind—about constructions of gender in the encounter between doctor and patient]*. In: Nordborg G. (ed.): Power and Gender. 13 contributions to feminist knowledge. Stockholm/Stehag: Symposium, 1997, pp. 1–129. (Available in Swedish only).

Hammarström A. *Why feminism in Public Health*. Editorial for the special issue on feminism in Public Health. Scand J Public Health 1999;27(4):241–244.

Harding S. *Feminism and methodology: Social science issues.* Bloomington: Indiana University Press, 1986.

Harrop-Griffiths et al. *The association between chronic pelvis pain, psychiatric diagnoses and childhood sexual abuse.* Obstet Gynecol 1988;71:589–594.

Hirdman Y. *Genussystemet—reflexioner kring kvinnors sociala underordning [The gender system: Reflections on women's social subordination].* Kvinnovetenskaptlig tidskrift 1988;3:49–63. (Available in Swedish only).

Hirdman Y. *Genusanalys av välfärdsstaten: en utmaning av dikotomierna [A gender-based analysis of the welfare state: Dichotomies pose a challenge].* Institute for Research on Working Life. Reprint 5, 1994. (English summary).

Holm MU. *Modrande och praxis: en feministfilosofisk undersökning [Mothering and practice: A feminist-philosophical study].* Department of Philosophy, University of Gothenburg; 1993 [Thesis]. (English summary).

Holter H. *Ny kvinnopolitisk situation—ny kvinnoforskning [A new situation for women's policy—new women's research].* In: Acker J, Baude A, Dahlström E, Forsberg G, Gonäs L, Holter H, Nilsson A. Kvinnors och mäns liv och arbete. Stockholm: SNS Förlage; 1992. (Available in Swedish only).

Hubbard R. *The politics of women's biology.* New Brunswick NJ: Rutgers University Press; 1990.

Hulley SB, Walsh JMB, Newman TB. *Health policy on blood cholesterol. Time to change directions.* Circulation 1992;86(3):1026–9.

Hägg K. *Kvinnor och män i Kiruna. Om kön och vardag i förändring i ett modernt gruvsamhälle 1900–1990 [Women and men in Kiruna: Gender and everyday life in transition in a modern mining community 1900–1990].* Department of Sociology, University of Umeå; 1993. (English summary).

Jacobs D, Blackburn H, Higgins M, Reed D, Iso H, McMillan G, Neaton J, Nelson J, Potter J, Rifkind B, Rossouw J, Shekelle R, Yusuf S. *Report of the conference on low blood cholesterol: Mortality associations.* Circulation 1992;86(3):1046–60.

Joint Work Environment Council for the Government Sector. *Reflections on Women in Working Life.* Stockholm, 1997. (In English).

Kannel WB. *Metabolic risk factors for coronary heart "disease" in women: Perspective from the Framingham study.* Am Heart J 1987;114:413–4.

Karanta M. Gymnasieutbildade: *Kvinnors inkomst 30 000 lägre än mäns [Secondary-school graduates: Women's incomes lower than men's by 30,000 Swedish Crowns]* Statistics Sweden's periodical VälfärdsBulletinen, No. 2, 1995. (Available in Swedish only).

Karlson BW, Herlitz J, Hartford M, Hjalmarson A. *Prognosis in men and women coming to emergency room with chest pain or other symptoms suggestive of acute myocardial infarction.* Coronary Artery Disease 1993;4:761–767.

Khan SS, Nessim S, Gray R, Czer LS, Chaux A, Matloff J. *Increased mortality of women in coronary artery bypass surgery: Evidence for referral bias.* Ann Int Med 1990;112:561–567.

Koblinsky M, Timyan J, Gay J, editors. *The health of women: A global perspective.* Boulder: Westview Press; 1993.

Kvinnofrid. Part A. *Swedish Government Official Reports 1995:60.* Stockholm: Ministry for Health and Social Affairs; 1995. (English summary).

Kvinnovetenskaplig tidskrift No. 3 1994: *Teoretiska positioner [Theoretical positions].* (English summaries).

Lagerlöf E. *Women, Work and Health.* OECD report, Ministry for Health and Social Affairs, Ds 1993:98, Stockholm; 1993. (In English).

Lalonde M. *A new perspective on the health of Canadians—a working document.* Minister of Health and Welfare, Ottawa; 1974.

Le Grand C. *Löneskillnaderna i Sverige: förändring och nuvarande struktur [Wage differentials in Sweden: Changes and current structure].* In: Fritzell J, Lundberg O, editors. Vardagens villkor. Stockholm: Brombergs; 1994. (Available in Swedish only).

Larsson G, Andersson M. *Violence in the family: morbidity and medical consumption.* Scand J Soc Med 1988;16:161–6.

Lundberg O. *Den ojämlika ohälsan. Om klass—och könsskillnader i sjuklighet [Inequalities in health: On class and gender differences in illness].* Institute for Social Research No. 11, Stockholm: Almqvist & Wiksell International; 1990 [Thesis]. (English summary).

Lundgren E. *Det får da vaere grenser for kjønn. Voldelig empiri og feministisk teori [Enough about gender: Violent empiricism and feminist theory].* Oslo: Universitetsforlaget; 1993. (Available in Norwegian only).

MacIntyre S. *The patterning of health by social position in contemporary Britain: Directions for sociological research.* Soc Sci Med 1986;23:393–415.

Medical Products Agency. *Information från Läkemedelsverket [Information from the Medical Products Agency]* No. 5 1993 Volume 4. (Available in Swedish only).

Meding B. *Epidemiology of Hand Eczema in an Industrial City.* Academic paper, University of Gothenburg, Gothenburg; 1990. (In English).

The National Public Health Commission. *Hur skall Sverige må bättre? Första steget mot nationella folkhälsomål [How can Sweden be healthier? A first step toward national public-health goals].* Swedish Government Official Reports 1998:43. Stockholm: Ministry for Health and Social Affairs; 1998. (Available in Swedish only).

Nordenfelt L. *On the Nature of Health. An Action-Theoretic Approach.* D. Reidel Publishing Company, P&M Vol. 26, Dordrecht, Holland; 1987.

Orth-Gomér K, Schenk-Gustafsson K. *Varför ökar ischemisk hjärtsjukdom hos yngre kvinnor? [Why is ischemic heart disease increasing among younger women?]* Läkartidningen 1992;89(21):1861–7. (English summary).

Puranen B. *Att vara kvinna är ingen sjukdom [Being a woman is not a disease].* Norstedts Förlag; 1994. (Available in Swedish only).

Riska E. *Kvinnors sjuklighet—den bortglömda siffran i hälsoforskningen [Women's illness: The forgotten quantity in health research].* In: Hägglund U, Riska E, editors. Kvinnors hälsa och ohälso. Åbo: Institute of Women's Studies at Åbo University; 1991. [Publication No. 7]. (Available in Swedish only).

Riska E. *Images of women's health.* Åbo: The Institute of Women's Studies at Åbo University; 1997.

Robert R, Uvnäs Moberg K. Hon och Han. *Födda Olika [Female and male: Born different].* Bromberg 1994. (Available in Swedish only).

Rubin G. *Traffic in Women.* In: Reiter, editor: Towards an Anthropology of Women, New York; 1975.

Rönnberg AK, Hammarström A. *Barriers encountered by women exposed to sexualized violence in their interactions with the health care system—a literature review.* Scand J Public Health 2000;28(3):222–229.

Sabo D, Gordon DF. *Men's health and illness: Gender, power and the body.* London: Sage; 1995.

Schei B. *Trapped in painful love. Physical and sexual abuse by spouse—a risk factor of gynecological disorders and adverse perinatal outcomes.* Trondheim: Tapir; 1990 [Thesis].

Schei B, Botten G, Sundby J. *Kvinnemedisin [Women's medicine].* Oslo: Ad Notam Gyldendal; 1993. (Available in Norwegian only).

Stenberg B, Wall S. *Why do women report "sick building symptoms" more often than men?* Soc Sci Med 1995;40:491–502.

Söderström M, Hovelius B, Prellner K. *Children with recurrent respiratory tract infections tend to belong to families with health problems.* Acta Pediatr Scand 1991;80:696–703.

Swedish National Board of Health and Welfare. *Sweden's Public Health Report 1997.* Stockholm 1998. (In English).

Twaddle A. *"Disease," "illness" och "sickness" på nytt. [A new look at "disease," "illness" and "sickness"]* In: Richt B, editor. Öppningar och farhågor. Fjorton humanister om hälsa, sjukdom och hälsofrämjande. University of Linköping, Tema Hälsa och samhälle, SHS 20; 1994. (Available in Swedish only).

Verbrugge L. *The twain meet: Empirical explanations of sex differences in health and mortality.* J Health Soc Behaviour 1989;30:282–304.

Waldron I. *Why do women live longer than men?* Journal of Human Stress; 1976;2(1)2–13 and 1976;2(2)19–31.

Wall S. *Epidemiologi för prevention [Epidemiology for prevention].* In: Kampen för folkhälsan. Om prevention I historia och nutid. Carlsson G, Arvidsson O, editors. Borås: Natur och Kultur; 1994. (Available in Swedish only).

Weaver W, White H, Wilcox R, Aylward PE, Morris D, Guerci A, Ohman M, Barbash GI, Betriu A, Sadowski Z, Topol EJ, Califf RM. *Comparisons of characteristics and outcomes among women and men with acute myocardial infarction treated with thrombolytic therapy.* JAMA 1996;275:777–782.

Westberg W-H. *Kvinnor och män märks. Könsmärkning av arbete—en dold läroprocess [Gendering of work and knowledge: Sex-marking—a hidden learning process]* Arbete och hälsa 1996:1. Solna: National Institute for Working Life and University of Stockholm; 1996 [Thesis]. (English summary).

Westlander G. Socialpsykologi. *Tankemodeller om människor i arbete [Social psychology: Models for thinking about people at work]*. Gothenburg: Akademiförlaget, 1993. (Available in Swedish only).

Widerberg K. *Vi behöver en diskussion om könsbegreppet [We need a discussion of the gender concept]*. Kvinnovetenskaplig tidskrift, 1992:4:27–32. (English summary).

Östlin P. *Working Life and Health: A Swedish Survey*. In: Järvholm B, editor. National Board of Occupational Safety and Health, National Institute for Working Life, Swedish Council for Work Life Research, Stockholm, 1996. (In English).

2

Differences between men's and women's health: The old and the new gender paradox

Maria Danielsson and Gudrun Lindberg

IN SWEDEN, LIFE EXPECTANCY has nearly doubled since the mid-nineteenth century (Figure 2.1) and it continues to increase today. In 1997 it was 81.8 years for women and 76.7 years for men, making Swedes among those populations with the highest life expectancy. The highest life expectancy is found in Japan. In 1996 Japanese women lived 1.1 years longer than Swedish women, while Japanese men outlived Swedish men by 0.5 year (OECD Health Data Base 1998). A comparison of different countries shows that economic development correlates with a country's survival rates. Thus, life expectancy in the poorest countries is only 40–50 years.

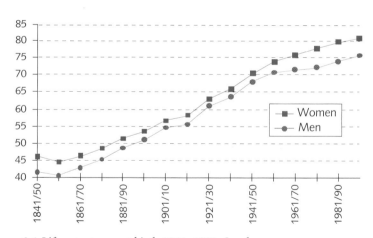

Figure 2.1 Life expectancy at birth 1841–1995. Sweden.

However, differences in life expectancy among the wealthy industrialized countries are closely linked to the distribution of wealth within each country, that is, how large a share of the resources goes to the worst-off members of society (Wilkinson 1992). Japan, for example, is a country with small gaps between income levels (Marmot & Davey Smith 1989). Among third-world countries as well, differences in life expectancy are more closely related to the distribution of wealth within each country than to differences in the overall wealth of different countries.

Health differences between social groups within a single country can be substantial. In the United States, for example, life expectancy for white women was 6 years longer than for black women (79.6 versus 73.9 years) in 1996, and white men lived an average of 8 years longer than black men (73.4 versus 65.2) (U.S. Department of Health and Human Services 1997). However, while black Americans show significant excess mortality relative to whites—attributed to their disadvantaged position in American society—black women still live longer than white men. Gender differences in longevity are thus greater than even the considerable differences in life expectancy between U.S. whites and blacks.

Compared with other European countries, Sweden shows small class-based differentials in the risk of an early death. Social class is defined in Sweden by people's occupations. Use of this type of measure shows larger mortality-risk differences between men and women than between occupational classes. Swedish data demonstrate that men with the lowest risk of an early death, high-level salaried male employees, are worse off than women with the highest risk of an early death, female unskilled workers. Thus gender differences are more salient than class differences in Sweden.

Why do women live longer than men? In an overwhelming majority of the world's countries, women have a higher life expectancy than men. There are some exceptions, such as India, Pakistan, Bangladesh and Iran (The World Bank 1993), which will be discussed further below. Women outlive men, yet their quality of life is often worse. They generally work more than men do, for less pay; they are more likely to be undernourished; moreover, they are subject to the hazards of childbirth. Could it be that women have a greater biological potential for survival than men, perhaps because the stresses of childbirth result in a selection of healthy women? Daughters may inherit genetic material that equips them to deal with stresses on the cardiovascular system. We know that female sex hormones lower mortality rates from cardiovascular diseases for women during their childbearing years. These hormones presumably do not afford sons the same protection. Men, on the other hand, can procreate even when they lack the favorable conditions –related, for example, to the cardiovascular system—that women need to bear children. From a public-health perspective, though, it is of primary interest to identify potentially modifiable social determinants of gender differences in health. Could it be that the lives of women throughout the world share certain characteristics that explain their greater longevity?

Although women live longer, they seem to be sicker than men. In Sweden, as well as in other countries, researchers have turned their attention to what is sometimes termed the "gender paradox" or "health paradox." While illness often precedes death, women live longer than men despite being sicker than men. A corresponding discrepancy is not found for class differences in health. In lower social

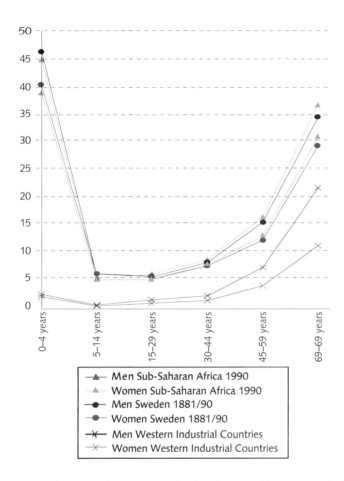

Figure 2.2 Death risks in the countries of Sub-Saharan Africa compared with Western industrialized countries, 1990, and with Sweden, 1881–1890. Number of deaths per 1000 inhabitants. (Present authors' arrangement of data from Murray Lopez 1995; SCB 1955.)

classes, both women and men have higher mortality and higher illness rates than more advantaged individuals. Gaining a better understanding of gender differences in health and of why illness and mortality do not go hand in hand in this case requires a closer look into what poor health actually means.

Comparing poor health

Studies of poor health are sharply limited by existing systems for recording illness and mortality. In most of the world, however, it is possible to estimate mortality for different age groups. Registries exist in the developed countries, and for other countries estimates can be made by comparing figures from one census to the next. Sweden is home to the world's oldest national registry system for individuals and causes of death, which offers a unique opportunity to study gender differences in mortality since the mid-eighteenth century. Figure 2.2 shows risks of dying at an early age. A hundred years ago such risks in Sweden were practically identical to the risks found today in sub-Saharan Africa. A high level of infant mortality was the primary cause for the very short mean life span in Sweden in the last century. It also accounts for the low average life expectancy in the world's poorest countries today. Figure 2.2 also shows that boys and men in all age groups 100 years ago and today have a higher risk of dying than girls and women of the same age.

There are limits to statistical comparisons of causes of death between countries, since in large parts of the world, such as the majority of the African countries, there is no systematic registration of such information. A longitudinal comparison of causes of death in Sweden, where records do exist, can also be difficult, since there have been changes over time in our understanding of what actually causes a person's death. The considerable improvements in survival rates in Sweden over the past 100 years that have resulted from increased prosperity are related to changes in the types of illnesses, and above all to a reduction in infectious diseases.

Naturally, it is even more of a challenge to measure the prevalence of disease. The first difficulty involves defining sickness. The historical perspective found in Chapter 4 shows the extent to which views on men's and women's health are culturally determined. One way of measuring illness is to look at how many people seek medical care, and for what reasons. Unfortunately, such estimates of illness can be biased, since they measure not only the prevalence of illness, but also access to medical care and the profile of illnesses the health care system is equipped to deal with. Since 1975, annual surveys asking people about their health have been conducted in Sweden; similar surveys are conducted regularly in a few other countries.

Shortcomings aside, Sweden has abundant data on the health of its population, compared with what is available in most other countries. Therefore, in the present chapter, Swedish data will be used to identify the components of the gender paradox. However, some historical and international comparisons will be made to illustrate the extent to which certain patterns of health among women and among men are consistent over time and from one place to another— regardless of whether these patterns are primarily cultural or biological in origin.

To illustrate the various components of the gender paradox, it is crucial to break down the patterns of death and illness by both gender and age group. In a country like Sweden, most women and men live to enjoy old age. Therefore, the overall causes of death reflect mortality patterns in old age, which are in fact quite similar for women and men and tend to be dominated by cancer and heart disease. What is more interesting is how premature mortality patterns and illnesses differ for women and men.

Infants

Today most children who do not reach their first birthday die before they are a month old. As shown in Figure 2.3, such early deaths are due primarily to birth defects or complications during childbirth or the immediate postnatal period, often related to premature birth. Sudden infant death syndrome generally occurs later, at about 2–3 months of age.

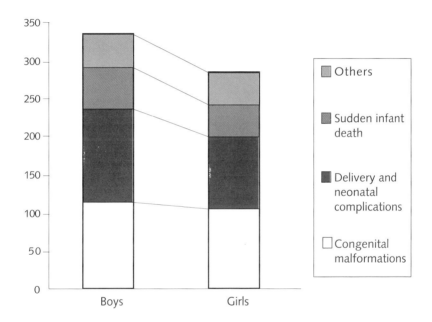

Figure 2.3 Causes of death during the first year of life. Number of deaths per year 1988–1996. Sweden. (Present authors' processing of the Causes of Deaths Register.)[1]

Boys show higher rates of mortality from all of these causes. Gender differences at such early ages are of particular interest, since they are presumably biological in nature and unlikely to reflect differences in social living conditions in Sweden today. Newborn boys, particularly if premature, tend to be less developed than girls at the same gestational age, which means, among other things, that their lungs are not yet adapted to life outside the womb. In addition, boys are more likely to suffer injuries during delivery, such as cerebral hemorrhage. More boys than girls are stillborn.

More boys than girls die of heart defects, one of the most common fatal congenital conditions found among newborns. The causes of birth defects are largely unknown. Only a few percent of the cases can be attributed to "external" effects from the mother on the fetus, stemming from factors such as drug or alcohol abuse, illnesses or medication.

Sudden infant death syndrome is the term used when an apparently healthy infant dies unexpectedly with no evidence of an underlying illness or other cause of death. Such deaths are not a new phenomenon. In the eighteenth century, records referred to "suffocation by nurse or mother" (Köhler & Jakobsson 1991). Such cases were given little attention until most other causes of death in late infancy were eliminated and sudden infant death became the most prominent cause of mortality among infants in the West (Peterson 1984). Sudden infant death syndrome is less common in the Scandinavian countries than in other Western countries. Mortality rates from sudden infant death in the United States and England, for example, are twice as high as in Sweden. Studies have regularly shown that boys are at a substantially higher risk than girls. The fact that sudden infant deaths occur most frequently among 2–3 month-old infants is probably due to weak breathing control at that age (Jakobsson & Köhler 1991).

Relatively little is known about the reasons for gender differences in health during infancy. Girls are born with two X chromosomes, one from each parent, while a boy has only one X chromosome, from his mother, and a much smaller Y chromosome from his father. Girls thus have a double set of genetic material that protects them against certain hereditary diseases. One could speculate that this may also have general significance for girls' higher rates of survival.

Ever since the eighteenth century, infant mortality has been higher in Sweden for boys than girls (Figure 2.4), although today's fatal diseases for infants are different from those in the past. In the mid-eighteenth century, 20 percent of all infants born alive died before their first birthday, and as late as the middle of the nineteenth century, 15 percent of all infants died. By comparison, only 0.5 percent of infants die in Sweden today. The decline has been sharpest for infant mortality during the latter part of the first year of life. Deaths during this period have been primarily due to infectious diseases. Gender differences have decreased continually since the mid-1700s.[2]

Social differences in Swedish infant mortality are very small, but not negligible. Smoking is more common among lower social classes and accounts for social differences in late infant mortality in Sweden, since it increases the risks of sudden infant death syndrome, low birth weight and stillbirth. The largest differences between social groups, however, are for fetal death, and these differences are not attributable to known factors connected with stillbirth, such as smoking, the mother's age or the number of previous pregnancies (Nordström 1995).

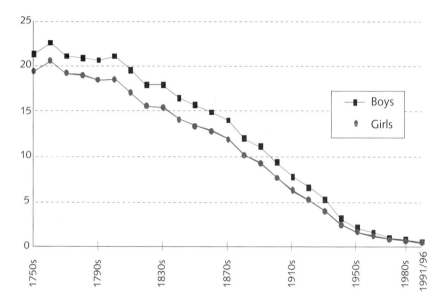

Figure 2.4 Infant mortality, i.e. mortality during the first year of life, 1751–1996 in Sweden. Number of deaths per 100 live births. (Present authors' processing of Statistics Sweden's population statistics.)

Children aged 1–14

Girls' and boys' physical health

Children in Sweden are in good physical health. Increased prosperity has meant higher birth weight, taller children and earlier onset of puberty, all of which are general measures of improved child health. In the 1910s the sons of salaried employees were 6 cm taller than sons of manual laborers (Nyström et al. 1987). In today's Sweden there are no longer any socioeconomic differences with respect to either children's adult height or girls' age at menarche (Köhler & Jakobsson 1991, Lindgren 1976).

Risks of death are lowest among this age group. Of the roughly 230 children who do die each year, about 30 percent die in accidents and about 20 percent from neoplasm. Gender differences in mortality among children are almost negligible today. Even historically, gender differences were small among children, with only slightly higher mortality for boys (Figure 2.5).

Infectious diseases used to be the primary cause of death. Since the mid-twentieth century, however, accidents have been the single most significant cause of death in this age group. One reason why the gender gap has narrowed is that accidents resulting in death have declined for both sexes. Since the accident rate among boys has traditionally been higher, this decline has affected mortality more for boys than girls. Compared with other parts of the world, the Nordic countries have very low rates of child mortality from accidents, which can be attributed to a particularly strong awareness of and commitment to child safety (Köhler & Jakobsson 1991). In contrast, children in Eastern European countries, such as Poland, the former Czechoslovakia, and Bulgaria, are about three times as likely to die as a result of an accident as are children in Sweden (Swedish National Board of Health and Welfare 1994).

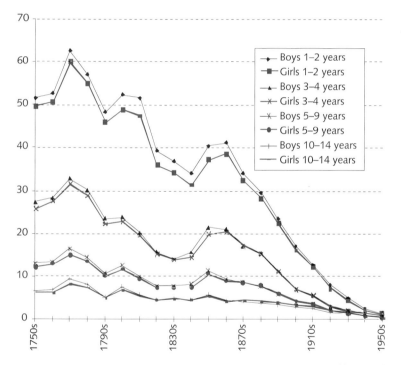

Figure 2.5 Changes in mortality for boys and girls 1–14 years old. Number of deaths per 1000 inhabitants. (Present authors' processing of Statistics Sweden's population statistics.)

The most common types of neoplasms among children are leukemia and brain tumors; the causes of these cancers are generally unknown. There is increasing success in treating cancer today, with cures in more than 70 percent of cases. Many children, however, develop lasting health problems as a result of the treatment (Köhler & Jakobsson 1991).

Allergies are the most common long-term health problems among children and young people. Ten to 20 percent of all children under the age of seven and 20–40 percent of all school-aged children suffer from some sort of allergy or hypersensitivity. Boys are affected to a somewhat greater degree than girls (Statistics Sweden 1994), except in the case of eczema, which probably results from an allergic reaction to the nickel content of jewelry. The tendency to develop allergies is inherited. Whether or not allergies actually develop, though, depends on external influences, that is, the extent to which the individual is exposed to allergy-producing substances. The relatively rapid increase in allergies throughout the Western countries is attributed to environmental changes, since genetic changes occur only over a very long period. However, there is still considerable uncertainty as to which environmental factors are responsible.

Aside from allergies, about 4 percent of all children between the ages of three and fifteen have some other long-term illness (Statistics Sweden 1994). Most prominent are diabetes and neurological diseases, such as convulsive disorders. Next to Finland, Sweden has the highest rate of diabetes in the world (Lithman & Kornfält 1991), and cases of diabetes among children and young people have increased by twenty percent in the last decade. Girls and boys are affected to the same extent. The cause of diabetes in children and young people (known as juvenile diabetes mellitus or Type 1 diabetes) is unknown.

Psychological health of girls and boys

In Sweden, then, the physical health of children is good and gender differences in morbidity are small. What about mental health? Does this pattern hold when we look at girls' and boys' mental well-being?

Estimates of mental and psychological disorders among children vary a great deal, ranging from 5 to 25 percent in various studies, which use different methods as well as different populations and age groups. Rates are lower in rural areas than in cities (Köhler & Jakobsson 1991).

Up to the age of twelve, considerably more boys than girls are treated at psychiatric outpatient clinics, but between the ages of twelve and nineteen girls are in the majority. Slightly more boys are hospitalized for psychiatric problems up to the age of fourteen. (Swedish National Board of Health and Welfare 1987). A public health report from the county of Värmland describes three peak ages for consulting such psychiatric clinics: Help is sought for five- and six-year-olds for their anxiety about starting school and for nine- to twelve-year-olds for depression and aggression. Boys predominate in these age groups. Among fifteen- to seventeen-year-olds, girls are referred to child psychiatric clinic because of anorexia and suicide attempts, while boys are treated for obsessive disorders (Center for Public Health Research 1994). Eating disorders, which affect primarily females, are discussed in Chapter 5.

Less serious psychological and psychosomatic symptoms are common among children and young people, and there are clear gender differences (Marklund & Strandell 1991). As many as 40 percent of girls in the fifth, seventh and ninth grades have headaches at least once a week, compared with 25 percent of boys. Twenty-four percent of girls frequently experience stomachaches, compared with 16 percent of boys. Headaches are equally common in all grades among boys, but increases substantially with age among girls, while stomachaches are more common in the lower grades among both boys and girls. Girls are also twice as likely to be depressed. Difficulty sleeping, however, is found with equal frequency among boys and girls. Studies from other European countries (Switzerland, Austria, Spain, Wales, Hungary, Finland and Norway) also indicate that girls report more psychological and psychosomatic problems than boys (Marklund 1997).

Boys are commonly thought to manifest more psychiatric disorders and psychosocial deviation than girls. If we ask boys and girls themselves how they are feeling, however, girls consistently report a larger share of psychological and particularly of psychosomatic problems, particularly in the teen years. Boys exhibit more aggression and acting-out behavior, and their psychological problems gain more attention and are thus more likely to be diagnosed than the more reserved behavior common among girls (Köhler & Jakobsson 1991).

Most psychiatric problems that appear in childhood disappear prior to adulthood. However, children with behavioral problems combined with social maladjustment and criminal behavior have a heightened risk of experiencing psychiatric difficulties as adults (Köhler & Jakobsson 1991).

The roots of psychological disorders may lie in difficult social circumstances, perhaps including experience of abuse, but such disorders may also stem from brain injuries, low levels of intelligence, and disabilities. Child abuse is a broad term that can encompass physical violence, neglect, verbal abuse, threats, and sexual abuse. Woman battering in the home also affects a child's psychological health, and this occurs in a large number of families. Violence against women in the family is discussed in more detail in Chapter 6.

Sexual abuse, which affects more girls than boys, has major implications for a child's future psychological health. Indeed, 25 percent of all teenagers who attempt suicide have been victims of sexual abuse (Center for Public Health Research 1994). It is difficult to ascertain just how widespread sexual abuse of children is, since this is one of the most taboo of human behaviors—particularly when it occurs between parent and child. Evidence indicates that it is two to three times as common for girls to be victims of sexual abuse as boys (Martens 1989). Usually the child knows the perpetrator, who is almost always a man in the case of a female victim, often her father or stepfather. When boys are abused, the perpetrator is equally likely to be a man or a woman (Martens 1989).

Largely owing to more public discussion of incest, the number of reported crimes against girls increased from about 200 per year at the beginning of the

1980s to 800 in the early 1990s. Reports of crimes against boys also increased somewhat in the 1980s, but since then they have remained stable for several years at about 150 per year (Martens 1992). However, experts suspect that 90 percent of all sexual crimes are never reported. It is extremely difficult to estimate how widespread incest is or whether it is increasing, since estimates depend on the willingness to report such crimes, which in turn is affected by public discussion of this problem.

When adults are asked whether they were subjected to sexual abuse in childhood, results tend to vary substantially depending on the design of a given study. In an oft-cited Swedish study of adults (18–70 years of age), 9 percent of women and 3 percent of men reported having been sexually abused as children. A similar study in Norway showed that 19 percent of women and 14 percent of men had been sexually abused, while a Danish study showed results of 14 percent for women and 7 percent for men. However, surveys underestimate the incidence of abuse. (Martens 1989)

It is difficult to compare psychological health longitudinally and across countries, since what is considered healthy or sick varies across cultures and over time. There are also differences in what is viewed as normal for girls and for boys. However, psychiatric disorders among children appear to be as common in Sweden as in comparable countries (Denmark, Canada, New Zealand) (Köhler & Jakobsson 1991).

Young people aged 15–24

Unlike childhood, there is a clear gender differential in the risk of dying during the late teens and early twenties. Between 1980 and 1991, on average more than twice as many boys as girls aged 15–24 died each year. As shown in Figure 2.6, suicide and accidents are the most common causes of death among young people. It is primarily these causes of death that are responsible for the excess mortality of boys.

Statistics from the eighteenth century show that even then there was a marked gender gap in mortality, with excess mortality among young men beginning at the age of 20 (Figure 2.7). Today the gender gap begins at a younger age—among young people between 15 and 19.

In contrast to other age groups, among people in their late teens and early twenties the risk of dying has remained relatively unchanged since the 1950s (Figure 2.7), although the causes of death have changed. Until the 1970s, deaths from illness declined, but there was an increase in deaths from suicide and traffic accidents. Since then, suicides and traffic fatalities have remained relatively constant, except for the most recent years, which have seen a decrease in traffic deaths among young men.

At all ages, it is more common for men than for women to die in traffic accidents, but this difference is most extreme among young people (Figure 2.8). If we

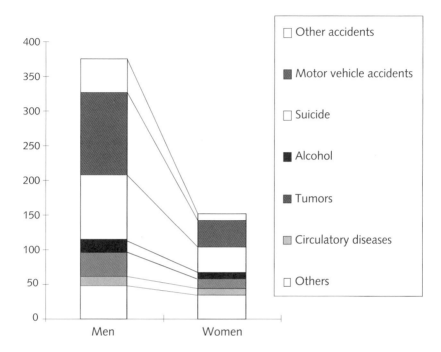

Figure 2.6 Causes of death among young people, 15–24 years, in Sweden. Average number of deaths per year 1987–1996. (Present authors' processing of the Causes of Death Register.)

look at traffic-related injuries, including those that are not fatal, it is clear that such injuries are heavily concentrated among young people, who have a rate three times as high as any of the older age groups (Swedish Institute for Transport and Communication Analysis, Statistics Sweden 1995). However, traffic-related injuries involving older people are more likely to be fatal.

Although suicide has a greater relative significance for the overall mortality of young people, it is more common among older individuals. Suicide is uncommon among children under the age of 15. However, it is not always easy to distinguish between suicide and accidents. A suicide may look like an accident, while some accidents may be the result of carelessness stemming from self-destructive tendencies. In many countries with relevant statistics—the United States, Canada, Mexico, Venezuela, Australia, Japan, and a number of European countries—young men (between 15 and 29) have a much higher rate of suicide than young women do (WHO 1989).

For both men and women, the risk of suicide increases with age. After the age of 75, however, there is a dramatic reduction in the rate of suicide among women, while the risk of suicide for men remains high. This pattern has been observed

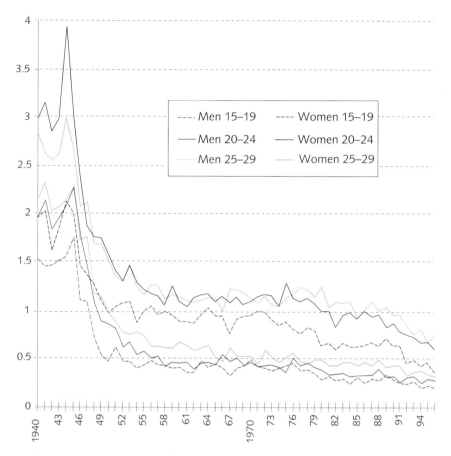

Figure 2.7 Change in mortality 1940–1996 among young people, 15–29 years, in Sweden. Number of deaths per 1000 inhabitants. (Present authors' processing of the Causes of Death Register.)

since the 1860s (Lindén 1993). Boys and men of all ages have always been more likely to commit suicide than girls and women. A discussion of gender differences in suicide follows on page 36.

Gender differences in morbidity among young people are also reflected in the fact that men are hospitalized 1.5 times more often than women for poisoning and injuries. Young women tend to be hospitalized for complications stemming from pregnancy and childbirth and for urinary tract and gynecological problems. In addition, young women are hospitalized more frequently for cancer and for diffuse symptoms. A larger percentage of young women than young men are hospitalized in the course of a given year (Sweden 1996, Swedish National Board of Health and Welfare, Hospital Discharge Register).

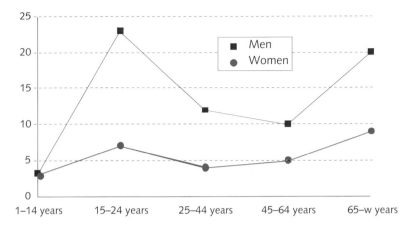

Figure 2.8 Deaths from traffic accidents in Sweden in various age groups. Average number of deaths per 100,000 inhabitants per year 1980–1996. (Present authors' processing of the Causes of Death Register.)

Between the ages of 16 and 24, equal numbers of men and women report having a long-term illness (1994/95). Young women are twice as likely to feel tired, anxious or fearful, to consume painkillers, tranquilizers or sleeping pills, and three times as likely to have headaches (Swedish Government Official Reports 1994: 73 1994). The gender distribution in reduced well-being for this age group is similar to that among children, as described above.

The groundwork for habits like smoking and alcohol use, which may, at least in the long run, affect one's health, is often laid during the teenage and young adult years. Since the 1970s, surveys of ninth graders (15–16 years old) have shown girls to be more likely to smoke than boys. Smoking declined substantially among boys during the 1970s (Andersson & al 1998). During that time there was also a large reduction in smoking among girls, but less than that among boys. Smoking started increasing again among this age group towards the end of the 1980s. In 1997, 12 percent of boys and 19 percent of girls aged 16–24 smoked on a daily basis. In addition, some men in all age groups used snuff, which is rare among women. Smoking is discussed in more detail on page 49.

Suicide

Suicide rates have changed a great deal in a historical perspective (Lindén 1993). Although records of suicide are problematic, it appears that suicide was uncommon in the eighteenth century. In the nineteenth century, suicide rates rose sharply among both men and women, reaching a peak among men around 1910–14 that has not been equaled since. Thus suicide is not a modern phenomenon. During World War I, the number of suicides by men fell by half. After the war, suicides increased gradually until 1967 and then decreased again slightly. Trends in suicide among women have been somewhat different, increasing throughout this century up to 1970, with the most marked increase occurring in the 1960s. During the past two decades, suicide has declined among women, but not as sharply as among men. Thus the gender gap in the risk of suicide has narrowed, but suicide continues to be more than twice as common among men. The most striking decline in recent decades has been among both men and women in late middle age, primarily reflecting a decrease in the number of drug overdose cases.

Drug overdoses and hanging are the most common suicide methods for both men and women (Allebeck & Beskow 1993). Gender differences are smallest for suicides by drug overdose, but here, too, men make up the majority of cases. It is almost exclusively men who shoot themselves or die of carbon monoxide poisoning in their cars, the next most common methods. Perhaps men's choice of successful suicide methods leads to their higher suicide rates. However, as we noted above, a sizable number of men also use drugs, the "female" method of committing suicide.

On the other hand, women attempt suicide much more often than men, generally using drugs or cutting themselves. Suicide attempts requiring medical care are about ten times as common as successful suicides. No one knows how many additional suicide attempts never receive medical treatment. Unlike successful suicides, attempts are most common among teenagers, young adults, and the early middle-aged. These attempts frequently occur at home, often as a desperate cry for help.

Considerably more people, perhaps ten percent of the population, have planned to kill themselves at some point in their lives, and even more have thought about suicide. A study in Västerbotten showed that suicide plans and thoughts about suicide were equally common among men and women (Salander et al. 1993). The gap between men and women in the rate of successful suicides may reflect the fact that women are more likely to seek help—sometimes, indeed, through a suicide attempt.

Suicide and suicide attempts often stem from relationship problems, in many cases separations. Divorced men, in particular, have a high suicide rate. A recent study conducted in the suburbs of Stockholm shows that single mothers have a disproportionately high rate of suicide attempts, which can be attributed to relationship difficulties as well as problems with money, work, and housing (Wasserman & Eklund 1993). Alcohol abuse is a significant underlying factor, particularly among men. Mental illness is not uncommon, but somatic disease may also be a factor.

There is no clear link between women's suicide and social class. However, women in certain occupational groups with high educational requirements, like journalism, library science, and medicine, tend to have higher suicide rates. With men there is clearly a social link; the highest rates of suicide are found among unskilled workers. However, men with managerial responsibilities tend to have higher suicide rates than other salaried workers (Stefansson & Wicks 1993).

Children and young people in the Third World

Most of the global population is made up of children and young people. One-third of the world's population is under the age of fifteen, compared with 19 percent in Sweden. Each year 96 million children are born, 90 million of them in the world's poorest countries. The number of children born per woman has dropped substantially. In wealthy countries, the average woman has two children, while in poor countries the average is four, but there are considerable variations: Chinese women have one or two children, but in Africa the average is at least six. The risk of death for mother and child increases when births follow in rapid succession and when the mother is very young. Fifty percent of women in Africa are married by the time they are eighteen. In Bangladesh 73 percent are married by the age of fifteen (United Nations 1991). Along with illegal abortions, complications related to childbirth are the most common cause of death among young women of childbearing age, as described in more detail in Chapter 3.

Child mortality is closely linked to the level of education among women. Countries that provide full schooling for boys but little for girls have a high rate of infant mortality. A single added year of schooling for girls means a two-percent reduction in infant mortality. Since girls are generally less highly valued and receive less education than boys, one woman in three in the world population is illiterate, compared with one man in five (Mackay 1994, The World Bank 1993).

In most countries, and in the entire Western world, boys have a higher mortality rate than girls. However, young girls have a higher mortality rate than boys in Pakistan, Bangladesh, India, China, Haiti, Panama, Mexico, Venezuela, and Peru (The World Bank 1993, United Nations 1991). This is due to discrimination against girls, which means among other things that in some countries girls are given less to eat than boys (United Nations 1991). Excess mortality among girls occurs more frequently in early childhood, after the newborn stage. There are also documented cases of newborn girls being killed. In many places, childhood for girls is curtailed in ways that do not affect boys to the same extent. Child labor, especially at home, and lack of schooling are examples of this. Moreover, girls often become mothers at early ages.

Malnutrition among girls also causes problems for childbearing, posing a danger to the child and the mother's own life. When malnutrition causes stunted growth, girls—who, moreover, may not be fully grown when they become pregnant—may have such a narrow pelvis that giving birth is problematic. Malnutrition also leads to anemia and to an increased tendency to bleed, which can be life-threatening during childbirth (The World Bank 1993, United Nations 1991).

Early middle age

Early middle age refers here to the period from the mid-twenties until the age of 45. During this period, most Swedish people are gainfully employed, and many also have children to care for. In 1998 a higher percentage of 25- to 44-year-old Swedish men were employed than women in that age group (82.6 and 77 percent, respectively), and slightly more men than women were officially unemployed (5.7 versus 5.3 percent). Virtually only women stayed at home (about 3 percent).

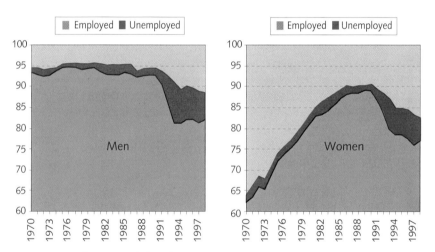

Figure 2.9 Changes in labor force participation among men and women 25–44 years, 1970–1998 in Sweden. Proportion (%) of the population in the labor force (employed and unemployed). (Present authors' processing of Statistics Sweden's Labor Force Surveys.)

During the 1970s, there was a decline in childbearing as large numbers of Swedish women were entering the labor market. Starting in the mid-1980s, however, the birthrate increased, although larger percentages of women than ever before were gainfully employed. Second only to Iceland, Sweden had the highest number of children per woman aged 15–44 in Europe, higher even than Ireland (Figure 2.10). In the second half of the 1980s, there was an increase in childbearing throughout Scandinavia, but not in other European countries.

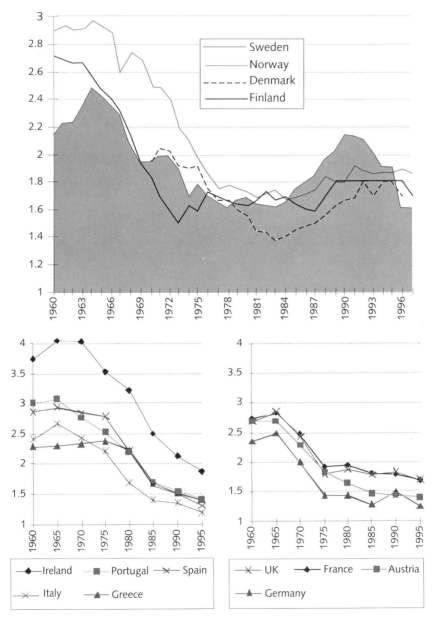

Figure 2.10 Change in the birth rate 1960–1997 in the Nordic countries and 1960–95 in a number of other European countries (World Health Organization 1999 and Nomesco 1996).

In Southern Europe, childbearing declined substantially in the 1980s, and these countries now have the lowest rates in Europe. Like Scandinavia, Central European countries saw a substantial decline in the 1970s, but in contrast to Scandinavia, rates in these countries continued to be low. Differences in fertility patterns in Europe reflect differences in life circumstances. The transition from an agricultural to an industrial and service-oriented society has doubtless brought with it a reduction in the number of children born. The increase in childbearing

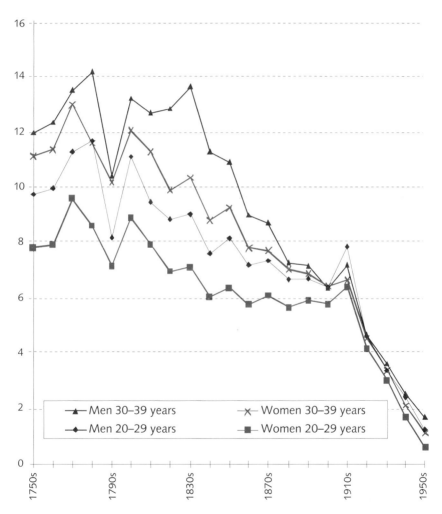

Figure 2.11 Changes in mortality rate 1751–1960, among men and women aged 20–29 and 30–39. Number of deaths per 1,000 inhabitants. (Present authors' processing of Statistics Sweden's population statistics.)

in Scandinavia in the 1980s is probably due to the fact that women have been able to combine gainful employment with family responsibilities. In the 1970s, a series of public policy reforms were enacted to enable parents to combine family and work life. Parental leave was prolonged and could, for the first time, be shared by both parents. At the same time, the system of childcare was expanded, making it easier for mothers of young children to work outside the home. Tax legislation was altered to the advantage of two-income families. Prior to this, joint taxation resulted in higher tax rates for married couples than for two unmarried individuals. For a long time, Sweden was also spared high general rates of unemployment. In the beginning of the 1990s, however, Sweden underwent an economic crisis, and unemployment rose to levels unseen in Sweden since the 1930s. The fertility rate has decreased substantially over the past decade, from 2.3 children per woman in 1986 to 1.6 in 1997. The greatest drop was found among women between the ages of 20 and 29. This means that young Swedish women are not getting pregnant when they cannot find work in the labor market. Instead, concern about the future and less favorable financial situations have caused them to postpone childbearing.

Although women used to have many children at great risk to their own health, Swedish women have had a lower mortality rate than men since the eighteenth century, even women of childbearing age (Figure 2.11).

The substantial decline in mortality rates that began in the mid-nineteenth century and lasted until the 1960s brought with it a decrease in the gender gap in mortality, since men's survival rates improved more than women's did. During the 1960s, mortality rates increased among Swedish men between the ages of 30 and 60 (Figure 2.12). This was a reversal in the trend of steady decrease for more than a century (apart from a peak among 15–34-year-olds in the 1920s).

Cardiovascular disease and accidents, the two most common causes of death, were the main reasons for the mortality increase between the ages of 30 and 60. Moreover, increased mortality was confined to male industrial workers, as mortality rates declined even in this period for male salaried employees. In contrast, mortality rates among women declined simultaneously among both salaried employees and manual workers (Diderichsen & Dahlgren 1991). Some of the reasons for this are discussed in Chapter 9.

Today twice as many men as women die between the ages of 25 and 44. Excess male mortality in this age range, as among younger people, is due mainly to a higher number of fatal accidents and suicides. However, alcohol-related causes of death, such as alcohol poisoning and cirrhosis of the liver, are also found in this group (Figure 2.13). Moreover, alcohol is involved in many fatal accidents and suicides. Further discussion of gender differences in alcohol use is found on page 45.

In 1996, twice as many women as men between the ages of 25 and 44 were hospitalized, not including hospital stays for routine childbirth (Swedish National

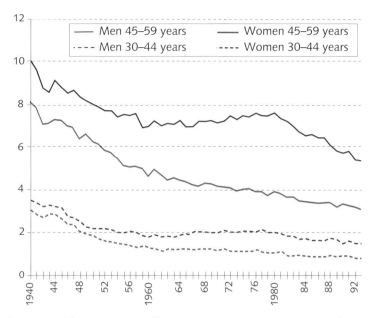

Figure 2.12 Changes in mortality rate 1940–1996, among men and women aged 30–44 and 45–59 in Sweden. Number of deaths per 1,000 inhabitants. (Present authors' processing of Statistics Sweden's population statistics.)

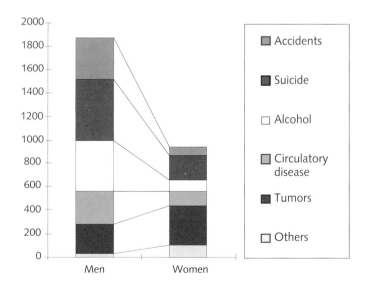

Figure 2.13 Causes of death in age group 25–44 in Sweden. Average number of deaths per year 1987–1996. (Present authors' processing of the Causes of Death Register.)

Board of Health and Welfare Hospital Discharge Register). This is due to complications from pregnancy and childbirth. Although maternal deaths in childbirth have largely been eliminated in Sweden, pregnancy continues to cause significant health problems for women, which are reflected in hospital statistics. Not including hospitalizations for complications from pregnancy and delivery, only about 10% more women than men are hospitalized. If we exclude treatment for gynecological problems as well (including urinary tract infections), we find that 6% more men are hospitalized than women. Men are more frequently hospitalized for injuries, poisoning, and psychological problems, many of which are alcohol-related. Women are more likely to be hospitalized for cancer.

Cancer mortality is also higher among women (Figure 2.14), since breast and gynecological cancers occur relatively early in life. Prostate cancer, which is common among men, tends to afflict primarily older men. Forms of cancer that are not biologically gender-specific show significant excess male mortality, largely because of tobacco and alcohol use.

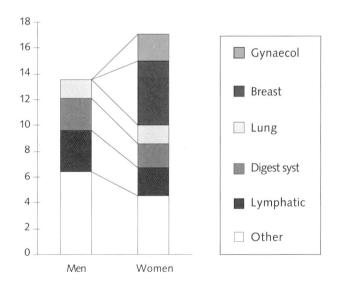

Figure 2.14 Cancer deaths in age group 15–44 in Sweden. Average number of deaths each year per 100,000 inhabitants, 1992–1996. (Present authors' processing of the Causes of Death Register.)

Alcohol

Surveys show that men consume twice as much alcohol as women, with men between the ages of 20 and 30 being the heaviest drinkers. About twelve percent of all Swedish men and five percent of women can be classified as heavy drinkers, defined as men consuming more than 125 cl of 40% alcohol per week and women more than 95 cl (Kühlhorn 1991). Alcohol abuse accounts for a large proportion of medical treatment. Fifty-three percent of men discharged from psychiatric hospitals in 1983 had been treated for alcohol abuse, compared with twelve percent of women discharged (CAN, FHI 1994).

No statistics are available on how common drinking was among women in the past, but it is likely that the gender gap used to be even larger than it is today. Liquor ration books were in use from the early 1920s to the mid-1950s, and were not issued to married women. Alcohol consumption was high in the nineteenth century, as reflected in liquor sales, but it declined sharply during World War I. Sales rose steadily after the war (except for a decline during World War II) and reached a peak in the mid-1970s, then dropped off again. Deaths from cirrhosis of the liver followed a similar curve from 1960 to 1990, which would appear to confirm that sales do indeed reflect actual consumption. Surveys show that consumption by women, particularly young women, increased more during the 1970s than men's consumption did. In recent years, no clear trend has been apparent in the leveling of alcohol habits between the sexes (CAN, FHI 1994).

Average alcohol consumption in Sweden is low relative to most European countries with comparable statistics. Since cirrhosis of the liver in Western countries is due primarily to alcohol, the death rate from this disease can be used as an indicator of excessive alcohol consumption. There has been a substantial rise in mortality in certain Eastern European countries like Hungary and Rumania, and a smaller increase in Poland and the former Czechoslovakia (WHO 1994). By the 1990s, a sharp decline in deaths from cirrhosis of the liver had occurred in Italy and France, down from a very high level in the 1970s. In all of these countries, women have a much lower mortality rate from cirrhosis of the liver, close to half that of men. Moreover, the trends are similar for women and men within each country. There are differences in alcohol consumption in the various Scandinavian countries, as shown in Figure 2.15 (note that the two graphs have different scales).

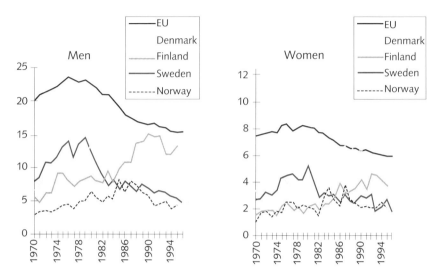

Figure 2.15 Changes in mortality from cirrhosis of the liver and other chronic liver diseases 1970–1996. Men and women under 65 years. Nordic countries and EU average. Number of deaths per 100,000 inhabitants, age standardized. World Health Organization 1999.

Late middle age

In late middle age—between the ages of 45 and 64—Swedish men continue to have a mortality rate about 60 percent higher than that of women, primarily because men are more likely to die of cardiovascular disease (Figure 2.16). A more detailed discussion of why men and women have different risks of cardiovascular disease is found in Chapter 8.

The improvement in mean life expectancy that has occurred in recent years can, particularly for men, be attributed primarily to a sharp reduction in mortality from cardiovascular diseases (Figure 2.17). This has also contributed to the recent decline in the gender gap in life expectancy. Between 1980 and 1996, mortality from cardiovascular disease declined by 47 percent for men aged 45–64 and by 38 percent for women in the same age group.

Cardiovascular mortality has been on the decline in the United States since the 1960s, and is decreasing in most European countries as well. There are some exceptions, however; deaths from cardiovascular disease are not decreasing in Greece and Hungary, for example. In most of Europe we are observing similar changes in mortality rates for women and men (WHO 1998). While cardiovascu-

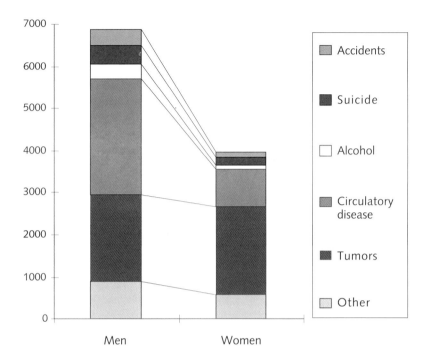

Figure 2.16 Causes of deaths in age group 45–64 in Sweden. Average number of deaths per year 1987–1996. (Present authors' processing of the Causes of Death Register.)

lar disease used to be more common among well-educated men, manual laborers are now more likely to be affected. A corresponding "social shift" has not taken place among women. Throughout this period, women in lower socioeconomic groups have continued to have higher mortality rates from cardiovascular disease than women at a higher social level (Vågerö & Norell 1989).

Approximately equal numbers of men and women die of cancer in late middle age (Figure 2.18). Setting aside specifically female cancers and prostate cancer, men have significant excess mortality from cancer, linked primarily to smoking. The same higher mortality rate from lung cancer is not found among younger men (Figure 2.14), which reflects the fact that smoking has increased among women. Higher rates of lung cancer among women are narrowing the gender gap in lung cancer mortality.

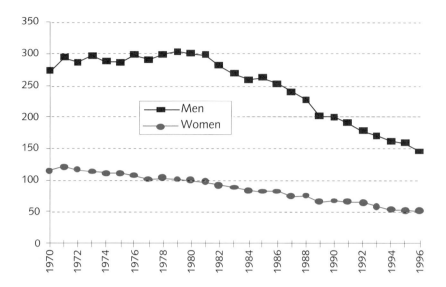

Figure 2.17 Changes in mortality from ischaemic heart disease 1970–1996. Age group 15–74 in Sweden. Number of deaths per 100,000 inhabitants. Age standardized. (Present authors' processing of the Causes of Death Register.)

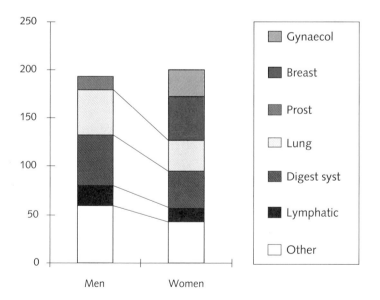

Figure 2.18 Cancer deaths in age group 45–64 in Sweden. Average number of deaths per 100,000 inhabitants per year 1992–1996. (Present authors' processing of the Causes of Death Register.)

Men and women in late middle age are equally likely to be hospitalized, but for different reasons. Men are twice as likely as women to be under treatment for cardiovascular disease. Women, on the other hand, are twice as likely to be treated for cancer or illnesses of the urinary tract or the sexual organs (Sweden 1996, Swedish National Board of Health and Welfare, Hospital Discharge Register).

During late middle age it is not unusual for illnesses to affect an individual's capacity to work, with health problems sometimes leading to early retirement, particularly among women. Gender differences are largest for early retirement brought about by ailments of the musculoskeletal system, which afflict twice as many women as men between the ages of 45 and 49. The next most common diagnoses are mental disorders, and here men are somewhat overrepresented. It is not uncommon for mental disorders to lead to early retirement even among young persons (Swedish National Social Insurance Board 1995), particularly manual laborers. The following table shows the relative share of manual laborers and salaried employees who took early retirement between the ages of 55 and 59 (averages between 1988 and 1993, according to the Statistics Sweden Surveys of Living Conditions).

	Men	Women
Manual laborers	18%	22%
Salaried employees	4%	8%

It is more common for manual laborers to take early retirement, partly because their jobs generally require more physical stamina. In addition, however, manual laborers are more likely to experience pain in the musculoskeletal system, as are women (see Chapter 7). Women also take more painkillers of all kinds than men do, but in particular anti-inflammatory medication, which is often used to relieve joint and muscle pain (Nordenstam et al. 1994).

Smoking

Trends in smoking habits are critical to an understanding of the illnesses that are of significance in Sweden today. Affecting tissues throughout the body, smoking is a major cause of illness. Lung cancer has been shown to be a common cause of premature death, afflicting almost exclusively smokers, but smoking increases the risk of other kinds of cancer as well. Further, smoking speeds up the aging process, leading to such conditions as arteriosclerosis, which in turn can cause coronary infarction as well as a number of common circulatory disorders. Smoker's cough, which results from chronic inflammation of the respiratory system, gradually leads to emphysema, an incurable condition that reduces the supply of oxygen to the blood. Moreover, smoking accelerates the process of bone calcium loss. These are the most important examples of diseases that are more prevalent among smokers, although the list is long.

Cigarette smoking increased greatly after World War II. In 1946, 50 percent of all men were smokers, as compared with only one in ten women (Magnusson & Nordgren 1994). In 1997, 17 percent of men and 22 percent of women between the ages of 16 and 84 smoked. More women than men under 75 smoke, while men nowadays make up the majority of smokers only in the oldest age groups. The percentage of male smokers has declined since the early 1970s, but smoking by women continued to increase until the end of the 1970s, when rates began to decline. The most obvious consequence of these trends is that the lung cancer death rate is continuing to rise substantially among women but is declining among men. Lung cancer begins to appear only after about twenty years of smoking, so a change in smoking habits does not affect lung cancer rates until decades later. Some studies also indicate that among heavy smokers, women run a greater risk of developing lung cancer than men (Risch et al. 1993).

An ex-smoker's risk of dying of a coronary infarction returns to the same level as that of a nonsmoker only a few years after he or she quits. Mortality from illnesses of the coronary vessels (including coronary infarctions) declined steadily among women throughout the 1970s and 1980s, in spite of an increase in smoking in the 1970s. Men's coronary mortality continued to rise until the early 1980s. Since then, however, it has declined more dramatically than the corresponding mortality rate for women, narrowing the gender gap (Figure 2.17). Trends in cardiovascular disease and smoking are not mirror images, since there are other significant factors (cf. Chapter 8). However, the reduction in the gender gap can be explained in part by the fact that men's smoking rates started to go down before women's rates did, and they declined more sharply.

The percentage of smokers varies substantially across social strata. In the 1960s, smoking was relatively evenly distributed among different classes. In the 1980s, when many people were giving up smoking, quitting was more common among more highly educated people, and fewer young people with higher levels of education were starting to smoke. As a result, 42 percent of relatively uneducated women between the ages of 16 and 44 smoked in 1992, compared with 20 percent of their more educated peers (Ramström 1993). The corresponding respective percentages for men were 30 and 13 percent. In many cases, success in quitting smoking involved using snuff instead. If we leave out those who changed to snuff, who were primarily men, there is no difference in the percentages of men and women who quit smoking (Ramström 1993).

The elderly

Most people in Sweden can expect to remain relatively healthy well into old age, as the age at which illness and a heightened mortality risk become more prevalent has steadily increased. In 1993 half of all deaths among women occurred over the age of 83 years, while half of the men who died were at least 78. Maximum human life expectancy has not changed, but more people are living longer and the risk of death has become largely concentrated within an increasingly narrow old age interval. Illness, too, is primarily concentrated among the oldest members of the population. Forty-seven percent of all hospitalization days for men in Sweden in 1993 involved men over the age of 70, and women over 70 accounted for 54 percent of women's hospitalization days (Swedish National Board of Health and Welfare, Hospital Discharge Register). In 1989, one quarter of all days spent in the hospital in Stockholm county involved individuals in the last year of their lives (Shin-Lindström 1994).

Women of all ages have a higher survival rate than men. Even among individuals who are over ninety years old, men run a greater risk of dying than women of the same age (Figure 2.19).

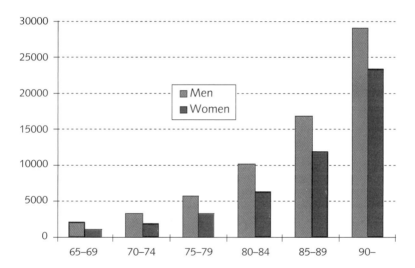

Figure 2.19 Gender differences in mortality among the elderly in Sweden 1996. Number of deaths per 100,000 inhabitants. (Present authors' processing of the Causes of Death Register.)

Cardiovascular disease is the dominant cause of death among men from their thirties on. For women, however, it is not until they reach their seventies that cardiovascular disease surpasses cancer as the most common cause of death. At older ages, cardiovascular disease is clearly the predominant cause of death. Since most people die in old age, half of all deaths, regardless of the individual's gender and age, can be attributed to cardiovascular disease, while one fifth are from cancer.

A larger proportion of men than women over the age of 65 are hospitalized. Nevertheless, the greater number of women in the elderly population (70 percent of people over 75 are women) means that most of the elderly people who are hospitalized are women.

In addition, the very oldest women are hospitalized for longer periods than men of the same age. Women over 75 are hospitalized for an average of fifteen weeks, compared with seven weeks for men (Stockholm county 1991), probably because these women have no relatives able to care for them at home. An average of 59 percent of men over 75, but only 23 percent of women of that age, are married or living with a partner (Statistics Sweden 1992).

Internationally, there are more women than men in the older age groups. In Sweden in 1990, there were 27 percent more women than men among individuals over the age of sixty, which is a considerably smaller gender difference than in most other industrialized countries. In Austria, for example, there were 68 percent more women than men, in West Germany 70 percent, in France 42 percent, in Spain 32 percent, in the United States 38 percent, in Poland 52 percent, and in the Soviet Union an exceptionally large 111 percent. Many men in these birth cohorts were soldiers in World War II, which is probably a major reason for the deficit of men.

Most other countries also show more women than men in this age group, often by between ten and twenty percent. In populous countries such as China there are nine percent more women, while in India the numbers of women and men are roughly equal (United Nations 1991).

There are a few countries, however, that differ markedly from the norm, having instead a deficit of older women. The largest deficits are found in the United Arab Emirates (-45 percent), Qatar (-63 percent), Kuwait (-23 percent), Bangladesh (-13 percent), Libya (-13 percent) and Ethiopia (-11 percent). The deficit in Tunisia, Pakistan, Sri Lanka, Nepal and Zambia is less than -6 percent. As we have already noted, these countries also have high relative mortality among girls (United Nations 1991).

Moreover, there are considerably more—about four times as many—widows than widowers throughout the world. Not only do women live longer than men, but women also tend to marry older men. It is particularly common for women in Africa and Asia to be widowed, since there are large age differences between African and Asian women and their husbands. In addition, men are more likely to remarry than women. Thus, at relatively young ages—under the age of forty—a larger percentage of women are married than men. In older age groups, it is considerably more common for men to be married than women (United Nations 1991).

Accordingly, older men who are in poor health frequently have a younger wife to care for them, while older women with health problems tend to be more dependent on their children, usually daughters or daughters-in-law, and/or on the health care system if it is available.

How healthy are older men and women in Sweden? Periodic interviews conducted by Statistics Sweden with a sample of the Swedish population show how older people view their own health:

A question asking whether respondents suffer from any long-term illness captures both serious and less serious illnesses. Older respondents usually respond affirmatively to this question, unless it is defined as referring only to serious conditions (Figure 2.20). More elderly women than men report having serious health problems stemming from a long-term illness.[3] In addition, more women than men in all age groups are under regular medical treatment for long-term illnesses.

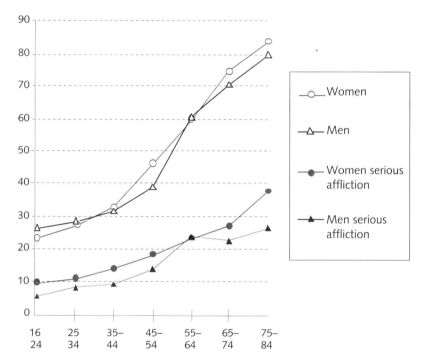

Figure 2.20 Proportion (%) reporting long-term illness and serious affliction by long-term illness. Sweden 1994/1995. Statistics Sweden. Survey of Living Conditions.

Although many people suffer from a long-term illness, they still tend to regard their health status as good. Between the ages of 65 and 74, slightly more than 50 percent of women and 60 percent of men report being in good health. Even among those aged 75 to 84, some forty percent of women and fifty percent of men view themselves as healthy.

Another way of measuring poor health is to ask whether an illness interferes with normal activities. The share of disabled persons[4] is greater among women than men in all age groups (Figure 2.21). Female manual laborers are particularly affected. Gender and social-class differences are especially noticeable among older people.

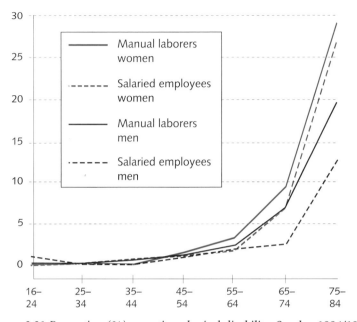

Figure 2.21 Proportion (%) reporting physical disability. Sweden 1994/1995. Statistics Sweden. Survey of Living Conditions.

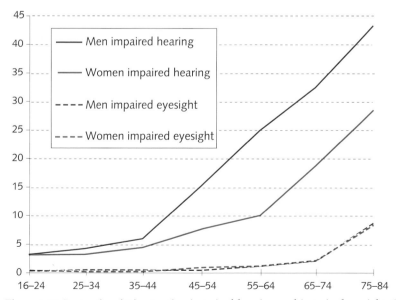

Figure 2.22 Proportion (%) reporting impaired hearing and impaired eyesight. Sweden 1994/1995. Sweden 1994/1995. Statistics Sweden. Survey of Living Conditions.

The most common long-term health problems reported in all age groups are illnesses of the musculoskeletal system, and this also holds true for the very oldest individuals, who commonly have ailments of the joints. Gender differences are most apparent for this type of illness. Men are more likely to report heart trouble, while women report more high blood pressure. Impaired hearing is another complaint that afflicts considerably more men than women, while gender differences in vision disorders are small, except among the very oldest group (Figure 2.22). There are particularly clear gender differences among older people when it comes to mental health, as shown in Figure 2.23 and discussed below.

Gender paradox

It appears, then, that while women are more likely to be ill than men, they nonetheless live longer. Since death is often preceded by a period of illness, it seems paradoxical that overrepresentation of morbidity and mortality do not coincide within the same population groups. There is no question that men die earlier than women. But in what respect do women experience illness more than men? Another important question is whether there are typical female and male patterns of ill-health that are similar in different areas of the world and over time.

Morbidity

Registries do not capture all the ramifications of illness, which include far more than just the health problems that may eventually lead to premature death. Further, illness is a concept with multiple meanings and dimensions. Since illness involves an individual's experiences in a specific situation, any attempt to measure it remains highly imperfect. It is impossible to determine objectively how much someone suffers from an illness.

Thus it is difficult to say with certainty whether women are sicker than men. In modern Sweden, there appear to be certain significant "spheres of suffering" that are widespread and differ substantially between men and women. First, the sphere of reproduction still causes considerable suffering, though maternal deaths are rare nowadays. This is reflected in the high hospitalization rate among women of reproductive age for complications related to pregnancy and childbirth.

The second sphere is that of musculoskeletal ailments, an area in which women appear to experience much more pain, symptoms and disabilities than men do. Besides reporting more musculoskeletal ailments, women are also more likely to be hospitalized for such problems. They also take more painkillers, especially anti-inflammatory medicines commonly used for pain in joints and muscles. Disability retirement due to musculoskeletal illnesses is much more common among women than among men. In a Swedish study of people over the age of 77, functional ability was evaluated using simple tests to determine, for example, a person's ability to pick up an object from the floor (Thorslund et al., 1993). Women showed an impairment in their functional ability more often than men.

These results would indicate that the gender difference in musculoskeletal illnesses cannot be explained entirely, if at all, by a greater propensity among women to report these conditions.

The third "sphere" is that of mental health problems, which are widespread and exhibit substantial gender differences (Figure 2.23). Anxiety, nervousness, and worry are very common, especially among older women. Men do not experience a similar increase in such symptoms as they age. It is also primarily older women who have difficulty sleeping. Gender differences in headaches are found mainly among younger people, with a large proportion of younger women having recurrent headaches.

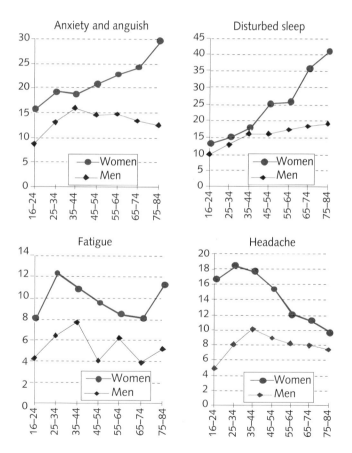

Figure 2.23 Proportion (%) reporting a) nervousness, anxiety and anguish b) fatigue c) disturbed sleep d) headaches during a two-week period. Sweden a), b) and c) 1994/1995 d) 1988/1989. Statistics Sweden. Survey of Living Conditions.

The complaints listed in Figure 2.23 are more common among manual laborers than among salaried employees (not shown in the figure), but these differences are smaller than the gender differences.

Women of all ages are more inclined to seek outpatient care for psychiatric problems (Stockholm county 1994). More sedatives, sleeping pills, and substantially more antidepressants are prescribed for women as well.

While it would appear that there is excess mental illness among women, men are hospitalized more frequently for psychiatric disorders. This is partly because considerably more men are treated for substance abuse, primarily alcohol problems. In addition, men are treated more often for schizophrenia, a seriously debilitating mental illness that afflicts relatively few individuals, but frequently requires long periods of treatment. Men develop schizophrenia at a somewhat younger age than women, and their illness often turns out to be more serious. Because of its early onset, many men have not yet established their own families, which might otherwise be a source of support for them. However, more women than men are treated for severe depression (affective psychosis) and for neuroses such as panic attacks, phobias and depression. (Neuroses are serious psychological disorders, but the personality remains more intact than in the case of a psychosis.)

It is difficult to say whether men or women suffer more from psychological disorders. It all depends on what is considered a psychological disorder—on what are viewed as normal feelings and behaviors for men and women, where the line is drawn between health and illness, who is doing the interpreting and so on. Based on the sources cited above, we could say that men and women seem to have different kinds of psychological disorders, or that they express mental illness in different ways. Men are overrepresented primarily in the cases of substance abuse, violence and suicide, but also among cases of serious psychosis. They are more likely to receive inpatient psychiatric care or to be imprisoned. Women experience more depression, anxiety and panic attacks, attempt suicide more frequently, have more headaches, and seek outpatient care more often.

Whether each of these observations truly reflects reality is uncertain. It may be that women express more nervousness and anxiety than men when they are interviewed, without necessarily suffering from these problems more than men do. Perhaps more attention is given to men's illnesses because their environment reacts strongly to antisocial behavior. Perhaps men fail to make use of available medical care because they are unwilling to seek help. All of these factors might contribute to distorting our measurement of mental illness.

However, these various sources appear to produce a pattern of consistent differences between men's and women's mental health. These patterns of female and male mental health, which reflect women's and men's culture, are closely linked to gender differences in physical health. It is essential to try to understand why this is so in order to understand the differences in men's and women's health, but that discussion exceeds the bounds of this chapter.

Since relatively few countries undertake comprehensive studies of the self-reported health of individuals, it is difficult to say whether similar gender differences in morbidity would be found in countries where the prevailing society differs substantially from that of Sweden.

Results from self-reported health surveys in Finland and Norway from 1986/87 and from a Danish survey in 1994 show gender patterns similar to those found in Sweden (Kjøller et al. 1995, Lahelma et al. 1993). As in Sweden, there were substantial gender differences for illnesses of the musculoskeletal system. In Norway and Finland, however, a substantially larger proportion of both men and women reported ailments of the musculoskeletal system than in Sweden. French surveys show similar patterns, finding that women are much more likely to report problems with backaches, nervousness, fatigue, headaches and depression (Ministère des Affaires Sociales et de la Solidarité Nationale 1984).

Mortality

It is easier in the case of mortality than of morbidity to determine which gender differences are constant and which are changeable by drawing international and historical comparisons. Ever since the mid-eighteenth century, women of all ages in Sweden have had lower mortality rates than men, with the exception of a few unusual years. National averages reveal little about gender differences within individual population groups, such as unmarried persons, orphans, and so on. Still, it is remarkable that throughout history girls and women in Sweden have consistently had higher survival rates, in spite of major changes in living conditions and types of illnesses.

Gender differences in mortality in Sweden have also been consistently small during post-infancy childhood, becoming apparent only in the teenage years. International data show that gender differences are small in children under the age of five in most of the world's regions, but there are exceptions, such as in India. Figure 2.24 shows male and female excess mortality in the age groups under 45 in six major world regions. What we term "established market economies" are industrialized countries not part of the Eastern bloc, while Eastern bloc countries in Europe are referred to as "former socialist economies in Europe."

India differs markedly from other countries in that girls and women have substantially higher mortality rates than males up to their thirties. Gender differences in China and the Middle East are also less favorable to girls compared with Western countries. The Middle East refers here not only to the countries generally included under that term, but also to North Africa, Pakistan and the central Asian republics of the former Soviet Union. In China it is primarily the youngest girls who have a lower survival rate. (Statistics do not indicate whether or not this excess mortality is concentrated among infants.)

Figure 2.24 shows that mortality among children under the age of five is much higher in the sub-Saharan countries of Africa than in other regions. The

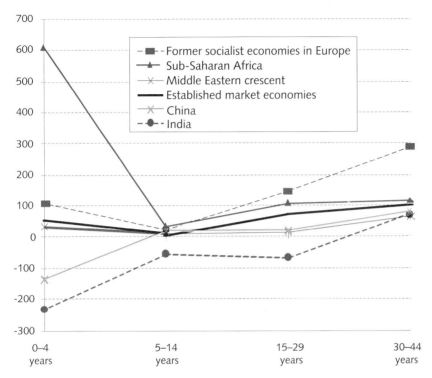

Figure 2.24 Gender differences in mortality in some large regions, 1990. Excess number of deaths among men relative to women, per 100,000 inhabitants aged 0–44 years. (Present authors' arrangement of data from Murray Lopez 1995.)

excess mortality among boys relative to girls is small, but owing to the extremely high mortality rate, as many as 600 more boys than girls die each year per 100,000 inhabitants. In the former socialist countries of Europe, excess male mortality is significantly greater than in market economies. Gender differences in Sweden reflect the pattern in other market economies.

Among individuals aged 45 and over, we consistently find excess male mortality in all regions (Figure 2.25).

Excess male mortality is largest in the former socialist countries, for both older and younger people. (We also find excess mortality among women in these countries compared with market economies, but on a smaller scale.) Interestingly, gender differences in China for this age group resemble those found in market economies. Patterns in India and the Middle East are different primarily for the elderly.

An important difference affecting mortality rates is men's greater risk of dying from injuries. As shown in Figure 2.26, this holds true for all regions of the world.

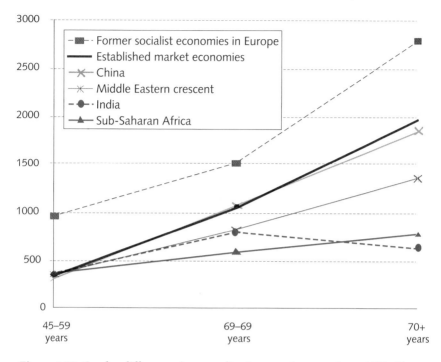

Figure 2.25 Gender differences in mortality in some large regions, 1990. Excess number of deaths among men relative to women per 100,000 inhabitants aged 45 and over. (Present authors' arrangement of data from Murray Lopez 1995.)

Wars contribute to the very high rate of injuries in sub-Saharan Africa, and they account for a large portion of the injury-related deaths in the Middle East. The high injury rate in the former socialist countries in Europe is due primarily to fatal traffic accidents and suicide. Homicide and violence cause a relatively large number of deaths in Latin America. Men have a higher risk of dying from all of these types of injuries—traffic accidents, violence, homicide, and suicide—in the regions mentioned above, with the exception of China, where the suicide rate is higher for women.

Cardiac deaths and lung cancer, both caused in large measure by smoking, are also more common among men than women in all regions of the world. Women have always been less likely to smoke than men throughout most of the world. Men in the former socialist countries have a particularly high mortality rate from cardiovascular disease and lung cancer, as well as accidents. A fifteen-year-old male in the former socialist countries in Europe has a 30-percent risk of dying before he reaches 60 (based on 1990 mortality risks), which is exceeded only by the sub-Saharan countries of Africa (Murray & Lopez 1995). An interesting but discouraging trend in Sweden is that while lung cancer remains twice as common

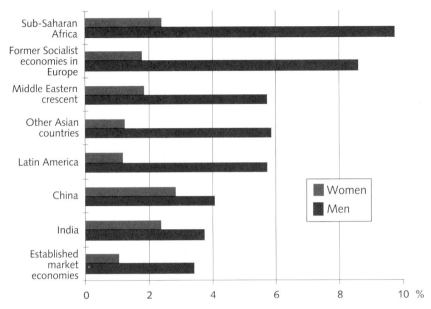

Figure 2.26 Risk of dying from accidents 1990 in age groups 15–60. All large regions in the world. (Present authors' arrangement of data from Murray Lopez 1995.)

among men overall, it is now equally common among men and women under the age of 54. This is because young women have not reduced their smoking to the same degree as young men have.

Is the gender paradox truly a paradox?

If we conclude that women are indeed more likely than men to be sick, is it then a paradox that women live longer than men? Since death is most frequently preceded by illness, we might expect men, who are more likely to die prematurely, to be more affected by illness prior to death. This presupposes that we see illness and death as homogeneous concepts and points along the same continuum. If we instead view illness as a composite term and keep in mind that men and women are affected by different illnesses that are differentially likely to lead to premature death, then the gender paradox is not really a paradox. Women's higher rates of illness include, for instance, ailments such as those affecting the musculoskeletal system that are hardly associated with increased mortality. The greater longevity of women despite higher rates of illness is undoubtedly related to these different patterns of illness.

The new gender paradox

What does a general measure like mortality, irrespective of cause of death, say about a population group? There are clear indications that certain groups are more susceptible to illness and death, almost regardless of the cause of illness. An obvious example is the correlation between old age and the risk of illness and mortality. Similar observations are made regarding the populations of rich and poor countries, as well as of different classes within a single country. Even in Sweden, where few suffer from malnutrition or dangerously unsanitary conditions, class differences do exist for illnesses and most causes of death. This class pattern is related to relative poverty; less privileged life circumstances lead to increased vulnerability and less control over one's own life, and this in turn is linked to psychosocial stress and less healthy lifestyles.

Worldwide excess mortality among men is persistent, except where women are subjected to particularly harsh discrimination. The impact of discrimination on women's health is far from insignificant. It is clear that improved conditions for women will improve women's and children's health and mortality rates. Countries with relatively higher mortality among women than among men are located along a belt of old traditional farming cultures stretching from North Africa and the Middle East to Pakistan, Bangladesh and India. These countries are characterized by an entrenched patriarchal system with varying degrees of discrimination against women (Caldwell & Caldwell 1994). Even in Sweden, where efforts to promote equality between the sexes are far-reaching, women are more likely to have lower paying jobs, lower levels of education, and less representation in organizations with influence over the distribution of resources between men and women, and so on.

Consequently, lower mortality rates among women do not imply greater privilege among women than among men. On the contrary, discrimination is present throughout the world, affording women less access to resources and less control over their lives. The fact that women nevertheless live longer than men is what we term the new gender paradox.

Notes

1   This figure shows gender differences in causes of death in terms of the number of deaths of boys and girls, respectively. An alternative would be to give the percentage of deaths per 100,000 births, for example. This would not appreciably change our results, since boys and girls are born in approximately equal numbers. We have chosen to use the actual number of deaths, since this is a more tangible measure. Similar reasoning applies also to Figures 2.3, 2.6, 2.13 and 2.16.

2   A reduction in the gender differential means that the absolute difference in mortality between the genders has declined, as illustrated in Figure 2.4 by the fact that the mortality curves for girls and boys become more similar. In epidemiological terminology, this corresponds to a reduction in risk differential. Similar comments throughout the text regarding changes in gender differentials refer to absolute differences unless otherwise noted. Relative differentials (relative risks) are not used here because, historically, mortality has substantially decreased among both sexes. This means that changes in relative risks between the sexes are

affected primarily by the large reduction in mortality for both males and females. Absolute differences are closer to what we generally perceive as differences when analyzing mortality curves of this type.

3   This refers to persons who have a long-term illness, health problems following an accident, a disability or other infirmity and/or take medication regularly.

4   Here disabled means unable to run a short distance, get on a bus without difficulty, and/or go for a short walk at a brisk pace. A severely disabled individual is unable to move from one place to another without help from another person or using a cane, etc.

References

Allebeck P, Beskow J. *Självmord 1970–88 [Suicide 1970–88]*. In: Beskow J, Allebeck P, Wasserman D, Åsberg M (Eds.): Självmord i Sverige. En epidemiologisk översikt [Suicide in Sweden: An epidemiological overview]. Only in Swedish. Stockholm: Medicinska forskningsrådet, 1993:53–67.

Andersson B, Grönberg K, Hibell B. *Skolelevers drogvanor 1997 [Drug habits of school-children in 1997]*. Only in Swedish. Stockholm: Centralförbundet för alkohol- och narkotikaupplysning, 1998.

Caldwell J, Caldwell P. *Patriarchy; Gender and Family Discrimination, and the Role of Women.* In: Chen CC, Kleinman A, Ware NC (Eds.): Health and Social Change in International Perspective. Boston: Harvard University Press, 1994:339–71.

CAN [Swedish Council for Information on Alcohol and Other Drugs] and Folkhälsoinstitutet [Swedish National Institute of Public Health]. *Alkohol- och narkotikautvecklingen i Sverige [Trends in Sweden with respect to alcohol and narcotics]* Report 94. Only in Swedish. Stockholm: Centralförbundet för alkohol- och narkotikaupplysning och Folkhälsoinstitutet, 1994.

Center for Public Health Research [Centrum för folkhälsoforskning LV]. Folkhälsorapport 1994. *Barns och ungdomars hälsa [The health of children and young people]*. Only in Swedish. Karlstad: Centrum för folkhälsoforskning, Landstinget Värmland, 1994.

Diderichsen F, Dahlgren G. *Klass och ohälsa i ett generationsperspektiv [Class and health from a generational perspective]*. In: Diderichsen F, Östlin P, Dahlgren G, Hogstedt C (Eds.): Klass och ohälsa [Class and health]. Only in Swedish. Stockholm: Tiden-Folksam, 1991, 1991:185–206.

Kjøller M, Rasmussen NK, Keiding L, Petersen HC, Nielsen GA. *Sundhed og sygelighed i Danmark- og udviklingen siden 1987 [Health and illness in Denmark: Developments since 1987]*. Only in Swedish. Copenhagen: Dansk Institut for Klinisk Epidemiologi, 1995.

Kühlhorn E. *Svensk alkoholpolitik—fakta och myter [Swedish policy on alcohol: Facts and myths]*. In: Atterstam I (Ed.): Hur mycket tål svensken?[How much can a Swede hold?] Only in Swedish. Stockholm: Forskningsrådsnämnden, 1991.

Köhler L. Jakobsson G. *Children's health in Sweden.* An overview for the 1991 Public Health Report. Stockholm:, 1991.

Lahelma E, Manderbacka K, Rahkonen O, Sihvonen AP. *Ill health and its social patterning in Finland, Norway and Sweden.* Helsinki: National Research and Development Center for Welfare and Health, 1993.

Lindén PA. Självmord 1750–1970 [Suicide 1750–1970]. In: Beskow J, Allebeck P, Wasserman D, Åsberg M (Eds.): *Självmord i Sverige. En epidemiologisk översikt [Suicide in Sweden: An epidemiological overview].* Only in Swedish. Stockholm: Medicinska forskningsrådet, 1993:27–52.

Lindgren G. *Height, weight and menarche in Swedish urban schoolchildren in relation to socio-economic and regional factors.* Ann Hum Biol 1976;3:501–28.

Lithman T, Kornfälth R. *Barns hälsa i Malmöhus läns landsting [Children's health in Malmöhus county].* Only in Swedish. Lund: Malmöhus läns landsting, 1991.

Mackay J. *Världens hälsa—atlas [World health atlas].* Only in Swedish?. Göteborg: Naturskyddsföreningens förlag, 1994.

Magnusson S, Nordgren P. *Om tobak. Bakgrund och kommentarer till tobakslagen [Tobacco: Background and commentary on tobacco legislation].* Only in Swedish. Stockholm: CE Fritzes AB, 1994.

Marklund U, Strandell A. *Europeiska skolbarns hälsovanor [Health habits of European schoolchildren].* Only in Swedish. Stockholm: Skolöverstyrelsen, 1991.

Marklund U. *Skolbarns hälsovanor under ett decennium. [Health habits of school children over a decade].* Only in Swedish. Tabular report. Health behaviour in school-aged children. A collaborative study. Stockholm: Folkhälsoinstitutet, 1997.

Marmot MG, Davey Smith G. *Why are the Japanese living longer?* BMJ 1989;299:1547–1551.

Martens PL. *Sexualbrott mot barn [Sex crimes against children].* Only in Swedish. Stockholm: Brottsförebyggande rådet, 1989.

Martens P. *Forskning om sexualbrott mot barn [Research on sex crimes against children].* In: Engwall V (Ed.): Brå-PM 1992:4 Sexuella övergrepp mot barn [Sexual abuse of children]. Only in Swedish. Stockholm: Brottsförebyggande rådet, 1992:21–35.

Ministère des Affaires Sociales et de la Solidarité Nationale. Secrétariat d'Etat chargé de la Santé. Institut national de la Santé et de la Recherche médicale. *La santé en France [Health in France].* Only in French. Paris: La documentation française, 1984.

Murray CJL, Lopez AD. *Global and regional cause-of-death patterns in 1990.* In: Murray CJL, Lopez AD (Eds.): *Global comparative assessments in the health sector. Disease burden, expenditure and intervention packages.* Geneva: WHO, 1995:21–54.

NOMESCO. *Health statistics in the Nordic countries 1996.* Nordisk Medicinalstatistisk Kommitté. Copenhagen 1998.

Nordenstam I, Wennberg M, Kristofersson K. *Svensk läkemedelsstatistik 94 [Swedish medical-products statistics 94].* Only in Swedish. Stockholm: Apoteksbolaget, 1994.

Nordström ML. *Effects of smoking on social differences in birthweight, late fetal death, and infant mortality.* Uppsala: 1995.

Nyström, Peck AM, Vågerö DH. *Adult body height and childhood socio-economic group in the Swedish population.* J Epidemiol Community Health 1987;41:333–7.

Peterson DR. *Sudden infant death syndrome.* In: Bracken MB (Ed.). Perinatal epidemiology. New York: Oxford University Press, 1984:339–54.

Ramström LM. *Sluta röka eller inte—vem gör vad och varför? [Quitting smoking or not—who does what and why?]* Only in Swedish. Stockholm: ITS Institute for Tobacco Studies, 1993.

Risch HA, Howe GR, Jain M, Burch JD, Holowaty EJ, Miller AB. *Are female smokers at higher risk for lung cancer than male smokers?* Am J Epidemiol 1993;138:281–93.

Salander Rhenberg E, Jacobsson L, Beskow J. *Självmordsbeteende och attityder till självmord i olika befolkningsgrupper [Suicide behavior and attitudes toward suicide among various population groups].* In: Beskow J, Allebeck P, Wasserman D, Åsberg M (Eds.) Självmord i Sverige. En epidemiologisk översikt [Suicide in Sweden: An epidemiological overview]. Only in Swedish. Stockholm: Medicinska forskningsrådet, 1993:121–35.

Shin-Lindström P. *Sjukvårdsutnyttjande under det sista levnadsåret [Medical care use during the final year of life].* Descriptive register study. Only in Swedish. Stockholm: HSNstaben, 1994.

Statistics Sweden [SCB]. *Historisk statistik för Sverige. 1. Befolkning. 1720–1950 [Population: 1720–1950].* Only in Swedish. Stockholm: Statens Reproduktionsanstalt, 1955.

Statistics Sweden [SCB]. FoB 90. Part 2. *Civilstånd och sammanboende [Marital status and cohabitation].* Only in Swedish. Stockholm: SCB, 1992.

Statistics Sweden [SCB]. *Levnadsförhållanden. Rapport 87. Barns hälsa 1988–89 [Children's health 1988–89].* Only in Swedish. Stockholm: SCB, 1994.

Stefansson CG, Wicks S. *Självmord i olika demografiska och sociala grupper 1960–1985 [Suicide among various demographic and social groups 1960–1985].* In: Beskow J, Allebeck P, Wasserman D, Åsberg M (Eds.): Självmord i Sverige. En epidemiologisk översikt [Suicide in Sweden: An epidemiological overview]. Only in Swedish. Stockholm: Medicinska forskningsrådet, 1993:79–96.

Swedish Government Official Reports [SOU] 1994:73. *Ungdomars välfärd och värderingar [Young people's well-being and assessments].* Only in Swedish. Stockholm: Civildepartementet, 1994.

Swedish Institute for Transport and Communication Analysis [Statens Institut för Kommunikationsanalys], SCB. *Trafikskador 94 [Traffic injuries 94].* Only in Swedish. Stockholm: SCB, 1995.

Swedish National Board of Health and Welfare [Socialstyrelsen]. *Barn och ungdomar inom psykiatrin [Children and young people in psychiatric care].* Only in Swedish. Stockholm: Socialstyrelsen, 1987.

Swedish National Board of Health and Welfare [Socialstyrelsen]. *Folkhälsorapport 1994 [1994 Report on Public Health].* Only in Swedish. Stockholm: Socialstyrelsen, 1994.

Swedish National Social Insurance Board [Riksförsäkringsverket]. RFV informerar. Statistikinformation Is-I 1995:4. *Sjukdomar som orsakat förtidspensionering [Illnesses leading to early retirement].* Only in Swedish. Stockholm: RFV, 1995.

Thorslund M, Lundberg O, Parker M. *Klass och ohälsa bland de allra äldsta [Class and ill-health among the oldest elderly].* Studie visar allmängiltigt samband [Study shows universally applicable links]. Only in Swedish. Läkartidningen 1993;90:3547–53.

U.S. Department of Health & Human Services. *Health in the United States 1992.* Hyattsville, Maryland: DHHS, 1993.

United Nations. *The World's Women 1970–1990.* New York: United Nations Publication, 1991.

Vågerö D, Norell S. *Mortality and social class in Sweden. Exploring a New Epidemiological Tool.* Scand J Soc Med 1989;17:49–58.

Wasserman D, Eklund G. *Självmordsbeteende och attityder till självmord i olika befolkningsgrupper [Suicide behavior and attitudes toward suicide among various population groups].* In: Beskow J, Allebeck P, Wasserman D, Åsberg M (Eds.): *Självmord i Sverige. En epidemiologisk översikt [Suicide in Sweden: An epidemiological overview].* Only in Swedish. Stockholm: Medicinska forskningsrådet, 1993:107–20.

Wilkinson RG. *Income distribution and life expectancy.* BMJ 1992;304:165–8.

WHO. *The health of youth.* Geneva: WHO, 1989.

WHO. *Health for all.* Copenhagen: WHO, 1994.

The World Bank. *World Development Report 1993. Investing in Health.* New York: Oxford University Press, 1993.

3

Reproductive health from an individual and a global perspective

Kajsa Sundström

Background

LITERALLY, THE TERM REPRODUCTION means replication. It is used in social science for repetitive work, e.g., domestic work or caring for children, and in the field of medicine for the repetition of life and reproduction of species. Human reproduction, the biological capacity and social opportunity to bring children into the world, is an essential part of human life. Parenthood—giving birth to, caring for and bringing up children—is a central task in the lives of both men and women. Reproduction is also important to society. Every religion and culture has rules regarding sexuality and childbearing, and every country has laws and institutions to protect families and safeguard the next generation.

Globally, there are large differences across and within countries in the state of reproductive health. Moreover, it was not long ago in Sweden that the same conditions prevailed as in poor developing countries today.

This chapter is devoted to the manifestations and conditions of reproductive life. Against the backdrop of our own history and the situation in other countries today, we describe the responsibilities of society, the individual and the health care system for promoting reproductive health.

Concept and definitions

The concept of *reproductive health* was introduced in the 1970s in the health care community. Analogous to WHO's definition of general health, reproductive health is not simply the absence of illness, but the state of complete physical, mental and social well-being in all areas associated with the reproductive system and its functions. Reproductive health services include prenatal and obstetrical care as well as advice on contraception, abortion services and the prevention of sexually-transmitted diseases. In this context the broad concept of health used by WHO is very appropriate, since the social and psychological aspects of sexuality and reproduction are closely intertwined with the physical.

Reproductive health is linked to the concept of *reproductive rights,* which refers to the right to determine one's childbearing. This is based on the 1968

United Nations Declaration of Tehran, which asserts that there is a human right of men and women to determine whether to have children, as well as when and how many (United Nations 1969). The United Nations also calls upon the governments of all countries to provide their people with the means to exercise this right through reliable contraceptives and access to abortion.[1]

However, this view of family planning and abortion as reproductive rights has been a source of controversy in international aid activities ever since the 1984 Mexico City conference on population (United Nations 1984). It was agreed at that conference that "abortion should never be used as a method of family planning."[2] This wording has had a major impact, effectively preventing the coordination of any family-planning activity with projects aimed at treatment and prevention of illegal abortions (Sundström 1993, Sen 1994).

Family planning, fertility regulation, abortion

Internationally, family planning is the prevalent term for birth control and contraceptive use. It refers both to the decision to plan one's childbearing and the methods employed. Family planning is generally used as a synonym for providing information on and services related to modern contraceptives. Furthermore, in some countries, family planning is used as a euphemism for specific government-run population projects, such as sterilization campaigns. Another disadvantage of using the term family planning in national or local aid programs is that "family" suggests that contraceptives should only be used by married couples, which automatically excludes young, single and divorced people.

WHO has recently sought to distinguish and define various components of reproductive health (WHO 1994). *Family planning* includes not only contraceptive measures aimed at avoiding unwanted pregnancies, but also help in achieving wanted pregnancies, for example through infertility treatments.

WHO defines *abortion* as a voluntary termination of an unwanted pregnancy, stressing the health aspect and skirting the issue of abortion as a reproductive right. Instead of speaking of legal and illegal abortions, WHO uses the term "unsafe abortion" when referring to the complications of criminal abortions.

Unsafe abortion is defined as "a procedure for terminating an unwanted pregnancy either by persons lacking the necessary skills or in an environment lacking the minimal medical standards, or both." Thus we can conclude that a *safe abortion* is a termination of an unwanted pregnancy by trained medical personnel in a medically safe environment.

Fertility regulation, according to WHO, refers to methods used to plan childbearing. This includes contraception and abortion—methods to prevent or terminate an unwanted pregnancy—as well as measures to protect fertility. Fertility regulation encompasses:

- the postponement of childbearing,
- breastfeeding,
- contraceptive use,

- the termination of unwanted pregnancies, and
- the treatment of infertility.

Sexual health

An important element in reproductive health is the opportunity for a gratifying sex life. In recent years the term "sexual health" has been introduced in the aid context, often in reference to "sexual and reproductive health" (Correa & Petchesky 1994, Germain et al. 1994). This is an important addition, since sexuality has frequently been ignored both in international family planning efforts and in women's health care in Sweden. However, the term is problematic, since it makes sexuality into a medical problem, something that needs to be prevented, treated or cured. WHO points out that it is impossible to develop a definition of sexual health that is acceptable to everyone, and recommends that it be considered part of reproductive health (WHO 1994).

At the 1995 U.N. conference on women in Beijing, several Western countries brought up the issue of women's sexual rights. The demands voiced by the European Union through its Spanish spokesperson were seen as too provocative for inclusion in the concluding document. However, the section on women and health did include a paragraph on women's human rights, which expressly stated that women have the right to decide freely on matters related to their sexuality, free of coercion, discrimination and violence.[3] Also included is the concept of sexual and reproductive health, along with a call for reciprocity and mutual respect in sexual relations (United Nations 1995).

Reproductive health

In sum, *reproductive health* can be defined to include *all aspects of sexuality and reproduction throughout men's and women's lives.*

Although strategies and priorities vary from country to country, the following basic elements are required for promoting reproductive health:

- gender equality and equal reproductive rights for men and women,
- providing sex education and information about sexuality and personal relationships in schools and society at large,
- prenatal and obstetrical care and encouraging all new mothers to breastfeed their babies,
- easily accessible contraceptive services for men and women, in accordance with people's needs and wishes,
- information and counseling for young people regarding sexuality and contraception,
- legal access to abortion, safe care for induced abortion, and post-abortion counseling and care,
- prevention and treatment of infertility, and
- measures to prevent the spread of sexually transmitted diseases.

Historical overview

The social history of reproductive health in Sweden over the last two hundred years is marked by major changes in human conditions in a time of dramatic social developments. Through legislation and economic commitments, society has assumed more and more responsibility for people's health. These developments have also been influenced by the efforts and commitment of certain individuals.

Pregnancy and childbirth

Ever since the establishment of the Kungliga Tabellverket—a national authority for vital statistics—in 1749, data have been available on the size, birthrate and causes of death of the Swedish population. Population statistics were compiled from data from all over the country, gathered by parish priests in church registries and records of home visits. In these 250 years of data, women's mortality rates associated with pregnancy and childbirth have decreased from 900 to fewer than five per 100,000 live births—a 150-fold decline. During this same period, infant mortality has gone down 30-fold, while child deaths during delivery have declined seven-fold relative to the time of King Gustav III in the mid-eighteenth century (Högberg 1985).

In the early eighteenth century, the physician Urban Hjärne, the president of Collegium Medicum, which was the health authority of that era, and Johan von Hoorne, Sweden's first obstetrician, called public attention to the dangers of child-birth. Criticizing the ignorance, carelessness and drinking of the women who served as lay midwives, von Hoorne started a program of training for midwives in Stockholm and, in 1719, published a textbook on midwifery. Collegium Medicum calculated that 60 percent of childbirth-related fatalities could be avoided if women received competent obstetrical care, and submitted a proposal to the Swedish Parliament in 1751 that each parish should have a trained midwife to assist women in childbirth. This marked the beginning of the midwifery system—although in some places the training and wages of a midwife were considered pro-hibitively expensive. It was not until the turn of the twentieth century that there was a midwife in every parish (Höjeberg 1991).

In the mid-nineteenth century, Sweden's mortality rate related to pregnancy and childbirth was as high as the rate in many developing countries today. Com-plications from abortion were a common cause of pregnancy-related death. The greatest dangers in childbirth were toxemia, infections and hemorrhaging. Weak-ness and a too-narrow pelvis resulted from deficiency illnesses, tuberculosis and rickets. Hard labor and many births in rapid succession also contributed to the high mortality rate. Childbed fever (post-partum blood poisoning) was particu-larly feared. This complication was most common when physicians delivered babies in maternity hospitals, owing to the heightened risk of infection from other patients.

Improved obstetrical care in rural areas led to a steady decrease in childbirth-related mortality from the mid-nineteenth century on. However, there was an increase in mortality from illegal abortions in the first three decades of the twentieth century (Högberg 1985).

At the beginning of the 1930s, maternal mortality reached a level of 300 per 100,000 live births. This was followed by a sharp decline, primarily because women's health generally improved and because women were bearing fewer and fewer children. Direct causes for the decrease included access to antibiotics for treating infections and a change in the 1950s to hospital deliveries, where better obstetrical care and facilities for performing cesarean sections and blood transfusions were available. Preventive prenatal care was also a significant factor. Finally, the current low mortality rate, fewer than five maternal deaths per year, is also related to the fact that illegal abortions no longer occur. Since the 1970s, as a result of changes in practices and legislation, safe and legal abortion care has been accessible in the public health services (Högberg 1985).

Early birth control

When Sweden was an agricultural society, there was strict social control of sexuality and childbearing. Premarital sex was punished, as was adultery. The law applied to both men and women, but while men could dispute the charges, women's guilt was evident when they became pregnant. Unwed mothers were disgraced and subjected to scorn and ostracism. They were required to wear a special kind of head covering known as a "whore's bonnet" and to sit exposed to public view on the "whore's stool" at church. It was hardly surprising that many poor unwed women gave birth in secret and left their children to die in the woods. Women did receive help from midwives, who could induce a miscarriage or see to it that the unwanted child died at birth or failed to survive the night (Höjeberg 1991).

In the eighteenth century, statistics showed a substantial decline in the population, resulting not only from war, hunger and disease, but also from the increased incidence of infanticide. Despite severe punishment, abortion and infanticide were appallingly common, especially among the very poor, but also to conceal an illegitimate birth. According to the 1734 criminal code, infanticide was punishable by death through decapitation; one-third of the people executed in the late eighteenth century were women convicted of infanticide (Högsberg 1983). In 1778, concern for the declining birth rate resulted in a bill, called the infanticide decree, to prevent women from terminating their pregnancies or killing their babies. It allowed a mother to deliver at a maternity hospital without giving her name or information on the child's name or descent.

Out-of-wedlock childbearing rose considerably along with the industrialization, increased mobility and migration to the cities that characterized the nineteenth century. There were a large number of unwed mothers in the regions where male migrant workers were employed, along the newly laid railways and the logging waterways of Norrland. Those who moved to the cities, where there were both a surplus of women and a shortage of jobs, ended up undertaking poorly-paid, often exhausting and filthy physical labor as maids, washerwomen, latrine workers or laborers in the textile or construction industry (Ohlander 1994). Unmarried women were often sexually exploited, and those who became pregnant were subject to immediate dismissal. Many of them were trapped in prostitution, while others chose to commit suicide by drowning rather than to live with the disgrace and misery that awaited an unwed mother. It was also common for women to risk their lives trying to induce abortion by taking substances like phosphorus. The suicide rate rose toward the end of the nineteenth century, and the large majority of those who took their own lives were pregnant women.

The need to conceal unacceptable sexual activity created a market for abortionists and "babyfarmers," who took in illegitimate infants, sometimes with the unspoken assumption that they would be left to die. The "infanticide decree" of 1778 allowed a child to be entered in the church registry with the mother listed as "unknown." Wealthier women could go away to give birth secretly, then pay a fee to leave the child with someone else. In cases of neglect or death, children with unknown parents were given little protection by society. It was not until 1915 that this bill was repealed, securing the right for a child to know his or her origins. The children of unwed mothers did not fare well, whether they were abandoned or not. A study in the early years of the twentieth century showed that children of unwed mothers had a mortality rate that was twice as high as other children, while the mortality rate of those whose mother was listed as "unknown" was four times as high (Högberg 1983).

Declining birth rates and traditional birth control

The early nineteenth century saw rapid population growth, since mortality rates were dropping and people were still having large families. At the end of the century, however, the country was plagued by poor harvests, unemployment and hunger; widespread emigration to America caused a shift from population growth to decline.

At the turn of the twentieth century, the average woman had four children, but childbearing soon declined precipitously. However, births were unevenly distributed among the female population. In the early part of the century and well into the 1930s, a large number of women remained unmarried and childless, while married women had large families. Before long, though, childbearing declined among married women, and in the 1930s the birth rate dropped to as low as 1.7 children per woman. Starting in the 1940s, the marriage rate increased and childbearing became more evenly distributed, while at the same time there was a noticeable decrease in the number of children per family.

How was it possible to limit the number of children a woman had, long before the age of modern contraceptives? As early as the end of the nineteenth century, some people were calling for limiting family size, but contraceptives were generally rejected as contrary to nature. In 1910, the political agitator Hinke Berggren gave a speech in Stockholm, in which he held up a condom and declared that the use of condoms was the only way to prevent hunger and misery among working-class people. The reaction to his speech was intense—parliament immediately passed a law prohibiting both the dissemination of information on and the sale of contraceptives, and Berggren was thrown in jail.

However, there were others who continued to provide information about contraception, and contraceptive use became more common. The most frequently used methods were coitus interruptus and condoms, which meant that men were in charge of contraception. Although these methods were often reliable, many women still lived in constant fear of unwanted pregnancy. Diaphragms were the only contraceptive for women, and they were introduced in Sweden, thanks primarily to the efforts of Elise Ottesen-Jensen, a pioneer in sex education. Starting in the 1920s, she defied the law on contraceptives, traveling around the country and lecturing on birth control to both men and women (Ottesen-Jensen 1986). Presenting the diaphragm as a way for women to embrace their sexuality without fear of pregnancy, she was instrumental in encouraging its widespread use. It was not until 1938 that the old contraceptive law was repealed, as part of a comprehensive social reform program.

Venereal diseases

Venereal diseases were widespread throughout Sweden in the eighteenth century. Although it was recognized that they were transmitted through sexual intercourse, little was known about the diseases themselves, and there were no effective remedies. Some experimentation was done using mercury as a treatment for syphilis, both externally and internally, but while this was sometimes effective to some degree, it frequently resulted in severe cases of poisoning. In the eighteenth century the Collegium Medicum put forward a number of farsighted proposals calling for isolating afflicted individuals in sanatoriums and preventing the spread of disease, but these measures were never put into effect. However, the need for hospital beds for treating venereal disease did lead to the expansion of county hospitals. From the beginning of the nineteenth century and throughout the better part of that century, more than half of those admitted to Sweden's hospitals and sanatoriums suffered from venereal diseases (Högberg 1983).

In order to limit the spread of venereal diseases, medical examinations were given to members of what we would today call "risk groups," including itinerant peddlers, sailors, soldiers, market women and wet nurses, as well as workers at inns and coffeehouses. Prostitution increased in cities, where opportunities for women to work were few, and with it the incidence of venereal diseases. Before long, efforts to control venereal diseases were concentrated on prostitutes and wet nurses, who were frequently unwed mothers and suspected of loose morals. In

1878, regulations were tightened to require that prostitutes undergo examination by a physician twice a week. If a prostitute failed to appear, she was picked up by the police and sometimes detained and forced to undergo treatment. Resistance to these regulations grew toward the end of the century, and this issue became a major focus of the women's movement of that era.

One of those who fought against these regulations was Karolina Widerström, who was the first woman physician in Sweden. In 1889, she opened her own gynecological practice in Stockholm. In view of the prejudice and hypocrisy that surrounded the issues of sexuality and women's ailments, it is no surprise that she won the trust of her female patients. Karolina Widerström regarded tuberculosis, alcoholism and venereal diseases as the major endemic diseases of her time, and she dedicated herself first and foremost to fighting the spread of venereal diseases. Her focus was on providing information on sexual matters, both for adult men and women and for young people, especially girls, through the schools, and she contributed to this effort by giving lectures and writing articles. She was a pioneer in public health, recognizing knowledge as the best protection against ill health (Andreen 1988).

Around the turn of the twentieth century, Karolina Widerström joined the group known as the abolitionists, who called for an end to the regulatory system to which prostitutes were subjected. In 1902, a statement on this issue was drawn up by a number of well-respected professors and teachers in the field of venereal medicine and introduced at a meeting of the Physicians' Association. It concluded that in order to safeguard public health and the family, the mainstay of society, it was essential to require continued regular examination of prostitutes and, if necessary, to isolate them in hospitals. It took courage for a woman to stand up to her male colleagues and teachers with an opposing view. Nonetheless, Karolina Widerström took the floor and criticized the Physicians' Association for failing to present an objective assessment of the issue. She accused them of underscoring the positive aspects of the present system and ignoring its defects. She questioned why coercive measures should be concentrated on the most vulnerable of women, prostitutes (Andreen 1988).

After years of further discussion, the controversial regulations were repealed. In 1919 they were replaced by the Lex veneris, which contained measures aimed at both men and women to reduce the spread of venereal infection. The wording of the law bears clear signs of Karolina Widerström's influence in requiring that instruction in sexual hygiene be conducted in the schools. Thirty years would go by before that recommendation was put into effect, but this was a first step.

Even after the passage of the Lex veneris, it was a long time before there was a decrease in the level of shame and secrecy surrounding venereal diseases. As late as the 1960s, when people were able to speak freely about sexuality, contraception and abortion, gonorrhea was still regarded as something to be ashamed of. Physicians had separate consultation rooms for treating venereal diseases, where patients tried to sneak in without being seen. The law required that the disease be treated. Those who had been infected or were suspected of being infected with gonorrhea could be forced—by the police, if necessary—to appear for treatment.

Today there is more openness on this subject, and knowledge of sexually transmitted diseases (STDs) has increased as new diseases have emerged. Although gonorrhea has nearly disappeared, cases of chlamydia, herpes and condyloma (genital warts) are on the rise, and AIDS has replaced syphilis as the most feared threat to sexuality, health and survival.

The danger posed by venereal diseases at the beginning of this century, perhaps most of all syphilis, is comparable to the AIDS situation today. Both cases involve a long-term, serious illness for which there is no cure. Their association with sexuality triggers feelings of guilt and shame, and reveals our prejudices with respect to sexual and interpersonal relationships.

The reform program of the 1930s

In 1930s Sweden, a country marked by economic depression, it was not poverty and unemployment, but concern about the falling birth rate that spurred social reform efforts. In 1934 Alva and Gunnar Myrdal wrote a book entitled *Population Crisis,* which caused alarm in society. They argued that social reforms to support the family would encourage people to have more children. A population commission was appointed to launch sweeping reform. Maternal and child health care were introduced as a public-health service, and since that time prenatal care for all pregnant women and health care for all children under school age have been cornerstones of the Swedish health-care system. There was no longer any charge for delivery care, maternal allowances were introduced, and housing loans were made available to young families. Child allowances were established in 1947, followed by free school lunches, nursery schools, youth recreation centers and day care.

An abortion act in 1938 determined that abortion was a crime, but could be permitted under certain conditions, including medical, eugenic and humanitarian grounds. The same year, the existing ban on the distribution of contraceptives was repealed. Before long, contraceptive services were being provided by the public health services, not only as part of postnatal care, but also to women who had never been pregnant. A recommendation was issued in 1942 calling for sex education in the schools, and sex education became a mandatory part of the curriculum in 1955. Employment legislation made it easier for women to work outside the home. In 1939 it became illegal for employers to dismiss women when they got married, became pregnant or gave birth. The efforts toward social reform in the spheres of sexuality, reproduction, family and working life that had begun in the 1930s continued, and each succeeding decade has brought new initiatives, laws and reforms (Table 1, page 80).

Contemporary reproductive history

Marriage and the family

When women of various ages were surveyed regarding cohabitation, childbirth and birth control over the past 50 years, it was clear that each age group had a certain ideal that most women sought to follow (Sundström-Feigenberg 1987). With each successive decade, women stayed in school longer, engaged in sexual activity earlier, and waited longer to get married and have children. A constant thread running through women's lives was the challenge of combining gainful employment with children and family responsibilities.

Women born in the 1920s went to primary school for six or at most seven years, then entered the work force. They considered themselves and were viewed by others as adults; the concept of the teenager had not yet gained currency. Young women worried about "getting in trouble," and if they became pregnant they "had to get married." They were expected to make the best of the situation, and quite a few of these marriages lasted for a lifetime.

In many respects the 1960s were a turning point. Women completed their basic schooling, they were sought after in the labor market, and opportunities were available for them to go to college and travel. Gender equality and gender roles were a topic of discussion, and the birth-control pill became available. Couples could live together without worrying about pregnancy, and more and more couples moved in together without getting married. Throughout the 1970s, informal cohabitation increased while marriage rates declined. It was no longer a matter of couples living together before marriage or of "trial marriage," but a completely new type of living arrangement.

The number of women bearing children out of wedlock increased, and attitudes toward unwed mothers changed. There was no reason to look down on women who had freely chosen to live alone with their children. While the marriage rate increased somewhat during the 1980s, many couples still move in together without getting married, whether or not they have children. Some of them marry sooner or later, for a variety of reasons—some when their children reach school age, some to demonstrate their commitment, some simply because, as one woman said, "We wanted to have a party."

Obstetrical care in transition

Prenatal and obstetrical care have improved dramatically over the last fifty years. The shift to hospital deliveries that took place in the 1950s meant a safer experience for the new mother. Since that time, virtually all mothers have delivered their babies at maternal hospitals attended by midwives. Two parallel developments were occurring in public health services for prenatal and delivery care, one being the improvement of medical technology, including effective anesthesia, the other a widespread desire for "natural childbirth" and methods of coping with pain without the use of technology. Both sides had their advocates among the women's movement, midwives and obstetricians. As a result, Parliament passed a resolution in 1971 affirming women's right to pain relief in labor and delivery, which was instrumental in the development of better methods of controlling and monitoring pain.

New technologies in prenatal care were introduced, such as ultrasound and amniocentesis aimed at detecting fetal abnormalities. In accordance with the parliamentary resolution of 1979 on parental education, expectant parents were offered classes and discussion groups to prepare them for birth and parenthood.

Delivery wards introduced high-quality electronic monitoring of the fetal heartbeat and the mother's contractions during labor. Efforts were made to improve pain management, techniques for inducing labor and intensive care for newborns. During the late 1970s and the early 1980s there was routine use of advanced electronic monitoring, which was met with opposition from feminist groups and midwives. In recent years the technological side has been tempered in favor of introducing "gentler" methods of delivering babies in a home-like atmosphere. Old routines, such as treating the newborn with silver-nitrate drops and adhering to a strict breastfeeding schedule, have been replaced by efforts to encourage early physical contact and nursing on demand. Every attempt is made to respect the parents' wishes regarding pain medication, method of delivery and newborn care.

Contraception and abortion

It used to be that women simply "got pregnant," and whether pregnancy was perceived as a punishment or a blessing, women simply had to accept their situation. Today we talk about "choosing" the right time to have a child, and we have, indeed, abundant means of planning our childbearing.

The modern contraceptives—birth-control pills and intrauterine devices (IUDs)—that became available in the 1960s meant that women now had more effective means of determining whether and when to bear a child. This did not appreciably affect the number of births, but first and foremost the timing of childbearing. Particularly noticeable was a trend toward delaying childbearing.

New contraceptives placed new demands on the health care system. Oral contraceptives required a prescription and the IUD required medical services before these methods could be used. In the past, birth control had been regarded as a private matter, and each individual was expected to assume the full cost of obtaining both information about contraception and the contraceptives themselves. The medical profession either perceived contraception as unimportant or opposed it for medical and moralistic reasons. Thus, many physicians refused to prescribe birth control pills for young, unmarried patients. It was not until the new abortion law was passed in the 1970s that more systematic efforts were made to provide information on contraception through the general health care system (Sundström-Feigenberg 1988).

The abortion law of 1938 was focused primarily on "exhausted mothers," those who had already given birth to several children. Often a physician was the one to suggest abortion if he considered it medically warranted or if the mother's health had been compromised by repeated pregnancies. Being young, single and abandoned by a fiancé was not considered adequate reason to have an abortion, and many women, especially young women, saw illegal abortion as their only option. At that time illegal abortions by far outnumbered legal ones. In the 1950s and the early 1960s, there were between 4,000 and 5,000 legal abortions each year. Illegal abortions during this time were estimated at about 15,000 annually.

Strict application of the law on abortion meant that in the 1960s many women went to Poland or paid for private clinic care to obtain abortions without long waiting periods or awkward questioning. Demands raised by women's groups and popular organizations such as the Swedish Association for Sex Education led to the appointment of a governmental committee to reconsider the abortion issue with the goal of relaxing the law's provisions. Attitudes toward abortion gradually changed within the health care system as well, and it became easier for young women to obtain abortions. While illegal abortions declined, the number of legal abortions among teenagers increased, which many saw as cause for concern.

In 1974, a new Abortion Act was passed, giving women the right to an abortion within the general health care system up to the end of the 18th week of pregnancy. After that limit, permission from the National Board of Health and Welfare is required. This law represented a substantial change, as it legalized abortion on demand and secured the woman's right to choose whether or not to terminate a pregnancy.

The 1974 Abortion Act was combined with a law making contraceptive services free of charge and subsidizing the price of contraceptives, the idea being that in legalizing abortion, society also had an obligation to make contraceptives equally accessible. Contraceptives should be the primary means of fertility regulation, with legal abortion as a last resort.

Combining employment and children

In the 1970s, a number of family-policy reforms were initiated that made it easier to combine employment with parental responsibilities. Separate taxation for married couples was introduced in 1972, based on the idea that every adult should provide for him- or herself. A system based on the man being the family breadwinner was abandoned in favor of having two earners in the household. Parental leave was extended, with the option of splitting it between the father and mother, and the childcare system was expanded. Divorce also became easier, eliminating the need for a woman to remain in a bad relationship for economic reasons. Reconfigured families, which may include children from former relationships as well as the current one, have resulted in new and intricate family patterns (Liljeström 1990).

Recent years have seen an increase in gainful employment among women, including those with small children. As women's participation in the labor market has increased, there has been continued discussion about equality and the division of labor between the sexes. Efforts to achieve equality have centered on offering both men and women the opportunity to devote themselves to their work and their children. Since parental leave with cash benefits may be shared between the parents, quite a few fathers take at least a few months off to stay home and care for a newborn.

In 1994, nearly as many women as men were in the labor force—80 percent of all women and 84 percent of all men aged 20 to 64. Seventy percent of the men, however, work full-time, while nearly 60 percent of the women have reduced working hours (Statistics Sweden 1995). Typically, women go from full-time work to vocational training, parental leave, part-time work, and back to full-time work (Elgqvist-Saltzman 1994).

Population trends

The number of births dropped steadily in Sweden beginning in the early 1970s, not least because more and more people were postponing childbearing and drawing the line at two children. This new pattern is reflected in the fact that the mean age of Swedish women at the birth of their first child was 23 in 1965, but 27 in the mid-1990s.

At the end of the 1980s childbearing began to increase again. The total fertility rate (the number of children a woman is estimated to have in the course of her reproductive life) declined to 1.6 in 1982, rising gradually to a level of 2.1 in 1992. Second only to Ireland, this was the highest rate in Europe, while countries like Italy, Germany and Hungary reported rates of between 1.3 and 1.5 children per woman. One of the reasons for the high birth rate in Sweden was that more and more women were having a third child, which some view as a reflection of better conditions for families with children in Sweden in the past two decades (Hoem 1993). Family law, parental leave and the day care system have meant that employed mothers of two children do not have to choose between continuing to work outside the home and having another child (Hoem 1992, Ohlander 1994).

In more recent years, however, the birth rate in Sweden has decreased markedly, in 1998 falling to 1.5 children per woman. This is partly due to young women's postponement of childbearing, which in turn reflects the country's weakened economic situation, anxiety about unemployment and reductions in parental-leave compensation.

Reproduction in society and private life

The necessary conditions for good reproductive health for each individual are created by society and the health-care system, in the extent to which society makes it possible for people to fulfill their desires, hopes and plans for their sexual and reproductive lives.

Society

Reproductive health is strongly influenced by the society in which we live. Material standard of living, level of education, the overall health situation, job opportunities, restrictions on childbearing and birth control, and the availability and quality of health care—all of these things affect personal and private matters such as pregnancy, childbirth and child rearing. Society provides both protection and control through family-related legislation, social insurance, the job environment, prenatal and maternal health care, child care, etc. Reproductive health involves social spheres beyond the realm of medicine alone. It touches on ethical and existential issues like human rights, equality, how highly women and men are valued, as well as power and influence within the family and in society at large.

As we have seen, issues of sexuality and reproduction have been a focus of society's attention and action for a very long time. Venereal disease was a primary concern around the turn of the twentieth century. The 1930s saw a comprehensive program of reforms to protect families and children. At the same time, there was a push to develop and improve prenatal and obstetrical care and to expand counseling services on contraception and sexually transmitted diseases. For the last few decades, abortion, sterilization, sex crimes, fetal diagnosis, genetics and artificial insemination have been some of the major issues for study and legislative initiatives (Table 3.1).

Table 3.1. Social and political initiatives, laws and reforms of the twentieth century

1911 Law on contraception banning information on and sale of contraceptives

1915 Repeal of the 1778 law permitting unwed mothers to remain anonymous and the child to be registered as "mother unknown"

1919 Lex veneris, requiring physicians to report venereal diseases and to track down the source of infection as well as any sexual contacts, and establishing the right and obligation for men and women with known or suspected venereal disease to be examined and treated

1938 A restrictive abortion act, allowing abortion on medical grounds, because of eugenic risk (hereditary diseases) and for humanitarian reasons (rape, incest)

1938 Repeal of 1911 law on contraception

1938 Free prenatal and obstetrical care, maternal allowances and housing allowances for families with children

1939 Law prohibiting firing women from their jobs because of marriage, pregnancy or childbirth

1947 Child allowances for all children through the age of 16, paid to the mother

1955 Required sex education in schools

1964 Oral contraceptives registered as means of birth control

1971 Report submitted by governmental committee on abortion: Right to abortion, followed by heated public debate

1971   Parliamentary statement on right to pain relief during childbirth

1972   Joint taxation for husband and wife abolished—every adult is expected to provide for him- or herself

1974   Parental benefits: Parental leave for 180 days at 90 percent of wages; right to split leave between mother and father

1974   Abortion act permitting abortion on demand up to the 18th week of pregnancy. In addition, a law institutes contraceptive services free of charge in the public health system.

1974   Governmental subcommittee submits a comprehensive report on sex education in the schools

1976   Revised law on sterilization passed, prohibiting compulsory sterilization on eugenic, genetic or social grounds, and permitting men and women over the age of 25 to choose sterilization as a method of birth control

1976   Midwives authorized to prescribe birth-control pills

1979   Parliamentary resolution on education for expectant and new parents

1979   Report by committee on sexual offenses proposing legislative changes, including more rigorous punishment for rape, sexual coercion and sexual exploitation

1979   Homosexuality is removed from the Swedish National Board of Health and Welfare list of diagnoses and no longer considered a disease or disorder

1980   Committee on prostitution submits a report on the factors behind prostitution and sex-related violence

1980   Law passed establishing equality between women and men in the workplace

1983   Committee to evaluate 1974 law on abortion delivers its report: Family planning and abortion

1983   Committee on childbearing through artificial insemination recommends that donors not be allowed to remain anonymous, resulting in a 1985 law confirming the right of children to know their origin

1987   Law on cohabitation, regulating common property of unmarried, cohabiting hetero- and homosexual couples

1988   Parental leave, which was extended in 1978 and again in 1980, is set at 360 days, 270 of which are compensated at 90 percent of wages

1992   Act on equal opportunities for women and men

1993   Law on paternal month: One month of parental leave cannot be reallocated to the mother if it is not utilized by the father

1995   Law on registration and official recognition of homosexual relationships

1995   Compensation during parental leave is reduced to 80 percent, in 1996 to 75 percent, in 1998 back to 80 percent

1998   Act on violence against women, stating more stringent penalties, ban on female genital mutilation, and 1999 ban on purchase of sexual services.

A national family planning program

An example of a significant and successful social initiative in the sphere of reproductive health is the abortion-prevention program launched in connection with the 1974 legalization of abortion. Even prior to 1974, parliament set aside 1 million Swedish crowns annually for a total of five years to be used by the National Board of Health and Welfare on long-term efforts to provide education on sexuality and interpersonal relations, with the goal of preventing unwanted pregnancies. Special funds were also allocated to assist women's, youth and immigrant organizations in providing information on sexuality and birth control.

A community-based, three-year project on the Baltic island of Gotland was a key component in efforts to prevent abortion (Sundström-Feigenberg 1988). It focused on developing and testing methods of communication and providing information, and approached the abortion issue in the context of sexuality, gender roles and interpersonal relations. Training and education were fundamental components of this project, which included courses for people working in the fields of social work, schools and health care. The goal was to tackle the problem of unwanted pregnancies and to reach the public through professionals. Encouragement was given to cooperation and the exchange of experiences across professional categories. When working with teenagers, the aim was to convey a positive attitude toward sexuality. Similar projects were initiated in other Swedish counties between 1977 and 1980. Some of the lasting effects of these activities were a more open, relaxed attitude in society toward teenage sexuality and a general decline in teenage fertility over the period from 1975 to 1985 (Weinberg et al. 1995).

Midwives in the maternity health care system were trained to provide contraceptive services, and such training has since become a feature of basic midwifery training. In 1976, midwives were authorized to prescribe oral contraceptives and insert IUDs. State aid helped facilitate a rapid expansion of contraceptive services as part of the general maternal care system, with midwives as service providers. Government subsidies also aided in the establishment of a number of youth clinics that provided information and counseling for young people. Thus efforts to prevent unwanted pregnancies through sex education and contraceptive services developed into a national family planning program integrated with the maternal care system (Sundström-Feigenberg 1988).

In 1980, a government subcommittee was appointed to assess the outcome of the 1974 law on abortion and the associated prevention program. The committee report detailed abortion trends following legalization and confirmed that there was no increase in the number of abortions, and that illegal abortions had stopped entirely. Abortions were now performed at an earlier stage, which meant fewer risks and complications for women and less stress for medical personnel. The report showed that women were not using abortion as a means of family planning, and abortion-prevention efforts had resulted in a sizeable reduction in the number of abortions performed on teenagers (Swedish Government Official Reports 1983:31).

Teenage sexuality

Increasing numbers of teenage pregnancies are a growing social problem in many countries. A comparison of teenage pregnancy in the industrialized countries in the mid-1980s (Jones et al. 1985) shows substantial differences between the United States and European countries. Pregnancy figures for American teenagers are more than twice as high as in England, three times as high as in Sweden, and seven times as high as in the Netherlands. The level of sexual activity and the age at which teenagers become sexually active differ only insignificantly. Evidently young people in Europe are better able to protect themselves against unwanted pregnancies than their American peers (Kirby et al. 1991, Miller et al. 1992, Weinberg et al. 1995).

The drop in teenage abortions that has been observed in Sweden and to some extent in other Scandinavian countries has not taken place in the United States. In 1975, the abortion rate among teenagers in both the United States and Sweden was about 30 abortions per 1000 women. By 1981, the rate had decreased by 30 percent in Sweden, while it had increased in the United States by 43 percent (Jones et al. 1985). Social attitudes toward sexuality constitute the most significant factor behind these changes. Most parents in Sweden accept the fact that young people are sexually active, and expect them to take responsibility and protect themselves against unwanted pregnancy. This, in turn, stems from a long tradition of sex education in schools and a positive attitude toward sexuality. Moreover, in Sweden information on contraception is available to young people through the health care system and youth clinics throughout the country (Bygdeman & Lindahl 1994).

The individual

Reproductive health—sexuality and childbearing throughout one's life—is important for both women and men. For women, biological and physical functions related to childbirth are in the forefront. Giving birth and caring for children also challenge a woman's emotional resources and social competence. For men, biology is certainly an important aspect; fatherhood is linked to a man's masculinity and sense of self-worth. Moreover, sexuality, as part of what we call reproductive health, is an important part of people's lives whether or not they decide to have children.

Beyond physiological changes, social conditions and emotional factors, there is also an existential dimension. While pregnancy and childbirth inevitably lead to intense involvement in the present moment, they also bring up memories of one's own childhood and dreams for the future. The childbearing period, short as it is for many people, awakens a sense of the connections and kinship between generations. Childhood, sexual maturity, psychosexual development, protection of one's fertility, sexual life, birth control and the care of children and grandchildren are all part of reproductive life.

While the medical profession tends to overemphasize the reproductive functions and the childbearing period (Martin 1987), sexuality throughout life is equally important to an individual's health and well-being.

How we live our reproductive lives is undoubtedly more crucial to our well-being than are many other health domains. Whether we succeed in realizing our reproductive plans or instead encounter disappointments and setbacks can affect our health. And yet, health research devotes more attention to eating, drinking and exercise habits than to the issues of childbearing and child rearing or of combining parenthood with professional work.

Studies show that reproductive health contributes to subjective assessments of health. A survey of women of various ages describes the time when they were having children and "getting their lives together" as the most rewarding years (Sundström-Feigenberg 1987). A study of links between work absences and parenthood showed that men with small children were the healthiest group. Despite a dismal economy and the threat of unemployment, it was "clear that people are doing well—indeed, being with small children is what life is all about."

Allowing women to control their fertility by giving them access to legal abortion and reliable contraceptives has been of great significance for gender equality. Women's right to choose has affected relationships between men and women, particularly at a personal level. The balance of power within families has shifted, and equality has increased in day-to-day life. Today women can decide for themselves with whom they want to have sex as well as with whom they want to live or have children. They are not compelled to get married or remain in a bad relationship, whether for reasons of convention, morality or economics. And while a man no longer has control over a woman's sexuality or the number of children she will bear, he now has the advantage of knowing that when a woman chooses him, it is for his own sake and because he is the one she wants to be the father of her children (Sundström-Feigenberg 1987).

Medical care

Today, the health care system has assumed the position once held by the state, civil society and the church in matters of sexuality and reproduction. We deliver babies in the hospital, receive instruction in how to be good parents, go to a midwife or a physician if we need contraceptives, and consult a medical specialist for infertility treatments. Physicians and midwives in obstetric care exercise a great deal of control over the most intimate aspects of women's lives and make far-reaching decisions about what is best for the individual woman (Sundström-Feigenberg 1988).

Different aspects of reproductive health come into focus in different phases of life. Supporting people during various stages of their reproductive lives requires medical expertise and an awareness of the social conditions affecting them, as well as sensitivity and experience. In today's reproductive health care, there is a tendency to "medicalize" normal life events and to seek technical solutions to existential problems. The medical profession is well-meaning and overprotective, but also quick to criticize and even punish noncompliance with its advice and prescriptions (Martin 1987, Carlstedt 1992).

Sexuality in reproductive health care

Although sexuality plays a central role in people's lives, little attention is given to it within the women's health care system. Sexuality is ignored unless it relates to procreation, or if it deviates from what is considered the norm. Little is said about the darker side of sexuality, about sexualized violence, sexual exploitation or prostitution. Nor is sexuality affirmed as a mutually pleasurable and joyful aspect of life. Sexual health is seen almost exclusively in terms of the risk of unwanted pregnancy or sexually transmitted diseases; moreover, scant attention is paid to the sexual needs of gays or lesbians, the handicapped or the elderly.

In an article on sexuality as part of reproductive health, Dixon-Müller (1993) discusses the role sexuality has, or should have, in women's health care. The author points out that issues of sexuality and gender roles are seldom touched upon in women's health care and family planning programs, and suggests that attention should be given to other dimensions of sexuality beyond the risk of disease or pregnancy.

New lifestyles, new health problems

Society's changing attitudes toward sexuality and relationships and new patterns of family formation and childbearing raise new issues and problems in the sphere of women's health care.

Concerns about fertility

When women postpone childbearing for many years, it is important to safeguard their fertility until they are ready to become pregnant. In large part because of the risk of HIV, more information has emerged in recent years on sexually transmitted diseases (STDs). We are more candid and more knowledgeable about the risks and ways of becoming infected, and those who suspect they may be infected are anxious to get treatment for themselves and their partners. People want to protect themselves and their loved ones so that they will be able to have children when they choose to do so.

Preventing and treating STDs is an important and sensitive matter. Central measures in the control of STDs include screening to detect symptom-free infections at an early stage, providing information on how these diseases are spread, partner notification and treatment of infected individuals. Moreover, any STD puts a strain on a relationship, since it raises the issue of infidelity. Thus there is a substantial need for adequate information, support and counseling.

Childlessness

Women of all ages express disappointment over an inability to have children. In the past, however, childlessness was regarded differently than it is today. While people might well experience profound grief over a miscarriage or infertility, having children was not considered a right, but a gift, and childlessness simply had to be accepted.

Today, when we tend to assume that we can plan everything, it can be particularly hard to accept not being able to have children precisely as hoped. Women who have taken birth-control pills ever since becoming sexually active have not tested their fertility, and may not discover until they are in their thirties that having children is not as easy as they had thought. Childlessness is viewed as a defect or illness, and those struggling with infertility turn to the health services for help and are offered medical treatment to remedy the situation. Ever more sophisticated methods of treatment are made available.

Artificial insemination and in-vitro fertilization are the most recent additions to the arsenal of treatment options, and these methods represent a new type of approach to infertility. Other methods seek to repair damaged Fallopian tubes or induce ovulation using hormone treatments. After that, childless couples are on their own. With these two newer methods, however, the health care system has gone a step farther. No longer is the goal simply to ensure the necessary conditions for pregnancy, but through increasingly sophisticated medical technology the aim is to bring about fertilization itself—to create a child in the hospital.

Research and technology involving the manipulation of gametes obviously raise ethical questions. A governmental committee on artificial insemination and in-vitro fertilization has drawn up proposals for legislative regulation of such activity, primarily aimed at protecting children born with the help of these technologies. Parliament has determined that sperm donors may not remain anonymous, but must agree to meet their biological offspring if the children request such a meeting when they are older—although donors have no financial or legal obligations to those children. Legal limits have also been placed on egg donation, the use of surrogate mothers and freezing and storing embryos for a period of more than one year. These regulations, proposed by a committee on medical ethics in research, have been opposed by the medical community, which favors exempting research from such guidelines.

Perfect children and a happy life

In our society, it is a major investment to bring children into the world. We do our best to avoid risks and ensure that each child will be given every opportunity. The health care system offers blood tests and ultrasound examinations to detect any risks or abnormalities, leading us to believe that everything will be fine if we just use the latest technologies or perform another test. Fetal diagnosis is used to detect certain disorders or the propensity toward an illness in the unborn child.

Those who elect to use fetal diagnosis need to face the issue of selective abortion, i.e., an abortion because of chromosomal abnormalities found in the fetus. Most abortions in Sweden are not selective, but are performed because the pregnant woman and her partner find themselves unable or unwilling to become parents. The issue in selective abortion, on the other hand, is the condition of the specific unborn child. This is a difficult decision, and parents need to take into account their resources and their ability to bring up the child.

By making such options as amniocentesis available, the health care system contributes to the misconception that all risks can be avoided. However, most pregnant women are quite aware that there are no guarantees and that having children is a risky proposition. A committee on fetal diagnosis (Swedish Government Official Reports 1989:51) proposed that expectant parents, rather than physicians, should decide whether or not to use amniocentesis, and this should also apply to fetal diagnosis. Medical science has provided us with new tools, but their application should be subject to the political decision-making process after public debate on what kind of society we want to live in. The health care system should provide medical technologies and offer adequate information on their uses and limitations, but it should not be given unlimited authority over questions of fertility control and childbearing.

Premenstrual syndrome (PMS)

In recent years, PMS has been recognized as a major health problem that can cause mood swings, uncomfortable swelling and headaches. Researchers have tracked the regular hormonal changes that occur during the menstrual cycle and proposed a number of different treatments using medication. Remarkably little research has looked at PMS as it relates to women's work and life situations or compared symptoms found in different social classes, countries or cultures (Martin 1987).

Taking the medical view of the female body as a machine, medical experts seek to alleviate discomfort and mood changes through medication, reasoning that pills should be able to cure anger and protest, just as they do pain. Other clinical experts, however, see symptoms like depression, irritability and anger as a message to be decoded. End-of-cycle hormonal changes tend to break down a woman's psychological defenses, putting her more closely in touch with her emotions. If she lets her true feelings out, then she may also be able to change her situation (Martin 1987, Fredelius et al. 1994). Rather than branding women with PMS as sick, we should respect their monthly rhythms and offer them support in the life phase in which they find themselves.

Menopause

In our culture, menopause is often described as a period of decline and failure. Despite this attitude, which is reflected both in the medical literature and in society at large, women's own perceptions are quite different. Women who have already gone through menopause often describe their experience as a relatively easy transition. Younger, premenopausal women generally have a more negative picture of what awaits them.

Women who experience little difficulty frequently regard themselves as exceptions, although it is in fact unusual to have long-term, serious problems related to menopause. It is estimated that between 20 and 30 percent of all women perspire excessively and experience hot flashes for more than a short time. Women's health in middle age has more to do with their family situation and their working conditions than with a decline in hormone production (Carlstedt 1993).

Unfortunately, estrogen treatment has become a major issue in the treatment of menopausal women. Hormone replacement therapy for the relief of symptoms should certainly be a part, but a relatively limited part, of what the women's health services should offer menopausal women. Moreover, during middle age both men and women undergo changes as a normal component of the process of aging and social adjustment that require attention and understanding.

Abortion, a reproductive health issue

There are substantial differences worldwide in the state of reproductive health. In every country one can trace a characteristic pattern of family life, childbearing and fertility regulation. Women's health is influenced first of all by women's status in society, their economic independence and their ability to control their own sexuality and childbearing, but also by their access to and ability to utilize reproductive health services (Petchesky & Judd 1998, Sen 1994). The policies and practices related to abortion in a given society tell us something about women's status and control over their fertility. The abortion situation is also indicative of the quality of reproductive health care (Sundström 1993).

Abortion trends in selected countries

In Sweden abortion is a right, a safe and legal method of terminating an unwanted pregnancy. In Africa and Latin America it is a criminal act that poses a threat to women's health, fertility and even survival. In Vietnam and China, finally, it is more or less an obligation to society in the interest of meeting national population goals (Sundström 1993).

To show the range of reproductive health, let us turn to selected countries with different population trends, laws, religion and family patterns. Table 3.2 shows birth and abortion rates, as well as pregnancy- and childbirth-related mortality in these countries based on data from the 1990s (Henshaw 1990, The World Bank 1993, WHO 1995, WHO 1998, Henshaw et al. 1999).

These countries, chosen to illustrate regional patterns, represent different stages in demographic development. Birth rates have long been low in Sweden and what is now Russia; Vietnam and Brazil and even Bangladesh are in a phase of rapid change from high to low birth rates; and Kenya, like other sub-Saharan countries, still has a high birth rate.

The countries are listed in order of increasing maternal mortality. Classifying them by decreasing gross national product would result in nearly the same sequence. The exception is Vietnam, one of the world's poorest countries, which has maternal mortality and infant mortality rates comparable to or even substantially lower than many "transitional economies" in Eastern Europe or Latin America (Sundström 1996).

Table 3.2. Fertility and maternal mortality in six countries in the 1990s.

Country	MMR	TFR	TAR	GNP
Sweden	< 5	2.1	0.6	25,100
Russia	50	2.3	5.4	3,220
Vietnam	110	3.7	2.5	350
Brazil	200	3.0	2.3	2,940
Bangladesh	570	4.6	1.2	220
Kenya	600	6.0	0.9	340

MMR = Maternal Mortality Ratio: Number of deaths related to pregnancy and childbirth per 100,000 live births

TFR = Total Fertility Rate: Lifetime number of children per woman, according to current birth rates

TAR =Total Abortion Rate: Lifetime number of abortions per woman, according to current abortion rate

GNP=Gross national product per capita, in US $

Sweden

In Sweden, in the early 1990s, a woman on average had 2 children and 0.6 abortions. Many people are sexually active at an early age but wait years to have children. Reliable contraceptive methods are required to achieve no more than three pregnancies in a reproductive period that spans 30 years. Contraceptives are easy to obtain, and they are used for long periods both before and after childbearing. Abortions are performed under legal and safe conditions as part of the general health care system. All of this stems from an open, responsible view of sexuality and relationships in society, sex education in schools since the 1950s, parental acceptance of young people's sexuality, and private sexual relationships marked by gender equality. In contrast to 30 years ago, Swedish women faced with an unwanted pregnancy are no longer forced to choose between bearing children against their will and having an illegal abortion (Sundström-Feigenberg 1987).

Russia

In the former Soviet Union and most of its Eastern European satellite countries, abortion was legal from the 1950s on. There was limited access to sex education or contraceptive information and services, but induced abortions were provided free of charge in the public health system. Social conditions and women's multiple work load made it necessary to limit childbearing. Warning women of the risks of contraceptives, physicians instead offered them abortions, which themselves were frequently dangerous. In practice, abortion became the predominant method of birth control, resulting in notably high abortion rates (David 1992).

In later years, the quality of the health care system declined, and private abortions were common in the Soviet Union long before democratization occurred. The same gynecologists who performed abortions in poorly equipped general hospitals were able to offer safer abortions in their own private practices. The "commercialization" of health care was legalized in Russia in 1989, which meant that—just as before, but now legally—extra charges were levied for anesthesia, antibiotics and other services, also in public hospitals (Popov 1991).

Consequently, those able to pay can obtain both contraceptives and safe abortions, while health care for the poor is even worse than in the past. And in view of the increased cost of living and the scarcity of work and childcare, it is precisely the poor who find themselves needing more than ever to limit their childbearing. The average Russian woman has between two and three children and undergoes four to five abortions (Popov 1994).

Vietnam

In Vietnam, abortion is considered an obligation to society, an officially sanctioned way of meeting population goals. The 1980s saw the introduction of the so-called "policy of one child, or at most two." Couples were permitted to have two children, but those who stopped at one were afforded special treatment and offered rewards. Abortion and contraceptives were provided free of charge by the general health care system. However, the supply of contraceptives was limited, and in practice the IUD continues to be the only alternative to abortion.

At the end of the 1980s, population guidelines became stricter, and an intense propaganda campaign, directed primarily toward women, was launched aimed at limiting the number of children in each family. Volunteers were recruited to spread the message, and cars equipped with loudspeakers were sent into communities to urge women, by name, to use contraceptives. Women who had already borne two children were exhorted to have an abortion. The effect of this campaign was a declining birth rate and a substantially higher rate of abortion. At the beginning of the 1990s, the number of abortions performed each year exceeded the number of children born (Johansson et al. 1996).

Interviews on attitudes toward fertility and birth control indicate that both men and women recognize the importance of putting a stop to population growth. By tradition most people have a strong and well-founded desire for sons, and they look back with regret to the past, when women had many children.

Women complain about the side effects of the IUD, but such symptoms are vague. These complaints may rather reflect resentment of the need to use contraceptives at all (Johansson et al. 1998).

Brazil

In Brazil, as in most Latin American countries, abortion is a crime in the eyes of both society and the Catholic Church. However, the law is broken constantly—in Brazil the number of illegal abortions exceeds the number of children born. In every large city there are rows of clinics advertising "early pregnancy detection" or "comprehensive obstetrical care." What they actually offer are abortions performed by well-trained personnel under safe conditions. Women lacking the necessary resources turn to less professional abortionists. As a rule, neither type of procedure is prosecuted under the law, nor is the provider punished. Instead, women are punished by being subjected to expensive procedures, humiliating treatment and impaired health (Singh & Wulf 1991).

The birth rate in Brazil is relatively low, and abortions are common. On average, women have three children and three abortions during the course of their reproductive lives. Brazilian society is marked by rapid change, a growing social and economic gap between classes, migration to the cities, increased job opportunities for women, and changing sexual mores. Premarital sexuality, separations and divorce are becoming more and more common. Sex roles, however, remain traditional, and young women in particular are trapped in the double standards of the macho culture. A young woman is expected to maintain her chastity, while young men are excused for their strong sexual needs. A woman who seeks to protect herself by using contraceptives is branded as immoral, since she has shown that she is "expecting" to have sex.

In Brazil, the two main methods of contraception are birth-control pills, which can be purchased over the counter in drugstores and pharmacies, and sterilization, which is permitted only when performed in connection with other surgical procedures. Accordingly, sterilization is usually carried out following a Caesarean section, which is one of the reasons why Caesarean deliveries are far more common in Brazil than medically necessary. There is widespread distrust of the public health care system. Resources are inadequate and quality is low, while private medicine offers the most advanced diagnosis and treatment. Health care workers are dismissive and unfriendly toward women obtaining abortions—perhaps because of their own anxiety and uncertainty. Most women fear and avoid the regular hospitals, seeking other, unconventional solutions to their health problems. Abortion is always available to women who have money, but young, poor and uneducated women find themselves at the mercy of untrained abortionists and hazardous methods (Barbosa & Arilha 1993).

Bangladesh

The average woman in Bangladesh has four to five children and undergoes one abortion in her lifetime. The birth rate is declining, especially in urban areas and among women with better education and some degree of economic independence. Abortion is prohibited by law, but inducing an overdue menstrual period by "menstrual regulation" is permissible. Several non-governmental organizations (NGOs) have initiated training of service providers, e.g. paramedics in menstrual regulation. Decentralized reproductive health services, including family planning and menstrual regulation, are available at low cost through government facilities, even in rural areas. Many women want to limit the number of children they bear, and inducing a delayed menstrual period is culturally accepted by most people. Still, the health services are not utilized, and many women resort to unsafe procedures. The estimate of 800,000 abortions each year includes menstrual regulation and a considerable number of illegal abortions (Dixon-Müller 1988). Maternal mortality is high, and about 20 percent of the deaths associated with pregnancy and childbirth are due to unsafe abortions (WHO 1998).

The barriers to utilizing health services stem mainly from women's subordinate position in the family and society at large. Within the family, the man is in charge of decisions regarding sexuality and childbearing. Married women have neither economic nor sexual rights, and young, unmarried women are "protected" and required to obey their fathers in matters of sexuality and marriage. Even if a woman is aware that contraceptives and menstrual regulation are available and where they can be obtained, she may not be allowed to visit a public health center.

Kenya

The highest birth rates and the highest maternal mortality ratio are found in sub-Saharan Africa. In Kenya, it is both common and expected for women to marry and have children at an early age. Women have an average of six children, and it is not unusual for a woman to have all her children before the age of 25.

Although abortion is prohibited by law, the termination of unwanted pregnancies, which used to be performed mainly when women had already given birth to many children, has become common in recent years among teenagers as well (Coeytaux 1988). Illegal abortions are particularly frequent in cities, where young people have come to study or work. Girls are expelled from school if they become pregnant. Many of these girls get married, fulfilling the expectations of their parents and society. Unwed mothers often leave their child with their own parents and move to the city to look for work. There is inadequate maternity and obstetrical care, as well as insufficient treatment for complications from abortion (Kizza & Rogo 1990). Between 30 and 40 percent of the extremely high maternal mortality rate is associated with abortion, although the number of abortions is small relative to births (Sundström 1993).

Reproductive health worldwide

Human conditions across various countries and differences in reproductive health highlight the injustice that exists between rich and poor countries as well as between the rich and poor of a given country. Our own history is marked by conditions similar to those prevalent in many countries even today. Parallels are evident between the poverty in Bangladesh today, a country plagued by repeated flooding, and nineteenth-century Sweden with its poor harvests and resulting hunger. Desperate women today take medicine designed to treat malaria in hopes of inducing abortion and end up dying before the medicine takes effect, just as, in Sweden, abused servant girls of the previous century used phosphorus to induce abortion. We hear of schoolgirls in Africa who are forced to quit school when they become pregnant by their teachers and are reminded of young, pregnant girls in Sweden who drowned themselves in the 1940s rather than bring shame on their parents.

Changes toward better reproductive health, which we have observed in Sweden and which are underway in many countries of the world, show that improvement is possible even in difficult conditions. The prerequisite is a favorable social and economic climate. In addition, however, efforts must be made to secure women's reproductive rights. This means access to education and the opportunity to plan one's childbearing, as well as the right to make one's own decisions and to retain control over one's own life. In Sweden, access to sex education, effective contraceptives, legal abortion and satisfactory reproductive health care have contributed not only to improved reproductive health, but also to increased equality between men and women.

Notes

1 The UN Declaration on Human Rights, issued in 1968 in Tehran, established a "basic human right for individuals and couples to decide freely and responsibly on the number and spacing of their children." The following year the UN General Assembly stated that governments and nations had a responsibility to "provide families with the knowledge and means to enable them to exercise this right."

2 Abortion was mentioned only once in the concluding document of the 1984 Mexico City population conference: "In no case should abortion be promoted as a method of family planning" (United Nations 1984). These words were repeated in the final document of the 1994 United Nations Conference on Population and Development in Cairo, although many considered this formulation to be unnecessary and harmful. It was approved in exchange for a paragraph asserting that women have the right to proper medical care in the case of an abortion (United Nations 1994).

3 The "Platform for action" from the United Nations' Fourth Women's Conference in Beijing, September, 1995, contains the following comments on women's human rights in Chapter IV, Strategic objectives and actions (United Nations

1995):"96. The human rights of women include their right to have control over and decide freely and responsibly on matters related to their sexuality, including sexual and reproductive health, free of coercion, discrimination and violence. Equal relations between women and men in matters of sexual relations and reproduction, including full respect for the integrity of the person, require mutual respect, consent, and shared responsibility for sexual behavior and its consequences."

References

Andreen A. Karolina Widerström. En levnadsteckning [Karolina Widerström: A biography]. Stockholm: Norstedts, 1988. (Available in Swedish only).

Barbosa RM, Arilha M. The Brazilian experience with Cytotec. Studies in Family Planning, 1993; 24:236–240.

Bygdeman M, Lindahl K. Sex education and reproductive health in Sweden in the 20th century. Report for the International Conference on Population and Development in Cairo 1994. Stockholm: SOU (Swedish Government Official Reports) 1994:37.

Carlstedt G. *Kvinnors hälsa—en fråga om makt [Women's health: A question of power]*. Stockholm: Folksam/Tiden, 1992. (Available in Swedish only).

Coeytaux FM. *Induced abortion in sub-Saharan Africa: What we do and do not know.* Studies in Family Planning 1988;19:186–90.

Correa S, Petchesky R. *Reproductive and Sexual Rights: A Feminist Perspective.* In: Sen G, Germain A, Chen LC (Eds.): *Population Policies Reconsidered. Health, Empowerment and Rights.* Boston: Harvard School of Public Health, 1994, pp. 107–123.

David HP. *Abortion in Europe, 1920–91: A public health perspective.* Studies in Family Planning 1992;23:1–22.

Dixon-Müller R. *Innovations in reproductive health care: Menstrual regulation policies and programs in Bangladesh.* Studies in Family Planning 1988;19:129–140.

Dixon-Müller R. *The sexuality connection in reproductive health.* Studies in Family Planning 1993;24:269–82.

Elgqvist-Saltzman I. *Declines and green hills: Competence development in a life perspective.* In: Bjerén G, Elgqvist-Saltzman I (Eds.): *Gender and Education in a Life Perspective. Lessons from Scandinavia.* Brookfield: Avebury, 1994.

Fredelius G, Klein Frithiof P, Ursing I. *Kvinnoidentitet—Dynamisk kvinnopsykologi i ett livsloppsperspektiv [Women's identity—Dynamic female psychology from a life-course perspective].* Stockholm: Natur och Kultur, 1994. (Available in Swedish only).

Germain A, Novorojee S, Pyne HH. *Setting a New Agenda: Sexual and Reproductive Health and Rights.* In: Sen G, Germain A, Chen LC (Eds.): *Population Policies Reconsidered. Health, Empowerment and Rights.* Boston: Harvard School of Public Health, 1994, p 27–46.

Henshaw SK. *Induced abortion—a world review, 1990.* Family Planning Perspective 1990; 22:76–89.

Henshaw SK, Singh S, Haas T. *The incidence of abortion worldwide.* International Family Planning Perspectives, 1999, 25(Supplement);30–38.

Hoem, B. *Recent changes in family formation in Sweden.* Research reports in Demography 71, 1992. Stockholm University.

Hoem, J.M. *Public policy as fuel of fertility: Effects of a policy reform on the pace of child-bearing in Sweden in the 1980s.* Acta Sociologica 1993;19–31.

Högberg U. *Svagårens barn. Ur folkhälsans historia [Children of hard times: A public-health history].* Stockholm: LiberFörlag, 1983. (Available in Swedish only).

Högberg U. *Maternal mortality in Sweden.* Umeå: Umeå University Medical Dissertations. New Series No 156, 1985.

Höjeberg P. *Jordemor. Barnmorskor och barnaföderskor i Sverige [Midwives and new mothers in Sweden].* Stockholm: Carlsson Bokförlag, 1991. (Available in Swedish only).

Johansson A, Hoa HT, Tuyet LTN, Bich MH, Höjer B. *Family planning in Vietnam. Women's experiences and dilemmas.* J Psychosomatic Obstetrics and Gynecology 1996;17:59–67.

Johansson A, Hoa HT, Lap NT, Diwan VK, Eriksson B. *Population policies, son preference and the use of IUDs in Vietnam.* Reproductive Health Matters 1998;6(11):66–76.

Jones EF, Forrest JD, Goldman N, Henshaw SK, Lincoln R, Rostoff JI, Westoff CF, Wulf D. *Teenage pregnancy in developed countries: Determinants and policy implications.* Family Planning Perspective 1985;17:53–63

Kirby D, Waszak C, Ziegler J. *Six school-based clinics: Their reproductive health services and impact on sexual behavior.* Fam Plann Perspect 1991;23:6–16.

Kizza AP, Rogo KO. *Assessment of the manual vacuum aspiration (MVA) equipment in the management of incomplete abortion.* East African Medical Journal 1990; 67:812–822.

Liljeström R, Kollind A-K. *Kärleksliv och föräldraskap [Love life and parenthood].* Stockholm: Carlsson Bokförlag, 1990. (Available in Swedish only).

Martin E. *The Woman in the Body: A Cultural Analysis of Reproduction.* Open University Press/Milton Keynes, 1987.

Miller BC, Card JJ, Paikoff RL, Peterson JL (Eds.). *Preventing adolescent pregnancy: Model programs and evaluations.* Newbury Park, California: Sage Publications, 1992.

Myrdal A, Myrdal G. *Kris i befolkningsfrågan [Population crisis].* Stockholm: Bonniers, 1934. (Available in Swedish only).

Ohlander A-S. *Women, children and work in Sweden 1850–1993.* Report for the International Conference on Population and Development in Cairo 1994. Stockholm: SOU (Swedish Government Official Reports) 1994:38.

Ottesen-Jensen E. *Livet skrev [Life wrote the story].* Stockholm: Ordfront, 1986. (Available in Swedish only).

Petchesky R, Judd K (Eds.). *Negotiating Reproductive Rights. Women's perspectives across countries and cultures.* London, New York: Zed Books Ltd., 1998.

Popov AA. *Family planning and induced abortion in the USSR: Basic health and demographic characteristics.* Studies in Family Planning 1991;22:368–377.

Popov AA. *Family Planning and induced abortion in the post Soviet Russia of the early 1990s.* Centre of Demography and Human Ecology, Moscow 1994.

Singh S, Wulf D. *Estimating abortion levels in Brazil, Colombia and Peru, using hospital admissions and fertility survey data.* International Family Planning Perspective 1991; 17:8–13.

Sen G. *Development, Population and the Environment: A search for balance.* In: Sen G, Germain A, Chen LC (Eds.): *Population Policies Reconsidered. Health, Empowerment and Rights.* Boston: Harvard School of Public Health, 1994, p 63–74.

Statistics Sweden (SCB). *Women and men in Sweden. Facts and figures 1995.* Stockholm: Statistics Sweden, 1995.

Sundström-Feigenberg K. *När livet var som bäst—Kvinnor i Sundbyberg berättar om samlevnad, arbete och barn [Fertility and social change—Sundbyberg women on living together, work and children].* Lund: Studentlitteratur, 1987. (Available in Swedish only).

Sundström-Feigenberg K. *Reproductive health and reproductive freedom: maternal health care and family planning in the Swedish health system.* Women & Health 1988;13:35–55.

Sundström K. *Abortion—a reproductive health issue. Background paper for a World Bank Best practices paper on Women's Health.* Stockholm, SIDA, Washington, The World Bank 1993.

Sundström K. *Abortion across social and cultural borders.* Demography India, 25: 1996; 93–103.

Swedish Government Official Reports (SOU) 1983:31. *Familjeplanering och abort— Erfarenheter av ny lagstiftning [Family planning and abortion: Experiences with the new legislation].* Betänkande från 1980 års abortkommitté. Stockholm: Socialdepartementet, 1983. (Available in Swedish only).

Swedish Governmental Official Reports (SOU) 1989:51. *Den gravida kvinnan och fostret—två individer. Om fosterdiagnostik och aborter [The pregnant woman and the fetus: two individuals. On fetal diagnosis and abortion].* Stockholm: Justitiedepartementet, 1985. (Available in Swedish only).

United Nations. *Human Rights 1969.* New York: United Nations 1969; 144–150.

United Nations. *Report of the International Conference on Population, 1984, Mexico City.* New York: United Nations, 1984.

United Nations. *Program of action of the International Conference on Population and Development, 1994, Cairo.* New York: United Nations, 1994.

United Nations. *Platform for action. Fourth World Conference on Women, 1995, Beijing.* New York: United Nations, 1995.

Weinberg MS, Lottes IL, Shaver FM. *Swedish or American heterosexual college youth: Who is more permissive?* Arch Sex Behav 1995, 24:409–437.

WHO. *WHO's current technical definitions related to reproductive health.* Progress in Human Reproduction Research, No 30, 1994. Geneva: World Health Organization, 1994.

WHO. *Complications of abortion. Technical and managerial guidelines for prevention and treatment.* Geneva: World Health Organization, 1995.

WHO. *Unsafe abortion. Global and regional estimates of incidence of and mortality due to unsafe abortion with a listing of available country data.* Third edition, (WHO/RHT/MSM/1997.16) Geneva: World Health Organization, 1998.

The World Bank. *Investing in Health.* World Development Report 1993. New York: Oxford University Press, 1993.

4

Gender inequalities in health:
An historical and cultural perspective

Karin Johannisson

THE CONCEPT OF GENDER underwent intensive reconsideration during the nineteenth century.[1] The view of the female body as an underdeveloped version of the male body was replaced by the *two-body model*, which regarded the male and the female body as different in every respect. This theory of two separate entities was not a result of new medical discoveries, but rather a cultural construct (Laqueur 1994). It reflected two middle-class social ideals: the strong masculine body and the weak feminine body, corresponding to the division of labor in an increasingly industrialized society that made a sharp distinction between the (male) productive sphere and the (female) reproductive sphere.

Before long, the two-body model left its mark on the concepts of health and illness as well. While health was seen as the hallmark of the normal male body, women were characterized by cyclical changes, instability and constitutional weakness. Ill health was seen as a more normal condition for the female than the male body. These models came to have a profound influence on our perception of gender-specific body identities in Western countries.

The modern health paradox—also referred to as the gender paradox—points to this striking fact: women are sicker than men, but they live longer. Women go to the doctor more often, consume more medication and are more frequently absent from work because of illness. They report having more health problems than men do. Gender differences are particularly great when it comes to restlessness, anxiety, insomnia, headaches and fatigue. At the same time, however, women possess more vitality in the root sense of the word, that is, they have a greater capacity than men for sustaining life (Hammarström & Hovellius 1994). Biological models alone cannot explain this paradox. It is important to consider cultural, social and psychological factors, as well as each individual's life situation, identity, roles, body image and self-image.

It is helpful in this context to introduce an historical perspective. History creates distance, revealing an overall pattern and enhancing our understanding of ourselves and our ability to identify underlying structures that affect how we think and act. It also shows how what we see as "natural" or innate is often related to culturally determined attitudes with respect to our bodies. Historical experience and a long-term perspective enable us to identify patterns in gender-specific illness. Since the female body is represented as a deviation from the male norm, it will be our focus in the following sections. We examine the interaction between biology, life circumstances and societal roles.

It is important, first of all, to examine women's ill health in terms of biomedically demonstrable illness. Even limiting ourselves to this narrow medical dimension, however, we also need to consider how academic medicine has interpreted female ill health relative to women's own perceptions. In doing so, it is helpful to keep in mind the distinction introduced in recent years between measurable/objective ill health (disease) and experienced/subjective ill health (illness). Much of the ill health typically experienced by women appears to be situated in this difficult but rich terrain between the objective and the subjective.

Second, women's ill health must be considered in the light of women's lives, since their lives as well as their bodies differ from those of men. Divergent life circumstances lead to different ways of experiencing and dealing with illness. Being sick opens the individual up to feelings of weakness and vulnerability. It requires establishing lines of communication linking the body, the self and society. Moreover, illness can provide certain benefits, such as rest, escape, comfort and power.

But women have also been assigned the role of being sick—which is the third aspect of women's ill health. Historically, women's illnesses appear to have resulted not only from medical and social factors, but also from cultural circumstances. This corresponds to some extent to certain theories of femininity created by a culture that needed to believe in them.

The female body and nineteenth-century society

Around the turn of the century—a period defined here broadly to include the period from about 1870 until the beginning of World War I—there was as much excess illness among women as there is today. Women went to the doctor more often, took more medication, and were seen as sickly, weak and delicate. It was not unheard of for housewives, mothers and daughters to spend weeks, months or indeed their entire lives in bed. Women found themselves in physicians' consultation rooms, on analysts' couches, in psychiatric clinics and at health spas. Women's gender identity and minds were in a state of confusion; they suffered from pain, anemia and migraine headaches. There were women who seemed to need to be sick, to compensate for the lack of another role in life, to affirm their femininity, to counteract their feelings of dissatisfaction, or to escape from married life and repeated pregnancies.

Such patterns of illness were strongly linked to social class, highlighting the complex relationship between gender and class and reflecting a certain social structure, with two distinct feminine ideals. (Of course, this relationship is equally complex for men. While the male body was depicted as constitutionally strong, it was not supposed to be characterized by brute strength. Here we see the influence of both Darwin's theory of evolution and the age-old dichotomy between body and mind. Indeed, some biologists at the turn of the century claimed to have identified a particularly weak body type common among students and intellectuals.)

While women of the working class—whose role was both to work and to reproduce—were described as strong, vigorous and sexual, middle-class women were depicted as weak, fragile and asexual. Middle-class women's activities were, in the main, centered around the home, where they were expected to serve as the nurturing hearth of family life, emanating love, providing care and seeing to social obligations. Men represented the mind, the intellect and production; women represented emotion, nature and reproduction. The man's sphere was the public arena, the woman's was private life. Determining gender differences in biological and scientific terms became a pressing concern for turn-of-the-century middle-class society, a society based on rationality and a certain division of labor that saw itself confronted with the threat of an emerging women's-liberation movement.

In *The Descent of Man, and Selection in Relation to Sex* (1871), Charles Darwin defined the "natural" gender differences in physical and mental capacity. Through natural selection, men had surpassed women not only in physical size and strength, but also in terms of energy, intellect and creativity. The areas where women had the advantage—in their superior intuition, perception and imitative abilities—were those that, according to Darwin, were characteristic of the lower races and thus of a bygone and lower stage of civilization (Darwin 1871). Women, then, had remained at a lower rung the evolutionary ladder, since their energy was needed for reproduction. While their own development remained stunted, the species as a whole benefited. Similar evolutionary reasoning was found in most textbooks in the fields of gynecology and sexology at the turn of the century. The scientific community used such theories in attempting to prove that women's subordinate position was biologically determined.

Scientists worked primarily with three models to explain gender characteristics. After the turn of the century, a fourth model was developed, a psychological model that defined the specific nature of women in terms of a more fragile psyche and certain personality types (e.g., the hysteric, the neurotic, the phobic, the depressive). It was claimed that subjective physical symptoms were psychogenic in nature, i.e., originating in women's minds.

Three models of the female body

The first might be termed the *anatomical-physiological* model. This model viewed women's anatomy and physiology as different from men's in almost every respect. Women's bodies were seen as having a fundamentally different structure from men's bodies. Their nervous and vascular systems, lungs and spleen, skull and brain were different.

Physiological differences were also scrutinized. Women's digestion was observed to be different from men's, their blood vessels were more constricted (with the exception of the blood supply to the pelvis), their secretions and their breathing were different. Women's blood was thinner, with a higher water content and lower calcium levels. Differences could also be observed at the microlevel, for example, in cells and tissues; when men were ill, their bodies tended to toughen up, "while women's tissues were more likely to take on a liquid state, as in dropsy and mucous discharge (catarrh)" (Kress 1905).

A pathology was developed that presented female biology as a closed system, in which each part affected every other. Unlike men's illnesses, women's ailments were not localized and clearly delineated, but vague and general. Women's symptoms seemed just as indistinct and blurred as the picture of women that was presented: soft, watery and fluid, in contrast to the "toughness" that characterized men. Here conceptions of what was male or female apparently led to the assumption that toughness and softness were gender-specific biological characteristics.

The second model might be termed the *gynecological* model. Here we find the image of the uterus as an unstable, energy-sapping organ, as well as a focus on menstruation, which early on resulted in the medical community viewing female characteristics in terms of illness. The constant change inherent in reproductive cycles demonstrated that, in contrast to men, women lacked control over their own bodies.

There was another aspect to the gynecological model as well, which might be termed the "gynecologizing" of women: the view that the uterus and the other reproductive organs influenced every other organ of a woman's body, and that every female complaint could be reduced, directly or indirectly, to a gynecological problem. Thus any imbalance, change or infection affecting the reproductive organs might lead to pathological reactions somewhere else in the body—in the head, eyes, teeth, heart or skin. Pain, vomiting or migraine headaches could be interpreted as genital reflexes.

Equally important was the fact that the gynecological model offered an explanation for women's mental disorders. Hysteria and insanity were seen as the result of functional disturbances in the uterus that were transmitted to the brain by the nervous system. Psychological ailments, then, could be treated by performing gynecological surgery. Based on extensive asylum case studies, gynecologists concluded that hysteria, mania (psychosis) and melancholy (depression) could be corroborated by finding pathological gynecological changes.

The third primary model of the female body and female pathology was the *neurological* model. This model posited that women were more fragile than men, not because of their reproductive organs, but because of their particularly sensitive nervous system. This fragility found expression in the diagnosis of neurasthenia. The elasticity of the concept of neurasthenia made it possible to link it with a number of existing theories of female pathology. This diagnosis paved new ground in introducing cultural and psychosocial factors—overexertion, alienation and a sense of emptiness—to explain disease. The concepts of neurasthenia, neurosis and nervousness became new code words for women's ill health.

The reduction of women to their biological nature was followed, in turn, by an overemphasis on medical treatment. A specific pathology of women's ailments was developed, which was applied not only theoretically (women's illnesses were seen as having different causes and taking a different course than men's), but also therapeutically (women required a different sort of treatment than men) and socially (illness was a more natural state for women than for men). Illnesses were regarded as specific to women if they could be directly or indirectly related to gender and the psyche; sometimes these aspects were closely linked, as in the diagnosis of hysteria. Nervousness, neurosis and insanity were seen as more characteristic of women than men, as was the tendency for thoughts and ideas, restlessness and anxiety to be expressed in the form of physical symptoms. The overriding importance of sexual difference for disease and ill health was a fundamental part of fin de siècle medical theory.

Gender-specific illness: women

Throughout history up to the 1940s, illness meant primarily infectious diseases. Individual diseases (unless they were linked to mortality) could only be tracked when they showed up in hospital records.[2] Statistics were compiled by gender beginning in 1891, but until 1900, data were compiled for only a small part of the population, principally the lower classes. A recurrent problem for historical analysis of illness is that members of the upper social strata were long under the care of private physicians and thus excluded from health statistics (a particularly difficult problem for studying sexually-transmitted diseases). Epidemics of infectious diseases were dramatic, but since they struck unpredictably, figures could vary widely from year to year. Thus the figures listed below are primarily indicative of trends.

That said, hospital statistics selected randomly from the years 1901 and 1911 show tuberculosis and diphtheria to be the dominant diagnoses among women, closely followed by diseases of the reproductive organs.

Table 4.1. The ten most common diagnoses for female patients in Swedish hospitals in 1901, with comparable figures for 1911. Number of hospitalizations.

	1901	1911
Diphtheria	2,899	3,750
Tuberculosis	2,807	4,655
Diseases of the reproductive organs	2,635	4,544
Sexually-transmitted diseases		
(gonorrhea, syphilis)	1,356	1,835
Cancer	1,233	1,604
Rheumatism (acute and chronic)	1,098	1,281
Scarlet fever	985	3,699
Inflammation of the skin	971	1,158
Chlorosis (a type of iron-deficiency anemia)	940	777
Neurasthenia	739	1,193

Source: Official Swedish statistics. Health and medical care, Tables 22a, 16a.

Along with infectious diseases and diseases of the reproductive organs, we see a high incidence of cancer. While not specific to women, cancer was widely regarded as a women's disease, probably because the types of cancer that typically affect women—breast cancer and cancers of the reproductive organs—were easiest to diagnose. Despite the fact that autopsies became more common and microscopic analysis was introduced to clinical medicine in the early 1900s, for years international statistics showed a female mortality rate from cancer that was hardly in keeping with the actual gender ratio. Swedish statistics confirm that a somewhat greater number of women than men were treated for cancer throughout this period, but they do not show higher mortality rates among women. Interestingly, the *fear* of cancer, sometimes to the point of phobia, was common among women as early as the 1870s.

There is also clear excess female illness in the cases of chlorosis (a type of iron-deficiency anemia) as well as neurasthenia, hysteria, St. Vitus' dance (chorea) and Graves' disease. Some excess illness among women is also found for gastric catarrh, gastric ulcers and heart defects.

A study of schoolchildren's health from 1885 offers valuable insight into the health of young girls at that time. Among other things, it indicates that the majority of the more than 3,000 girls studied—who were students at girls' schools and thus members of the upper classes—were classified as sickly. The most common ailments were chlorosis (35%), headaches (36.1%), appetite loss (12%), and scoliosis (curvature of the spine) (10.8%); in addition, the girls suffered from nosebleeds, nervousness and scrofula (a clinical manifestation of tuberculosis). A sup-

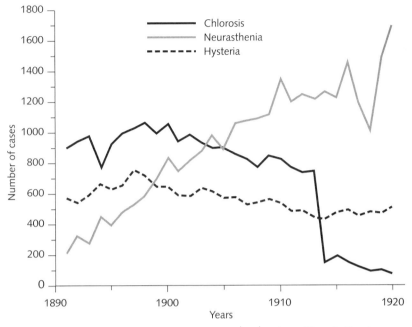

Figure 4.1 Chlorosis, neurasthenia, and hysteria. Number of hospitalizations 1890–1920. (Source: Official Swedish statistics. Health and Medical care.)

plementary investigation seems to confirm that the majority of Sweden's school-girls were sickly; it determined that 61.7% were sick over an extended period.[3]

It is notable that the three rather vague diagnoses of chlorosis, neurasthenia and hysteria are prominent in the picture of overall female illness. All three of them disappeared—dramatically, in the case of chlorosis—after World War I.

The term *chlorosis* appears as an endemic disease in Swedish health-care statistics from the mid-nineteenth century on, but in the 1880s, as its incidence increased sharply, it came to be regarded as primarily afflicting girls and women (figure 4.1). In 1891, when Swedish hospital statistics first reported cases of chlorosis by gender, over 86% of the patients treated (894 of 1,029 cases) were women. This remarkable gender imbalance is reflected in international statistics as well. The physiological background of this illness was well known—reduced hemoglobin levels and/or a decrease in the number of red blood cells. The name comes from the Greek word "chloros," meaning green, from the greenish complexion typical of this illness (also referred to as "greensickness"). Chlorosis was found at every level of society, but particularly among upper- and middle-class girls between the ages of 14 and 20. Its symptoms were vague: pallor, fatigue, headaches, eating disorders, menstrual problems and depression.

Neurasthenia was introduced around 1880 as a general diagnosis that covered a number of diffuse nervous complaints, or what are termed functional nervous disorders. Its symptoms included unusual fatigue, weakness, indeterminate pain, headaches, depression and insomnia. This illness was believed to afflict first and foremost the upper classes, but there was some dispute on that issue. This was also true of its overrepresentation among women; recorded diagnoses of this illness among men were one-third lower, on average, and the gender gap widened appreciably during the first decades of the 1900s.

While *hysteria* had long been regarded as a classic women's illness, its incidence seemed to increase dramatically during the last decades of the nineteenth century. Whether it was linked to gynecological or neurological models, it manifested the very horizon of expectation with regard to femininity and culturally constructed female gender. The incidence of hysteria appears to have been relatively stable during the decades around the turn of the century, but there is no doubt that a large number of cases remained unreported. Women accounted for the vast majority of hysteria diagnoses, as one might expect, but Swedish statistics did show a small percentage of men diagnosed as suffering from hysteria as well (1901: 9.8 percent).

Gender-specific illness: men

While research in the past decade has devoted substantial attention to the female body, less is known about notions concerning the male body. Given that the male body was regarded as the norm, it is difficult to establish specifically male biological models. (The very concept of "specifically male" seems a bit odd, for example, as the focus of a medical specialty called "andrology" or "men's health.")

Men's health, like women's, can be viewed in a number of ways. One obvious approach is to look at mortality statistics. Excess male mortality in infancy and early childhood has been a well-known phenomenon since the seventeenth century. Swedish mortality statistics also show relatively constant excess male mortality in terms of mean life expectancy (Sundbärg 1970). The gender difference in mean life expectancy amounted to about five years in 1850, as compared with three years at the turn of the century. This temporary reduction in the gender gap was clearly related to a decline in men's alcohol consumption.

Sweden's draft registration statistics offer an invaluable source of information on (young) men's health. The "causes for disqualification" from service illustrate a striking range of male illness: deafness, blindness, mental illness, heart defects, hernias, spasmodic conditions, illnesses of the musculoskeletal system, skin diseases, dwarfism and general weakness.[4] Short stature was linked, directly or indirectly, to a number of deficiency diseases. In 1900, nearly 26 percent (9,986 of 38,742) of eighteen-year-old males were barred from military service for health reasons.

Hospital statistics show the following illnesses to be most common among men:

Table 4.2. The ten most common diagnoses for male patients in Swedish hospitals in 1901, with comparable figures for 1911. Number of hospitalizations.

	1901	1911
Tuberculosis	3,097	3,925
Diphtheria	2,556	4,043
Sexually-transmitted diseases (gonorrhea, syphilis)	3,097	2,621
Inflammations of the skin	1,789	2,081
Rheumatism (acute and chronic)	1,330	1,361
Hernias	1,218	3,063
Cancer	1,017	1,552
Alcoholism	974	1,374
Inflammation of the lungs	969	1,300
Scarlet fever	869	3,346

Source: Sweden's official statistics. Health and medical care, Tables 22a, 16a.

When we examine men's health in a larger cultural context, we can distinguish historically several types of illnesses. Since a great deal of research remains to be done in this area, we offer here only a few general remarks:

First of all, *illnesses stemming from overindulgence* typically affect men, *gout* being a prime example. Well known throughout history as primarily a men's illness, during the eighteenth century gout became something of a badge of distinction for men. Its link with prosperity was in keeping with the self-image of the rising middle class. The biological cause of this illness (deposits of uric acid in the joints) was discovered in the nineteenth century, just as gout was losing its status as a class marker. The fact that gout sufferers were "men who led a luxurious and indolent life, who ate a great deal, drank strong wine and malt liquor and exercised little" ran counter to the ideal of disciplined and healthy masculinity that took hold in the late nineteenth century (Berg 1903). The link between cardiovascular disease and indulgent living in general, and a specific male personality type (type A) in particular, is a relatively recent twentieth-century phenomenon.

Men are substantially overrepresented among those suffering from *sex-related diseases*. Of particular interest are gender- and class-specific explanatory models of how infection is transmitted. While it was believed that among the upper social classes it was men who exposed women to infection (in keeping with the concept of the monogamous middle-class wife), it was thought that the path of infection was reversed among the working class (reinforcing the image of the sexually-charged lower-class woman as a carrier of disease).

Sex-related illnesses include not only infectious diseases, but also ailments associated with sexual function. While diagnoses such as nymphomania, kleptomania and hysteria were introduced for women's disorders, with regard to men there was particular concern about the ill effects of masturbation, as well as for the diagnoses of *satyriasis* (hypersexuality) and *spermatorrhea* (involuntary discharge of semen). The incidence of gynecological surgery rose dramatically toward the end of the nineteenth century, but during the same period there were also a number of horrific operations performed on men's genitals (Dally 1991). At the same time, it is interesting to note that in the intense interest in hermaphroditism that prevailed at the turn of the century—reflecting efforts to establish scientific criteria for determining biological gender—surgical procedures on men's sexual organs were avoided. Feminine characteristics, however, could be removed from the male-defined body (Lietoff 1995). Attempts at introducing the term *andrology* (from the Greek *andros* = man) as a counterpart to *gynecology* (from the Greek *gyne* = woman) were unsuccessful. Men's sexual organs and ability to reproduce, unlike women's, were not regarded as a proper focus of study; as late as the 1970s, this field was subsumed under the more general designation of urology.

Nervous disorders represent a third aspect of men's ill health. Here, the diagnosis of *hypochondria* is of particular interest. As early as the eighteenth century, hypochondria was fashionable among men, associated with selectivity and upper-class refinement. At that time, hypochondria did not signify, as it does today, an exaggerated fear of illness, but was instead regarded as a biological illness rooted in the highly sensitive nervous system of the diaphragm (Johannisson 1995). The concept of hypochondria also offered a male counterpart to female hysteria. There was disagreement as to whether men could suffer from hysteria; some physicians did consider it possible.

Another illness of interest from the perspective of gender is *neurasthenia*. While in Sweden this was largely a female diagnosis, it was originally seen as characteristic of urbane, intellectual men. It was unique among psychiatric diagnoses in that male patients tended to accept it willingly, indeed sometimes happily. Neurasthenia also offers interesting opportunities for examining explanatory models in terms of gender and class. A systematic analysis of 167 cases reported around the turn of the century in American medical journals shows that this disorder was directly related to an individual's gender and class.[5] (See Table 4.3.)

This analysis is interesting in that it reveals certain value judgments and social stereotypes—the hardworking white-collar worker, the dissolute laborer and the central role of the reproductive organs in women's lives. Thus the large percentage of neurasthenia cases among working-class men that are attributed to sexuality or substance abuse—in other words, caused by their own behavior—reflects a class stereotype typical of that era and marked by the influence of social Darwinism. Similarly, the fact that overexertion is seen as more typical of the intellectual

Table 4.3.

Neurasthenia: causes	Middle class	Working class
1. Men	%	%
Overexertion	69	26
Sexual excesses	20	41
Substance abuse (alcohol, tobacco, drugs)	10	29
Genetic	10	0
Other	6	9
2. Women		
Diseases of the reproductive organs	49	40
Overexertion	7	26
Substance abuse	14	14
Genetic	23	12
Other	14	12

man than of manual laborers reflects the era's view of physical strength. Among women, overexertion is seen as a more common cause of neurasthenia in the working class (when middle-class women are perceived to be suffering from overexertion, it is because they are required to care for ill family members). Furthermore, it is worth noting the relative unimportance of genetic causes among working-class women and men. For women, the reproductive organs are seen as the most significant factor in causing neurasthenia.

Another type of nervous disorder found in men are *war-related neuroses.* The psychological symptoms that occurred after World War I among war veterans raised a number of issues. How were these symptoms to be diagnosed and classified, and what should they be called? There was a whole range of disorders confronting medical scientists, from neurasthenia (a diagnosis for officers that seemed preferable to less "manly" diagnoses such as hysteria, cowardice or desertion) to the newly-coined condition referred to as *shellshock.* This diagnosis unleashed an intense debate, both within the medical profession and in the arena of social policy, since—as a recognized medical diagnosis—it entitled sufferers to a military pension and threatened to bankrupt the nations involved in the war (Showalter 1991).

A fourth area for the study of male illness is that of *occupational medicine.* Since men were overrepresented in heavy-industry jobs, they were particularly affected by industry-related ailments—although female textile workers, for example, were widely exposed to dust, which is one explanation for excess female mortality from tuberculosis. The data paint a dismal picture of workers ravaged by various kinds of lung diseases, eye injuries, and ulcerous conditions. In turn-of-the-century Sweden, nearly 50 percent of deaths among younger industrial workers could be attributed to illnesses of the respiratory organs. High-risk occupations also included upholstering and jobs that involved handling fireworks or working with dyes. Railroad engineers, telegraph operators, violinists and office workers were exposed to less serious types of risk (Almquist 1919).

Fifth, men suffered from *alcohol-related ailments*. Such illnesses were the eighth most common cause of hospitalization among men, while they account for a relatively insignificant number of women's hospital stays. During the first half of the nineteenth century, alcohol consumption had reached enormous proportions (in 1829, per-capita consumption was estimated to be 46 liters; the average adult male drank a third of a liter of schnapps per day). Although consumption declined dramatically, it remained high at the turn of the century. While alcohol consumption is not specifically reflected in mortality statistics, the fact that 56 percent of the Swedish population voted in favor of an absolute ban on alcohol in a 1909 referendum is indicative of the significance of the alcohol problem (Elmér 1975).

Female illness in society

Gender research in the last few decades has shown the importance of gender—sex in social terms—as a system of power relationships, in establishing norms and values with respect to male or female, and as a model for an individual's gender identity and attitudes toward the body.

Seen in a historical framework, gender-specific illness can only be understood within its overall cultural context and as it relates to one's life. In order to identify the relevant cultural and existential structures, it is important to consider a variety of levels: political, scientific and structural; personal, biological and social; and the conscious, unconscious and subconscious. This holds true for both sexes, but we are concerned here primarily with women, since they are defined as *the other*—a deviation from the implicit norm.

A first level is the societal. Social change always puts strain on traditional social roles. The industrialized and urbanized society that had emerged by the late nineteenth century assigned middle-class women a restricted, passive role. The stereotype of the middle-class woman as virtuous, passive and nurturing became increasingly inflexible. At a time when the world around them was signaling independence and self-realization, new ambitions and opportunities, women found it more and more difficult to conform to traditional expectations. Urban life, new economic structures and new behavioral patterns left their mark on families and family dynamics. Servants were no longer available, as the role assigned to middle-class women became increasingly hollow. Women were having fewer children, starting to work outside the home, living longer, and marrying later. Despite these fundamental social, economic and demographic changes, training in family dynamics and gender roles remained static. In a changing society, women were routinely socialized to assume a confining and limiting kind of femininity.

Being ill could be a way of taking the role of the weak, dependent woman to an extreme, or it could offer a surrogate role to women lacking other content in their lives. Historically, subjective female illness was characteristic of those groups disconnected from an active role in life, who had only limited opportunities to transgress the limits of the behavior expected of women. From nineteenth-century upper-class women to the middle-class housewives of the 1950s, sickness was a refuge for women who watched the monotonous passing of time and saw their lives slipping away. Perhaps this was the real content of their malady: sorrow over lost opportunities?

A second level involves cultural factors. Women's ailments developed as a response to certain theories of femininity, i.e., to the cultural construction of a certain female ideal. While the medical view of women as constitutionally fragile and traditional gender patterns that rewarded female weakness did not in themselves make women sick, these things did affect women's self-image and legitimized illness as an accepted form of feminine behavior. If women were told that they were weak—if weakness was part of how they defined themselves—it was only logical for them to respond by showing weakness. Patterns of perceiving and communicating physical pain were deeply ingrained. Young girls learned an emotional language in which tears signaled pain, and concern and consolation were expected in return. Adult women, on the other hand, were expected to be long-suffering. Throughout pregnancy and childbirth, they were to endure pain and illness, even to risk their lives, while at the same time they were expected to serve as the family's emotional mainstay. Nevertheless, it was boys, rather than girls, who were taught to handle pain. Women of the nineteenth century reached adulthood with a poorly developed sense of self and limited opportunities for self-realization. They were ill-equipped to deal with the role of housewife, mother and nurturing center of the family that adult women were expected to fulfill. Tension and conflict between the roles of girl/woman and mother/woman, along with the incapacity to develop a strong sense of self, meant increasingly inadequate means of emotional expression. Openly expressed anger was seen as unfeminine and vulgar; it was only through illness that behavior that deviated from the norm, emotional outbursts and suppressed aggression were allowed expression.

A third level is the realm of medicine. Women are an object of medical treatment in connection with menstruation, pregnancy and menopause, but we are referring here also to the general conception of the female body as an unstable biological system, an object requiring control and monitoring. Cyclical changes, instability and fragility, along with the sensitivity of the reproductive organs and the nervous system, seemed to justify reducing women's problems to a matter of medical treatment.

The medical community offered women descriptions and designations of illnesses, permitting them to classify their symptoms or choose their neuroses. The relationship between doctor and patient, moreover, reinforced a patriarchal structure, in which one party was in a position of superiority, while the other was subordinate. Being ill allowed women to revert both to the role of a helpless child and to a hyperfemininity capable of bringing out men's protective instincts. In addition, however, it led to depression and self-flagellating physical illness.

Fourth, there is the biological level, which involves such significant factors as having several children within a short period of time, the aftereffects of childbirth and sexually-transmitted diseases, heightened exposure to tuberculosis and other infections, and unpredictable hormonal systems. It is reasonable to assume that the frustration and limitations that characterized women's lives at the turn of the century resulted in high levels of anxiety and depression, which in turn affected their physical well-being. Indeed, modern immunological research has demonstrated that long-term depression weakens the immune system. Based on the more sophisticated knowledge available today in the fields of genetics, endocrinology, neurophysiology and developmental biology, it is clearly possible to construct gender-specific biological models (Fausto-Sterling 1992).

One argument against biological considerations as the deciding factors in gender-specific illness is the fact that women's life expectancy has consistently been greater than men's. This fact has perplexed feminist researchers (who have not been able to reconcile greater life expectancy with less favorable life circumstances), demographers (who have been inclined to see life expectancy solely in terms of living standards—the higher the standard of living, the longer the life expectancy) and biologists (who have focused on searching for biological components).

Fifth and final is the existential level. Illness can be both an expression of depression and a strategy for channeling that depression. Modern instruments for analyzing the connections between existence and health, in terms of how individuals experience their situation and the opportunities they have to affect it, are highly relevant in this context.

This discussion may appear to be of little relevance in today's world. Women have moved into the labor force. They have access to education and jobs, as well as the right to vote and to express themselves freely. They can move about as they choose in the public arena. The sharpest contours of the class-based society have been worn down by the rapid expansion of the welfare state in our century.

We can construct two main lines of interpretation for the understanding of culturally determined female illness today. It goes without saying that these explanations do not preclude biological components or biomedical models.

The first of these focuses on stress, encompassing chronic fatigue and pain syndromes such as fibromyalgia. The second centers on the conflicting roles assigned to women. Performance expectations, frustration and anxiety leave their mark on the body in the form of aches, pains and eating disorders. Thus the sharp increase that has occurred in the incidence of anorexia and bulimia can be interpreted as a response to an extremely control- and achievement-oriented culture. As early as the 1940s, Viola Klein (*The Feminine Character*, 1948) pointed out that women had taken on several new roles without really shedding the old ones. Women are expected to be all things at once—girl and woman, maternal and professional, emotional and rational, nurturing and efficient.

Arguing against the latter hypothesis is the intriguing fact that women who combine several roles seem to be healthier than women with fewer roles.[6] This supports the idea that women's illness needs to be interpreted in a broader cultural context, in which existential problems profoundly affect one's relationship to the body, health and illness.

In view of women's longer life span, we should also discuss the apparently paradoxical question of whether illness may constitute an investment in health. Being a patient or being ill seems to be more closely linked to the traditional female role than to the male role. To express illness is to admit to feelings of weakness and vulnerability. Illness is a language that creates communicative links and stimulates active listening to the body's signals.

Male health and culture

For a more thorough understanding of *men's* relationship to health and ill health, we need to know more about how culture has shaped the concept of masculinity, male gender identity and male self-image.[7] Age-old patterns—reflected in Darwin's discussion in *The Descent of Man, and Selection in Relation to Sex*—have shown men's gender identity to be based on strength and power. Simply put, this means that illness, indicating physical weakness, was less permissible for men than for women. Of course, there were exceptions to this rule. During the eighteenth century, sexually-transmitted diseases were seen as a sign of the aristocrat's indulgence in life's pleasures. Among members of the middle class, it was considered a sign of masculinity to show one's refinement by exhibiting hypochondria. That such behavior ran counter to male stereotypes is indicative of the complex relationship between class and gender.

Within nineteenth-century middle-class culture, there was intense interest in the healthy male body. Physical exercise and athletics were seen as an integral part of one's training in the moral ideal of masculinity. Achieving a healthy body meant being in control; it was a sign of the male virtues of self-discipline, rationality and a fighting spirit. There were a number of different male types and ideals: the *striving civil servant and family provider*, motivated by a sense of duty and a zeal for efficiency, housed in a clean and healthy body; the *gentleman*, characterized by intellectual refinement and a well-kept and well-groomed body; the *masculine nature-loving romantic*, enthralled by the new male ritual of mountain climbing, and seeing in the challenge of polar expeditions a synthesis of physical and moral courage; the *macho athlete*, reflected in the era's renewed interest in such sports such as boxing and wrestling; and, finally, the antithesis: the *dandy*, who flirted with androgyny and erotic excess within the framework afforded by urban life.

These masculine types reflected social codes that deemed it less acceptable for men than for women to be sick or under medical treatment, to admit to experiencing pain, or to talk about illness. Moreover, they all expressed a physical ideal revolving around—or challenging—the concept of disciplined strength. Sometimes this ideal was undercut by depression or overexertion, diagnosed as neurasthenia or hypochondria. This may be why the neuroses afflicting soldiers who fought in World War I were not only of medical significance, but also culturally important. Experiences in the trenches and the horrors of gas and grenade attacks gave rise to a more ambiguous kind of masculinity, with the "stronger sex" manifesting symptoms traditionally ascribed to women.

The subject of gender and health is as elusive as it is important. It is a well-established fact that gender roles are socially constructed. The next step is to show how notions of masculinity and femininity affect scientific theories and our understanding of illness, treatment, as well as patients' own experiences.

Historically, women have been described as prisoners of their biology. Along with their reproductive role, women's anatomy, physiology and genetic makeup tend to assign them a passive role and the responsibility for caring for and nurturing others. Increasingly, menstruation, pregnancy and menopause have been regarded as medical problems and equated with illness. Based on biology—which, in turn, affects women's psyche and intellect—women have been represented as unstable, emotional and subject to cyclical fluctuations. For a long time—until 1923—the biology argument was influential in denying women in Sweden the right to high-level positions in public service (for example, as judges, chief physicians or professors). The medicalization and demedicalization of the female body have been governed by the dictates of the labor market.

Gender-specific biological models have played an important role in the context of ideology and labor-market policy. It is women's bodies that have been reshaped, altered and reduced to mere biology. The ideal has ranged from weak and fragile (1880s) to potent and fertile (1910–1920); from slim and capable (1930s) to healthy, well-adjusted and wifely (1950s); from the strong and liberated woman (1970s) to a likely reappearance of a more feminine body ideal and a more pronounced gender dichotomy in the early years of the next millennium.

The question of how health and ill health are molded by sex and gender, culture, class, existence and physical ideals is a challenging one for future research.

Notes

1   This article is based primarily on Johannison, K. *Den mörka kontinenten—Kvinnan, medicinen och fin-de-siècle* [The dark continent—Women, medicine and the turn of the century]. Stockholm: Norstedts, 1994; Johannisson, *När sjukdom behövs*, Medicinens öga [When we need to be sick—a medical view]. Stockholm: Norstedts, 1990; Johannisson, *Folkhälsa—det svenska projektet från 1900 till 2:a världskriget* [Public health—the Swedish project from 1900 until World War II], Lychnos: Årsbok för idé- och lärdomshistoria 1991.

2   A gender-related historical and statistical morbidity analysis covering the period 1750–1900 was conducted by Jan Sundin, Tema H, University of Linköping ("Dödlighet och sjuklighet bland män och kvinnor i Sverige 1750–1900" [Mortality and illness among men and women in Sweden 1750–1900]).

3   *Läroverkskomiténs betänkande* (Report by the committee on secondary schools). Bil. E. Report to the health study, published by Axel Key. Stockholm, 1885.

4   *Bidrag till Sveriges officiela statistik (fr. 1911 Sveriges officiella statistik) [Contribution to Sweden's official statistics]*, Health and medical care 1890–1920. I. Report from the Council on Medicine entitled "Summary of reports on physician's examinations of draftees" and "Reasons for rejection."

5   Gosling, F.G., Ray, J.M. *The right to be sick—American physicians and nervous patients, 1885–1910*, Journal of social history 1986:4. Since physicians occasionally list more than one cause of illness, percentages total more than 100.

6   See, for example, a study on the incidence of male and female absences from work, Department of Social Medicine, University of Linköping (Per Bjurulf, Gunnel Hensing, Kristina Alexandersson).

7   One notable contribution to the growing body of literature on this topic is Mangan, J.A., Walvin, J. *Manliness and morality: Middle-class masculinity in Britain and America, 1800–1940*. Manchester: Manchester University Press, 1987.

References

Almquist E. *Om yrken och näringar [About occupations and industries]*, In: *Allmän hälsovårdslära [General health care theory]*, 2nd edition. Stockholm: 1919. (Available in Swedish only).

Berg H. *Gikt [Gout]*. In: *Läkarebok [Medical book]*. Göteborg: 1903. (Available in Swedish only).

Dally A. *Women under the knife—a history of surgery*. London: Hutchinson Radius, 1991.

Darwin C. *The descent of man, and selection in relation to sex*. 1871: reprint London 1982, 326–27.

Elmér Å. *Från fattigsverige till välfärdsstaten [From an impoverished Sweden to the welfare state]*, 6th edition. Stockholm: 1975, 32–33. (Available in Swedish only).

Fausto-Sterling A. *Myths of Gender: Biological theories about women and men*, 2nd edition. New York: HarperCollins, 1992.

Hammarström A, Hovelius B. *Kvinnors hälsa och ohälsa ur ett könsteoretiskt perspektiv [Women's health from a gender-theory perspective]*. Nordisk medicin 1994:11, 288–91. (Available in Swedish only).

Johannisson K. "Kroppens retorik—exemplet hypokondri" [The body's rhetoric—the example of hypochondria]. In: Åsberg C (Ed.): *Talets gåva [The gift of speech]*. Stockholm: Norstedts, 1995. (Available in Swedish only).

Kress G. *Människans könslif [Human sex life]*. Stockholm 1905, 35–36. (Available in Swedish only).

Laqueur T. *Making sex—body and gender from the Greeks to Freud*. Cambridge: Harvard University Press, 1990.

Lietoff E. *Hermafroditen—en studie i biologiska kriterier för kön i svensk läkarvetenskap kring sekelskiftet 1900 [Hermaphrodites: A study of biological sexual criteria in Swedish medicine around the turn of the century 1900]*, Dpt of the History of Science and Ideas, Uppsala University, 1995. (Available in Swedish only).

Showalter E. "Male Hysteria." In: *The female malady—Women, madness and English culture*. London: virago Press, 1991, 167–94.

Sundbärg G. *Bevölkerungsstatistik Schwedens 1750–1900 [Population statistics for Sweden 1750–1900]*. Skriftserie 3. Stockholm: Statistiska centralbyrån, 1970. (Available in Swedish only).

5

Gender differences in mental health

Tore Hällström

DETERMINATION OF THE EXTENT OF mental illness requires making a clear distinction between health and illness. This task has been greatly facilitated by diagnostic criteria developed over the last quarter century and now commonly used in the fields of both psychiatric treatment and scientific research (ICD-10 1992, DSM-IV 1994). In addition to applying academic definitions of illness, of course, we can also ask people how they would assess their own health. Responses vary substantially, depending on how the question is posed.

Statistics Sweden's report on health and medical care in Sweden indicates that 1.9 percent of men and 3.2 percent of women consider themselves to be mentally ill (Statistics Sweden 1992). The same source, however, shows that as many as eight percent of men and seventeen percent of women are suffering from anxiety, restlessness or fear at a given time. Such problems increase as people age, particularly among women. Insomnia is more common among women than men and increases with age for both sexes (see Figure 2.23, Chapter 2). It is unclear to what extent these percentages correspond to the prevalence of mental disorder in a clinical sense. While figures on the prevalence of mental illness are clearly valuable, they should be supplemented with data on incidence and lifetime risk to provide a more complete picture of the dynamics of health changes.

In terms of methodology, one of the best studies of a population's psychiatric health is the Lundby study, which showed that the risk of becoming mentally ill before reaching the age of sixty was as high as 43 percent for men and 73 percent for women (Hagnell 1970). The risk over a one-year period of falling ill, whether it be a first illness or a relapse, increases for men up to the age of 30, remains fairly constant until the age of 75, then increases again. Women have a higher risk than men between the ages of 15 and 60. There is a particularly large gender gap between 25 and 55 (Figure 5.1). By the time women are between the ages of 65 and 75, their risk has dropped to the level of that of men. After the age of 75, the risk of mental illness rises for women as well as for men.

The most common types of mental disorder among women are depression and anxiety disorders, while men are most likely to suffer from alcohol-related disorders. Population studies from Europe and the United States have shown that some three percent of men and seven percent of women are suffering from

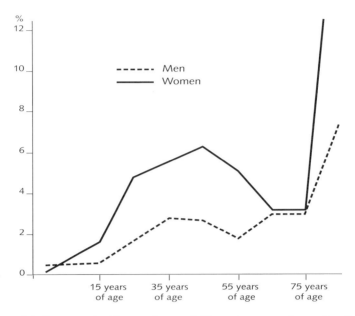

Figure 5.1 One-year incidence of mental illness by sex and age, Lundby study (Hagnell 1970).

clinical depression at any given time (or during a fairly short period, such as one month or one year). Lifetime risk is substantially higher, with estimates indicating that some 12 percent of men and 25 percent of women will suffer from depression at some time in their lives. However, the Lundby study indicates that the risk of becoming clinically depressed before the age of 80 may be even higher—28 percent for men and 49 percent for women (Rorsman et al. 1990). Bipolar affective disorder (manic-depressive illness) is far less common—lifetime risk amounts to between one and two percent, with no substantial gender difference.

Suicide in Sweden is two to three times as common among men as women. Rates are highest for both men and women between the ages of 45 and 64. For men, suicide rates are higher the lower their social class. For women, in contrast, there is no association between suicide rates and social status. Suicide attempts are 10–20 times as common as successful suicides, and occur most often among both men and women between the ages of 25 and 34. In every age range, women are more likely than men to attempt suicide. A Swedish study found the ratio of women's suicide attempts to men's to be 1.5 (Medical Research Council 1993).

Anxiety disorders are also substantially more common among women than men. Table 5.1 shows that the one-year prevalence of panic disorders, agoraphobia, social phobia and generalized fears is approximately twice as high for women (Eaton et al. 1991). Obsessive-compulsive disorder (obsessive thoughts or compulsive actions) is also somewhat more common among women.

Table 5.1. Prevalence of anxiety disorders and obsessive-compulsive disorder for men and women in the United States (Eaton et al. 1991, Blazer et al. 1991, Karno & Golding 1991).

Anxiety disorders	Gender	Prevalence (%)		
		One month	One year	Lifetime
Panic disorder	Men	0.35	0.58	0.99
	Women	0.69	1.22	2.10
Agoraphobia	Men			3.18
	Women			7.86
Social phobias	Men			2.53
	Women			2.91
Generalized	Men		0.94	
anxiety disorder	Women		2.41	
(not included under another				
DIS/DSM III disorder)				
Obsessive-compulsive	Men	1.13	1.42	2.03
disorder	Women	1.52	1.86	3.04

Gender differences are even more striking when it comes to eating disorders (anorexia nervosa and bulimia nervosa), with these conditions 10–20 times as likely to affect women as men. Among 20-year-old females, it is estimated that approximately one percent suffer from anorexia nervosa or have suffered from it in the past, while between one and two percent are afflicted with bulimia nervosa. The risk of developing anorexia nervosa is highest during the teenage years, and particularly high among girls aged 14–19. Bulimia nervosa generally shows up somewhat later, between the ages of 18 and 25.

Schizophrenia is the most important of the psychotic illnesses and is usually diagnosed between the ages of 15 and 30. In about one-fifth of all cases it develops quickly into a chronic disorder, and some 50 percent of cases show a variable course with fairly frequent episodes of deterioration. Roughly 30 percent of schizophrenics have a favorable prognosis. The risk of developing schizophrenia at some point in life is about one percent. At any given time, between 0.5 and 1.0 percent of people throughout the world suffer from schizophrenia.

Men and women have a similar risk of developing schizophrenia, but in other respects there are substantial gender differences. On average, women are diagnosed between three and four years later than men. Boys are more likely than girls to show symptoms long before developing full-blown schizophrenia. There are also certain differences in men's and women's symptoms. Men show more "negative" symptoms, such as emotional distance, lack of interest and involvement, and general passivity. The prognosis is better for women, with respect to treatment as well as the individual's ability to function in society. Schizophrenic men are more likely to remain unmarried than their female counterparts, and less likely to have children. A study conducted in the Stockholm region of individuals with long-term functional psychoses, where schizophrenics account for 70 percent of all cases, showed that 64 percent of these individuals lived alone (Borgå 1993). Two-thirds of them were unemployed and three out of four lived in their own apartments. Women had more favorable living conditions than men in every respect, except that their incomes (corrected for diagnosis) were lower.

Changes in the incidence of psychiatric illnesses

Results of the Lundby study show that cases of mild and moderately severe depression increased sharply between 1947 and 1972 (Hagnell et al. 1982). During this period, the risk for men nearly tripled, while it doubled for women. The risk of developing a serious case of depression was cut nearly in half for both men and women during the same period. This increase in mild and moderately severe depression may overestimate the true change in incidence of such cases, since the concept of depression was expanded during this time as antidepressants were introduced and shown to be successful in treating even milder types of depression. The decline in cases of severe depression may be the result of a tendency to seek help at an earlier stage, before psychotic or other more severe symptoms develop.

The ratio of men's suicides to women's declined gradually in Sweden from 4.4 in the 1920s to 2.8 between 1961 and 1970. Suicides among men increased until 1971–75, then decreased somewhat. Women's suicides increased until 1976–79, after which they declined as well (Medical Research Council 1993). Regarding suicide attempts, several studies have shown a marked increase in various industrialized countries during the 1960s.

The incidence of anorexia nervosa has been increasing in the Western industrialized countries at least since the 1950s. There has been an even more dramatic increase in bulimia nervosa, although it did not occur until the 1970s. The 1980s saw a shift in the types of symptoms manifested by anorexia nervosa sufferers, with increasing numbers of patients showing signs of bulimia within two years of onset, in the form of compulsive eating and vomiting.

The course of schizophrenia appears to have become milder during the present century, with acute psychotic episodes more commonly followed by recovery (Bleuler 1974). However, the risk of developing schizophrenia seems to have remained unchanged.

Gender differences in use of medical resources

With the exception of inpatient psychiatric care, women seek out and receive treatment for mental disorders more often than men at all levels of the mental-health system. A study conducted of primary care in Tierp showed that women accounted for 55 percent of those seeking medical care during a given period, in 20 percent of these cases because of psychological problems. The corresponding percentage of men seeking psychological care was 14 percent (Kebbon et al. 1985).

This gender difference has been corroborated by a study of primary care in the Stockholm region (Stefansson and Svensson 1994).

An individual's first contact with outpatient psychiatric care most frequently results from those conditions that carry the highest lifetime risk and have the greatest clinical significance: depression, agoraphobia, panic disorder, social phobia and an inability to respond appropriately to crisis situations. The presence of a severe personality disorder increases the likelihood of contact with the psychiatric-care system.

Most psychiatric disorders under outpatient treatment at any given time are conditions with a high recidivism rate or a high risk of developing into a chronic disorder. This is borne out by statistics from a psychiatric outpatient clinic in the greater Stockholm area, which show that women make up 71 percent of patients treated. Patients with anxiety syndromes were most common (34 percent), followed by affective disorders (27 percent), psychoses (23 percent), responses to crisis (10 percent), borderline-personality disorder (6 percent) and eating disorders (2 percent). Alcohol abuse was present as an underlying factor in 8 percent of cases, while brain damage was a factor in 4 percent of cases.

A study conducted in Östergötland county showed that more women than men were absent from work for psychiatric reasons—2.1 percent as compared with 1.3 percent over the course of a year (Hensing et al. 1995). An analysis of prescriptions issued in Stockholm, Gothenburg and Malmö between 1986 and 1988 showed that fully 40 percent of prescriptions written by primary-care physicians were for psychopharmacological drugs, while the corresponding percentages for prescriptions written by internists, psychiatrists and other physicians were 12 percent, 25 percent and 20 percent, respectively (Wessling et al. 1991). These distributions were the same for both men and women. However, relative to the population, such drugs were prescribed nearly twice as frequently for women as for men. A similar gender difference is also found in Statistics Sweden data (Statistiska centralbyrån 1992) on the use of tranquilizers and sleeping pills (Table 5.2). Moreover, substantially more women than men undergo psychotherapy, whether through the public health-care system or on a private basis. In 1991, for example, 82 percent of patients at the Institute for Psychotherapy in Stockholm were women.

At any given time, there are approximately equal numbers of men and women in inpatient psychiatric care facilities. A large proportion of these patients—38 percent in 1988—are suffering from schizophrenia. Women made up less than half of the total, which reflects the more favorable prognosis for female schizophrenics. Alcohol abuse accounted for seven percent of patients, of whom 25 percent were women. Patients with affective disorders and neuroses together made up 14 percent of the total, two-thirds being women. It should be kept in mind, however, that a large proportion (46 percent) of these individuals under inpatient care were over the age of 65.

Table 5.2. Treatment with psychopharmacological drugs over a two-week period 1988–89, in percent. Figures do not include institutionalized individuals. (Statistiska centralbyrån 1992)

Type of medication	Use	Men	Women	Total
Tranquilizers	Regular	1.4	2.9	2.2
	Sporadic	1.3	2.4	1.8
Sleeping pills	Regular	1.4	2.9	2.2
	Sporadic	2.2	4.9	3.5

Treatment of schizophrenia is more successful with women than men. This holds true for family therapy (Spencer et al. 1988) as well as for psychopharmacological treatment, where women require lower weight-corrected doses of neuroleptics (Seeman 1992). Of those patients suffering from long-term functional psychoses, about half are under inpatient psychiatric treatment during the course of a given year. Men and women are admitted at the same rate, but men remain in treatment for twice as long (Borgå 1993).

Clinical psychiatric research has not shed a great deal of light on gender differences. Clinical descriptions of schizophrenia, for example, are based on data from a patient base made up of two-thirds men. Since many academic analyses do not distinguish by gender, it is often impossible to draw gender-specific conclusions.

Causes of higher rates of depression and fear-related disorders among women

Genetic factors

Genetic predisposition is an important factor in bipolar affective disorder (manic-depressive illness). Genes play a much less important role in most types of unipolar depression, although there are subgroups with a more pronounced genetic component. So far it has not been possible to identify an x-chromosome-linked gene associated with an increased likelihood of developing depression.

There are a number of studies in the field of behavioral genetics that are relevant in examining the importance of negative life experiences in adulthood for subsequent mental health. The results of these studies provide a framework for assessing the notion that we are passively "exposed" to events that may affect us positively or negatively. As adults, we all have at least some choice in our lifestyle and environment. Recently, however, twin studies have shown that these choices are probably influenced somewhat by genetic factors.

A study of 890 identical (monozygotic) and 1425 fraternal (dizygotic) twins of both sexes showed that family environment and genetic factors explained approximately the same amount of variation in the number of psychosocial stressors during a specific observation period (20 and 23 percent, respectively). These stressors were divided into two groups: network events, which primarily affected someone in the person's network of friends and relatives, and personal events, which primarily affected the individual him- or herself. It was shown that by and large family environment explained network events, while genetic factors explained personal events (Kendler et al. 1993). Such factors as personality traits, temperament and social environment may mediate genetic influences on personal life events.

A study of female twins (Kendler et al. 1991) looked at various ways of coping with problems in life. Three coping stratagems were examined: turning to others for help with a problem, solving the problem on one's own, and denying the problem. The first two methods proved to be effective and associated with low levels of anxiety and depression. Both of these were best explained by the influence of genetic factors, which in each case explained about 30 percent of the variation in coping behavior. Denying the problem was a poor way of dealing with the situation and led to high levels of anxiety and depression. Here the family environment explained 19 percent of the variation in coping behavior, while genetic factors were insignificant.

Early negative experiences

An upbringing characterized by a lack of love and an excess of control is a risk factor for depression. Since girls have not been shown to be more likely than boys to experience such an environment, nor to be more sensitive to it, this factor cannot explain the gender gap in depression.

There are many studies examining whether losing a parent at an early age (whether through death, temporary separation or divorce) is associated with depression in adulthood. Most recognized epidemiological studies indicate that experiencing the death of a parent in childhood does not increase the risk of depression later in life (Tennant 1991). An extensive study of twins showed that both parental separation and parental death predict the development of panic disorder, while only parental separation predicts clinical depression and generalized anxiety (Kendler et al. 1992). Since parental separation can be assumed to occur equally in the lives of boys and girls, and girls have not been shown to be more vulnerable in childhood, there is no clear link between parental separation and the higher rates of depression and fear-related disorders found among women.

Girls are much more frequently the victims of sexual abuse than boys. A number of studies have shown a link between sexual abuse in childhood and psychological disorders of various kinds later in life (Bifulco & Brown 1991, Mullen et al. 1993). Girls who have been sexually abused are also more likely to be exposed to other negative experiences, such as parental conflict and divorce and psychological and physical abuse. One study that controlled for the negative effects of such other factors showed that suicidal behavior (suicidal impulses and acts) occurred nine times as often among women who had been exposed to sexual abuse that included genital contact, as compared with women who had not been sexually abused (Mullen et al. 1993). Among the subgroup who were victims of the most serious sexual abuse, including actual intercourse, suicidal acts were 26 times as likely as one might otherwise expect.

A significant mediating factor is how experiences of sexual abuse affect a woman's ability to relate to men later in life. Both sexual abuse and other early negative experiences have been shown to increase the likelihood that a woman will choose to remain single or, if she does marry, that her marriage will end in divorce (Bifulco & Brown 1991), and in these cases depression is a common outcome. However, if a woman succeeds in establishing a lasting marriage, there is no increased risk of depression despite sexual abuse or other negative events in childhood.

While sexual abuse is obviously a risk factor for depression and suicidal tendencies, we cannot rule out the role of other factors such as genetic makeup. A father's antisocial personality disorder or alcohol dependence increases his daughter's risk of both sexual abuse and genetic predisposition toward depression. Further studies may be able to determine the extent to which sexual abuse early in childhood constitutes a direct psychosocial cause of depression among women.

Phobias are learned behaviors in which conditioning occurs in two-thirds of all cases. Modeling is present in 15 percent of cases, meaning that a child's parent models fear behavior. Modeling is particularly common—occurring in about 30 percent of cases—in producing two phobias that frequently appear in childhood: fear of animals and fear of blood. The child usually takes on the fear of his or her mother, and since it is probably easier for girls than boys to identify with their mothers, modeling may be one reason why certain phobias are more common among women.

Interactions of biological, psychological and sociocultural factors during adolescence

Two personality traits—self-esteem and neuroticism—are associated with the risk of developing depression. During puberty, self-esteem increases for boys while it decreases for girls, largely owing to differences in how boys and girls view their physical development. Teenage girls are more likely to assess their bodies negatively, probably because girls are under particular pressure to be thin. Satisfaction with one's physical appearance is more closely tied to self-concept and self-confidence for female than male teenagers. These issues are discussed in more detail in the section on the causes of eating disorders.

A study has shown that teachers tend to be more critical of teenage boys than girls, but their criticism of boys is expressed more generally, while girls are criticized more specifically for their intellectual failings. At the same time, boys are offered more specific encouragement, but girls are praised in general terms. Girls were more likely than boys to blame themselves for poor achievement in school and tended to give up rather than to work harder. This is one example of how a social pattern interacts with other factors to produce in some teenage girls a learned sense of helplessness.

Boys' and girls' socialization and identity development take different paths (Hammarström & Hovelius 1994). Boys find their own identity mainly through achievements of various kinds. Relationships (with other boys) are largely competitive. A girl's identity development is more closely related to an intensive relationship with her mother (or her closest caregiver). Girls develop within a framework of relationships that reinforce a sense of belonging and the ability to function as part of a network. These developmental and psychological differences between the sexes probably stem from interactions among biological factors, i.e., differences in men's and women's brain structure, as well as from the effects of sociocultural learning experiences.

During the teenage years, girls develop an ability to communicate, to recognize others' needs and to encourage and support other people in a way that distinguishes them from boys. They appear to be more sensitive to such events as a parental divorce. Girls' heightened interpersonal sensitivity may also make them more aware of the potential benefits of certain reactions to such events. For example, the threat of parental conflict may be averted if the parents focus instead on the difficulties their children are experiencing.

Boys and girls appear to develop divergent cognitive-response styles when faced with problems (Nolen-Hoeksema 1987). Men distract themselves by engaging in physical activity. Women are less physically active and tend instead to obsess over the causes of their problems to the point of making themselves sick. This type of behavior can have a negative effect on a girl's ability to solve problems and lead to a sense of helplessness and failure, as well as bringing up unpleasant memories. It should also be noted, however, that there is much that remains to be learned about how men and women deal with life's problems.

Women's reproductive functions and depression

Since the earliest times, women's psychological vulnerability has been linked to puberty, menstruation, pregnancy, childbirth and menopause, but on the whole the explanatory value of these factors is quite small. The role of puberty in the development of eating disorders will be discussed below.

Premenstrual syndrome (PMS) occurs in the luteal phase of the menstrual cycle and is characterized by affective and behavioral changes and/or somatic symptoms. These symptoms continue for a period ranging from a day or two up to two weeks. Forty percent of menstruating women experience mild premenstrual symptoms that have no effect on their ability to function, but between two and ten percent report more severe symptoms that impair their ability to work to varying degrees. Since even severe cases of premenstrual syndrome are transitory, PMS does not meet the standard of clinical depression, so it is not a factor in the excess psychiatric illness we find among women.

Most women manifest a mild affective instability immediately after giving birth, but these symptoms generally disappear quite rapidly. Between 10 and 15 percent of new mothers develop clinical depression, which probably accounts to some extent for women's higher rate of depression. However, this factor's explanatory power is limited, not least because it has been shown that men, too, have a higher incidence of depression shortly after the birth of a child. Postpartum psychosis is so rare (1–2 cases per 1,000 births) that it is only a marginal factor in women's higher rates of psychiatric illness.

Menopause-related depression used to be regarded as quite common. However, several population studies have shown that there is no excess depression during menopause (Hällström 1973, McKinlay et al. 1987).

Social factors in adulthood

Whether women more frequently experience unfavorable life events is a matter of some dispute, and may indeed be a question of definition. It has been shown that men and women have approximately the same likelihood of encountering negative events that affect them personally or someone close to them. However, women respond to negative events in their lives with more depressive symptoms than men at a comparable level of stress. Such events quadruple women's risk of depression during a six-month period (Cooke 1987). Various methods have been used to quantify the degree of negative stress during a given period of time, for example by assigning points to certain life events and arriving at a total score. However, such point totals account for only about 10 percent of the variation in the incidence of depressive symptoms.

In fact, there are probably two reasons why women are subjected to more psychosocial stressors than men. One is that women are more frequently married to an alcoholic, a child or spouse abuser, or a criminal. Consequently, women are more frequently victimized than men in their marriages through the tacit or explicit threat of violence, abuse or rape. The second reason is that women tend to be emotionally involved with a larger group of people than men are, so they are more affected by negative events that occur within their network of friends and acquaintances. Moreover, women tend to experience negative events affecting others in their families as more stressful than those directly related to themselves, while for men the opposite is true.

It is possible, though, to counteract the negative effects of psychosocial stress factors. One population study has shown, not surprisingly, that the number of negative life events increased gradually for women as they had more children (Samuelsson & Hällström 1987). However, the risk of developing depression or a fear-related disorder was unrelated to the number of children a woman had, which may have several possible explanations. One reason why the results of this Swedish study are at odds with English and American findings may have to do with Sweden's relatively well-organized system of childcare.

Several studies have shown that a lack of emotional support increases women's risk of developing depression (Brown & Harris 1978, Hällström 1987). Married men are more likely than women to report that their partners understand them and to have only their wives as confidantes, while wives tend to have one or more other close friends, usually other women. Women attach particularly great importance to the quality of their interpersonal relationships. As a rule, women are more likely than men to assume responsibility for offering support to others, showing solidarity, enhancing the status of others, helping, caring, rewarding, mediating, understanding and accepting those around them. When women themselves receive too little support or lack someone to confide in, their vulnerability to depression increases. Women show greater sensitivity than men to marital problems, which increases their vulnerability to depression and anxiety. The fact that marriage provides greater protection to men than to women may explain why women are significantly more likely to initiate divorce proceedings. Happily married women are less depressed than other married women, but still five times as likely to be depressed as their husbands. After the death of older men, their widows experience a long-term improvement in their psychological health, while the reverse is true for widowers. The emergence of psychiatric symptoms puts men at a disadvantage, since mentally ill men are more isolated than women and more likely to be found at the lowest levels of society. It is less common for men to become mentally ill, but when they do, the social consequences are more severe.

How employment affects a woman's mental health is a complicated question, since it depends not only on working conditions, but also on such things as childcare arrangements, her reasons for working and her husband's attitude toward her job. The psychosocial work environment, measured in terms of the percentage of people with high-stress jobs, worsened in Sweden during the 1980s (Krantz 1994, Lundberg 1995). High-stress jobs are those that are psychologically taxing and provide little opportunity for people to make decisions, which makes it difficult for them to deal with the psychological demands of their jobs. The percentage of high-stress jobs for women increased during the 1980s from 15 to 21 percent, six times the increase for men. In the 1980s, 15 percent of women went from no job or a low-stress job to a high-stress job. This change has occurred primarily among women in low- and midlevel public-sector jobs in the areas of health care and education, with nurses and orderlies among those most affected.

An American study of how work, marriage and related problems affect the incidence of depression showed that married women with few marital problems and little job-related stress were least depressed (Aneshensel 1986). Housewives who did not work outside the home but were dealing with major marital difficulties were more than five times as likely to be depressed (Table 5.3). Employed women with marital problems and stressful jobs had a lower risk of depression than housewives who did not work outside the home. Housewives with children reported being substantially more depressed than childless housewives. Women working outside the home who had good childcare arrangements experienced minimal depression, while women whose husbands took on their share of responsibility for the children were even more satisfied than childless employed women, doing almost as well psychologically as their husbands. This study showed men to be relatively unaffected by problems relating to their children and childcare arrangements. A weakness of this study is that it is based on cross-sectional data, confounding efforts to determine cause and effect. For example, it may be that depression causes women to quit their jobs.

Table 5.3. Relative risk of depression among various groups of women (Aneshensel 1986).

Group	Relative risk
Married women with few marital problems and little job stress	1.0
Married women with few marital problems and high job stress	1.4
Single women with little job stress	1.6
Housewives with few marital problems	2.1
Single women with high job stress	2.3
Married women with major marital problems and low job stress	2.6
Single unemployed women	3.4
Married women with major marital problems and high job stress	3.6
Housewives with major marital problems	5.5

Women with professional careers are a particularly vulnerable group. In Sweden, highly educated women have been shown to have a higher risk of suicide than other women. The reverse is true for men, with upper- and middle-class men having the lowest incidence of suicide (Medical Research Council 1993). Female executives report that they need to perform better than their male colleagues in order to be considered just as good, which is the most common cause of stress for such women (Frankenhaeuser 1993). Women in managerial positions are more competitive and push themselves harder than their male colleagues. Male executives are frequently married to women who have organized their own work around their husband's careers and relieve their husbands of most household responsibilities. In contrast, a woman with a career is often married to a man who is also pursuing a career, so that she can rarely count on any substantial help at home. Managerial positions are designed by and for men who demonstrate their commitment to their jobs by working overtime, traveling on business and working at home in the evenings and on weekends.

Gender integration in the workplace has been shown to be a significant factor in psychological problems among both men and women that make them unable to work (Hensing et al. 1995). Absences related to mental health were highest, for both sexes, in occupations where employees of one sex predominated, and lowest where men and women were represented in fairly equal numbers (Figure 5.2). Women working in occupations with an overwhelming male majority were most likely to miss work because of psychological problems, while men working in extremely female-dominated jobs had the highest corresponding absentee rate of all men. As there are a number of possible explanations for this finding, this question deserves further study.

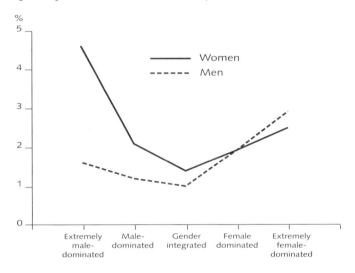

Figure 5.2 Incidence of absenteeism owing to psychological disorders, as related to gender integration in the workplace (Hensing et al. 1995)

Women's higher rates of eating disorders

We have not yet found a necessary and sufficient cause for the development of anorexia or bulimia nervosa, although a number of factors have been linked to an increased risk of developing an eating disorder. Some are condition-specific, in that they increase the likelihood of an eating disorder without affecting the risk of developing other mental disorders. These factors may be able to explain symptoms and gender distribution, as well as the higher incidence of such disorders in the industrialized countries and the differences in the rates of eating disorders across different cultures. Non-specific risk factors increase the risk not only of eating disorders, but also of other psychological problems.

Risk factors can also be general, in the sense that they affect all women and thus may explain women's higher rates of eating disorders in particular or, more generally, women's higher rates of a variety of psychological disorders. Other risk factors are individual-specific and may explain why a certain individual develops an eating disorder or another psychological problem. Below we shall focus on the possible causes of eating disorders.

Biological factors

Twin studies show that the restrictive form of anorexia nervosa tends to be associated with a genetic predisposition (Treasure & Holland 1989), although we do not know just how this predisposition is mediated. The increase in cases of anorexia nervosa over the last few decades demonstrates that sociocultural factors are also important. Whether genetic factors can explain the large gender gap is uncertain.

After puberty, women have a greater tendency than men to gain excess weight, although they eat less. The anabolic principle governing how women's bodies store nutrients constitutes a biological advantage. A pregnancy requires 100,000 additional calories, while breastfeeding consumes 1,000 per day. During puberty, women's physiological makeup clearly comes into conflict with the prevailing ideal of a trim body.

Serotonin is a transmitter in the brain that, among other things, helps to regulate the intake of carbohydrates and protein (Spigset 1990). Serotonin activity declines when healthy women diet, an effect that is not observed when men restrict their intake of food, and a reduced level of serotonin activity can lead to a strong craving for carbohydrates. Moreover, there is a link between low serotonin levels and difficulty with impulse control. Both of these mechanisms may explain why compulsive eating is more common among women than men. Individual differences in serotonin level prior to dieting may constitute an individual-specific risk factor for developing bulimia nervosa. However, the role of serotonin in the incidence of eating disorders is a controversial and as yet unsolved question.

Negative childhood experiences

Girls are substantially more likely to be subjected to sexual abuse than boys. The more serious the abuse and the longer it continues, the higher the risk of mental illness and other psychological disorders later in life. Patients with eating disorders report more sexual abuse than women in the general population, but no more than women with other psychiatric illnesses.

Cultural factors

The ideal of gender equality has increasingly gained ground in Western-influenced cultures during the past quarter century. This has brought changes in the roles of both men and women, but social pressure on women to become more like men has clearly been greater than the reverse. This is particularly striking in the case of young people. Traditionally, a teenage girl, particularly in the upper classes, was expected to be dependent and passively conformist, as well as to delay sexual activity. Today, however, girls are rewarded for seeking independence, achievements of various kinds, early sexual activity and becoming involved in the job world. Both of these ideals still exist more or less side by side, which in itself leads to a conflict that may constitute a general risk factor for psychological disorders among teenagers.

One significant explanation for the fact that eating disorders affect primarily women is that they, more than men, are expected to achieve today's ideal of a slim figure. Commercial pressure from the fashion industry, conveyed through ads in women's magazines, fashion reporting and a steady onslaught of dieting advice, focuses mainly on women. The cosmetics industry's stake in underscoring the importance of appearance is also a factor. The importance of a trim figure has steadily increased during the past 50 years. This also explains the increased incidence of eating disorders, the main components of the clinical presentation (weight phobia and appearance fixation), but also the gender distribution of eating disorders and the fact that they are found almost exclusively in "modern" Western societies.

The ideal of being thin, which increases the risk of eating disorders for all women, does not offer a clear explanation of why only a small minority of women actually develop eating disorders. However, there are certain risk groups where pressure to remain thin is particularly great since it is linked to success in competition. This applies, for example, to young people involved in athletics, ballet or modeling, groups that show a high incidence of anorexia nervosa and eating disorders in general. However, young women in these groups tend to be able to function well both physically and socially and to respond to advice from their coaches and teachers, so their prognosis tends to be better than that of clinical patients in general.

Some studies have looked at what happens when young women move from a non-Western society, where eating disorders are rare, to a Western country. Egyptian women studying in London are more likely to have eating disorders than comparable students in Cairo (Nasser 1986), while the daughters of Asian immigrants in England have an even higher incidence of eating disorders than white schoolgirls.

The interaction of biological, psychological and sociocultural factors in adolescence

The cultural ideal of a slim figure is difficult to reconcile with the rounded contours that develop during puberty and offer a biological advantage for pregnancy and breastfeeding. This conflict tends to make teenage girls dissatisfied with their physical appearance during puberty, while teenage boys more readily accept their body types. This conflict between the cultural ideal and biological reality can be viewed as a risk factor that increases the likelihood of eating disorders among young women. Women who suffer from anorexia nervosa often exhibit weak personality development and a strong bent towards perfectionism. It is not surprising that young women with these personality traits end up losing a great deal of weight in response to pressure from their environment.

Since the age of menarche has declined sharply during this century, many teenagers experience several years in which there is a discrepancy between their biological and emotional/cognitive maturity. This can also increase the vulnerability of young teenage girls who become involved with older boys. Accordingly, the new role of independence and early sexual activity for girls may combine with a lack of cognitive and emotional maturity to increase the strain. This may help explain not only women's higher rates of eating disorders, but also the increase in such disorders in Western societies and the fact that eating disorders occur almost exclusively in Western-influenced societies. This model, however, is speculative rather than empirically proven. It is compatible with a psychodynamic model of self-starvation as a means of postponing or avoiding physical maturity by regressing to a state of pre-puberty, which postpones the threat of independence, responsibility and sexuality posed by the adult world.

It has been shown that various kinds of negative events are overrepresented during the months immediately preceding the onset of an eating disorder. Thus such life events may trigger an eating disorder, but they may also lead more generally to disorders such as depression and anxiety. A study shows that teenage girls are more sensitive than boys to their parents' divorce. It is likely that young women are more sensitive to negative life experiences than young men are, as early as the teen years.

Individual causal factors vary from case to case. The sociocultural factors discussed above have changed over time, and their effects differ in different situations, which explains why eating disorders have been found to be most common at higher social levels and in urban areas. Some equalization has taken place, though, so that eating disorders are now found at approximately the same rate in all social groups.

A better prognosis for women who suffer from schizophrenia

Schizophrenia generally appears later in women, and they tend to respond better to treatment and show a more favorable prognosis than men. While the reasons for this are not entirely clear, we do know that there are gender differences with respect to both risk factors for schizophrenia and protective factors.

A genetic predisposition to develop schizophrenia is most commonly found in women, while childbirth-related injuries are more common among male schizophrenics. Myelinization occurs at a slower rate in the brain of the male fetus, which may make it more vulnerable to injury during delivery. Moreover, the female sex hormone estrogen may well provide biological protection for women through its neuroleptic-like effect on dopamine neurons in the brain.

There may also be psychosocial factors affecting one's predisposition toward or risk of developing schizophrenia, as well as offering protection against it. These may in turn interact with biological factors to affect the development of such disorders as schizophrenia. Some of these factors are found differentially in men and women. Looking at boys' and girls' relationships with their mothers, for example, we find that boys may have more trouble establishing close relationships, while girls are more likely to have difficulty with separation and establishing their own identity. The differing expectations placed on men and women by society may play a role in the worse prognosis for male schizophrenics. Schizophrenic men are under more pressure to live up to the expectations commonly placed on men— to achieve professional success, engage in competition and take on responsibility for a family. These demands are incompatible with the cognitive and emotional disturbances inherent in this disorder. Women may be better able to deal with their illness because of the more protective environment offered them by marriage—although this is a less significant factor than in the past, since being a housewife has increasingly become the exception rather than the rule. Because men tend to develop schizophrenia at an earlier age, they are more likely to miss important stages in their development, such as secondary education, vocational training and relationships with the opposite sex.

References

Aneshensel C. *Marital and employment role-strain, social support, and depression among adult women.* In: Hobfoll S (Ed.): *Stress, social support, and women,* pp.99–114. Washington DC: Hemisphere 1986.

Bifulco A, Brown GW, Adler Z. *Early sexual abuse and clinical depression in adult life.* Br J Psychiatry 1991, 159, 115–122.

Blazer DG, Hughes D, George LK, Swartz M, Boyer R. *Generalized anxiety disorder.* In: Robins LN, Regier DA (Eds.): *Psychiatric disorders in America.* New York: Free Press 1991.

Bleuler M. *The long-term course of the schizophrenic psychoses.* Psychol Med 1974, *4*, 244–254.

Borgå P. *Studies on long-term functional psychosis in three different areas of Stockholm County.* Umeå University Medical Dissertations, New Series No. 358. Umeå 1993.

Brown GW, Harris TO. *Social origins of depression: A study of psychiatric disorder in women.* London: Tavistock 1978.

Cooke DJ. *The significance of life events as a cause of psychological and physical disorder.* In: Cooper B (Ed.): *Psychiatric Epidemiology.* London: Groom Helm 1987.

Diagnostic and statistical manual of mental disorders, 4th edition. Washington DC: American Psychiatric Association 1994.

Eaton WW, Dryman A, Weissman MM. *Panic and phobia.* In: Robins LN, Regier DA (Eds.): *Psychiatric disorders in America.* New York: Free Press 1991.

Frankenhaeuser M. *Kvinnligt, manligt, stressigt [Female, male, stressful].* Only in Swedish. Höganäs: Bra Böcker 1993.

Hagnell O, Lanke J, Rorsman B, Öjesjö L. Are we entering an age of melancholy? Psychol Med 1982, *12*, 279–289.

Hagnell O. *The incidence and duration of episodes of mental illness in a total population.* In: Hare EH, Wing JK (Eds.): *Psychiatric epidemiology.* London: Oxford Univ Press 1970.

Hammarström A, Hovelius B. *Kvinnors hälsa och ohälsa ur ett könsteoretiskt perspektiv [Women's health from the perspective of gender theory].* Only in Swedish. Nord Med 1994, *109*, 288–291.

Hensing G, Alexanderson K, Åkerlind I, Bjurulf P. *Sick leave due to minor psychiatric morbidity: Role of sex integration.* Soc Psychiatry Psychiatr Epidemiology 1995, *30*, 39–43.

Hällström T. *Mental disorder and sexuality in the climacteric.* Stockholm: Scand Univ Books 1973.

Hällström T. *Social origins of major depression: The role of provoking agents and vulnerability factors.* Acta Psychiatr Scand 1987, *73*, 383–389.

The ICD-10 classification of mental and behavioural disorders. Clinical descriptions and diagnostic guidelines. Geneva: WHO 1992.

Karno M, Golding JM. *Obsessive compulsive disorder.* In: Robins LN, Regier DA (Eds.): *Psychiatric disorders in America.* New York: Free Press 1991.

Kebbon L, Svartling PG, Smedby B. *Psychiatric symptoms and psychological problems in primary health care as seen by doctors.* Scand J Prim Health Care 1985, *3*, 23–30.

Kendler KS, Kessler RC, Heath AC, Neale MC, Eaves LJ. *Coping: A genetic epidemiological investigation.* Psychol Med 1991, *21*, 337–346.

Kendler KS, Neale MC, Kessler RC, Heath AC, Eaves LJ. *A twin study of recent life events and difficulties.* Arch Gen Psychiatry 1993, *50*, 789–796.

Kendler KS, Neale MC, Kessler RC, Heath AC, Eaves LJ. *Childhood parental loss and adult psychopathology in women.* Arch Gen Psychiatry 1992, *49*, 109–116.

Krantz G. *Hälsoutvecklingen för nordiska kvinnor [Health trends among Scandinavian women].* Only in Swedish. Nord Med 1994, *109*, 284–287.

Lundberg O. *Kvinnors livsvillkor i dag [Women's living conditions today].* Only in Swedish. In: *Kvinn-o-hälsa.* Stockholm: Spris förlag 1995.

McKinlay JB, McKinlay SM, Brambilla DJ. *Health status and utilization behavior associated with menopause.* Am J Epidemiol 1987, *125*, 110–121.

Medicinska forskningsrådet. *Självmord i Sverige. En epidemiologisk översikt [Suicide in Sweden: An epidemiological overview].* Only in Swedish. Stockholm 1993.

Mullen PE, Martin JL, Anderson JC, Romans SE, Herbison GP. *Childhood sexual abuse and mental health in adult life.* Br J Psychiatry 1993, *163*, 721–732.

Nasser M. *Comparative study of the prevalence of abnormal eating attitudes among Arab female students of both London and Cairo universities.* Psychol Med 1986, *16*, 621–625.

Nolen-Hoeksema S. *Sex differences in unipolar depression. Evidence and theory.* Psychol Bull 1987, *101,* 259–282.

Rorsman B, Gräsbeck A, Hagnell O, Lanke J, Öhman R, Öjesjö L, Otterbeck L. *A prospective study of first-incidence depression. The Lundby Study, 1957–72.* Brit J Psychiatry 1990, *156,* 336–342.

Samuelsson S, Hällström T. *The distribution of adverse life events and impaired mental health in a female community sample.* In: Angermeyer MC (Ed.). *From social class to social stress.* Berlin: Springer Verlag 1987.

Seeman MV. *Addressing gender differences in schizophrenia and its treatment.* Contemporary Psychiatry, Nov–Dec 1992, 4–8.

Spencer JH, Glick ID, Haas GL, Clarkin JF, Lewis AB, Peyser J, DeMane N, Good-Ellis M, Harris E, Lestelle V. *A randomized clinical trial of inpatient family intervention, III: Effects of 6-month and 18-month follow-ups.* Am J Psychiatry 1988, *145,* 1115–1121.

Spigset O. *Serotonins rolle i normal appetittregulering og i patogenesen ved anorexi-bulimi [The role of serotonin in normal appetite regulation and in the pathogenesis of anorexia/bulimia].* Only in Norwegian. Nord Med 1990, *105,* 292–297.

Statistiska centralbyrån [Statistics Sweden]. Levnadsförhållanden. Rapport 76. Ohälsa och sjukvård 1980–89 [Living conditions. Report 76. Health and medical care 1980–89]. Only in Swedish. Stockholm: SCB 1992.

Stefansson CG, Svensson C. *Identified and unidentified mental illness in primary health care—Social characteristics, medical measures and total care utilization during one year.* Scand J Prim Health Care 1994, *12,* 24–31.

Tennant T. *Parental loss in childhood: Its effect in adult life.* In: Bebbington PE (Ed.): *Social Psychiatry.* London: Transaction Publ 1991.

Treasure JL, Holland AJ. *Genetic variability to eating disorders: Evidence from twin and family studies.* In: Remschmidt H, Schmidt MH (Eds.): *Anorexia nervosa.* Toronto: Hogrefe & Huber 1989.

Wessling A, Bergman U, Westerholm B. *On the differences in psychiatric drug use between the three major urban areas in Sweden.* Eur J Clin Pharmacol 1991, *40,* 495–500.

6

Violence against women: A social, criminal justice, medical, or public health problem?

Karen Leander, Maria Danielsson

Why focus on violence against women?

WHETHER VIOLENCE MORE PROFOUNDLY affects women's or men's health is a difficult question to answer. The consequences of violence for men's health are quite visible: more men than women are hospitalized as a result of violent injuries, and they are also more likely to die of such injuries. However, the health consequences of violence go far beyond what we see reflected in hospitalization and cause-of-death or criminal statistics. Violence against women is different in kind from violence against men. Perpetrators of violence are primarily men, whether their victims are women or other men. Violence against women frequently occurs in close relationships, continues systematically over a long period of time, and has different consequences for health and well-being than violence directed against men, which is often perpetrated by unknown men and tends to be of a more random and unsystematic nature. Moreover, sexual violence primarily affects women. Therefore, although the question of violence against men raises some related issues, we shall limit our discussion here to violence against women, that is, men's abuse of women and its repercussions for women's health. The social structures that permit and perpetuate violence will serve as the backdrop of the discussion.

Addressing the issue of violence against women

For more than twenty years, we have seen new, intensive efforts to increase awareness among the general public and decision-makers of how common coercion, violence, humiliation and abuse are within families, marriages, and the sexual sphere—in other words, in the most intimate and socially-sanctioned of human relationships. The victims in these contexts are primarily women and children. What distinguishes the debate that has taken place in the last few decades from earlier discussions is that we have come to view violence against women in the "private" sphere as a social problem with roots and *solutions* in the social system. The public discussion that has called attention to the issue of this violence represents a process of "social definition" (Hydén 1994, p. 4). In Hydén's analysis of violence against women within marriage, she points out that the insights of the women's movement in the 1970s and 1980s were crucial in Sweden in leading to a change in the public perception of violence against women.

Blackman, an American social psychologist who has examined the abuse of women, has described how a social problem is defined as it passes through various stages in public debate. First regarded as taboo, it is then discussed publicly, leading to political pressure and public reaction, after which programs of action are implemented, the scope of research expands, and experts appear on the scene (Blackman 1989). During this process, attitudes shift as to who is at fault, who is the victim and why, what has "gone wrong," the extent of the problem and who is responsible for seeing to it that appropriate measures are taken. According to Blackman, an important insight highlighted by researchers and other experts, such as workers at women's shelters and medical personnel, is the limited control that battered women have over the violent situation in which they find themselves.

A milestone in the effort to increase public awareness of violence against women was passed in Sweden in 1982, when the power of prosecutors was expanded to permit the prosecution of all assaults committed in a private area (thus including battering of wives or cohabiting partners in the home), even without the active cooperation of the abused party. In 1984 such provisions were extended to rape and other sexual crimes as well. Making such crimes equivalent to other violent crimes meant that private violence was collectively redefined as a public crime (Hydén 1994).

What is meant by "(men's) violence against women"?

> It appears that a significant shift has occurred within feminist thought over the decade. This is evident in the conceptualization of male violence against women, which moved from separate accounts of specific types of violence to an appreciation of male violence overall as being at some level a unitary phenomenon, and in the theoretical importance attached to violence—as well as other forms of male power—in the analysis of what different writers describe as patriarchal, male-dominated or male-supremacist society (Edwards 1987, pp. 15–16).

Various terms have been used to refer to violence committed against women simply because they are women, but not as random targets of violence. Liz Kelly uses the term *sexual violence* as a general term to cover "all forms of abuse, coercion and force" that the women in her English study experienced from men (Kelly 1987, p 59). There are several reasons why she chooses to use this particular term. First, it underscores the fact that the violence is committed by one sex (men) and directed against the other (women). Second, it is difficult to draw a clear line distinguishing between physical, sexual, and psychological violence, since one type of violence often involves aspects of another. Finally, the term can be linked to an analysis of sexuality as a system of power through which men try to control women. Any manifestation of violence that reflects male dominance and women's subordinate position can be viewed as sexual violence.

In Scandinavia, the term *sexualized violence* has been used as a collective term for a number of related phenomena. It generally includes "assault against women, rape, incest/sexual abuse of children, prostitution and pornography, seen as related because they are expressions of *the oppression of women*" (Folkhälsoinstitutet 1994a, p. 5, our translation).

The term *gender violence* has been used to indicate violations perpetrated "against people due to their gender identity, sexual orientation, or location in the hierarchy of male-dominated social systems such as families, military organizations or the labor force" (O'Toole & Schiffman 1997, xii).

This chapter focuses on "woman battering" and rape. The term woman battering or abuse is taken here to include violence in marriage as well as in non-marital cohabiting relationships, and has been defined as violence, frequently repeated, directed against a woman by her current or former husband, partner, fiancé, and so on —thus occurring between individuals whose relationship is an emotional one (Dahlberg 1989). Such assaults often become aggravated upon dissolution of a relationship.

In 1993, the Swedish government established The Commission on Violence Against Women (SOU 1995:60). The Commission's mandate was to propose changes in the legal, social, and health sectors. A National Center for Battered and Raped Women was opened in Uppsala in 1995. A new Government Bill (Regeringskansliet 1997/98:55) has led to the criminalization of the purchase of sexual services. This means that as of 1999, prostitution customers face the risk of criminal prosecution that can lead to fines or imprisonment up to six months. Further, the Bill outlines extensive allocations to the various public authorities, more stringent sanctions against female genital mutilation and sexual harassment in working life, a call for improved criminal statistics and gender perspectives in criminological research, an inventory of policing efforts, support to certain voluntary organizations, and a national crisis telephone line and other services for survivors of gender violence. The multi-agency campaign in Stockholm County—Operation Kvinnofrid [Women's Peace]—is working with European partners and other regions in Sweden.

A Commission on Sexual Offenses has also been appointed to review all the legal provisions on sexual offenses, focusing on the boundary drawn between the various specific offenses and the punishment for them, the extent to which the definition of rape should focus on consent versus force, and rape committed against children. The definition of rape was considerably expanded in 1984 to include acts previously defined as lesser sexual offenses, homosexual rapes as well as those committed by women, and a more subjective definition of what constitutes a threat. The legislative history emphasized that the core of the crime was the refusal of one person to respect another person's non-consent. Further, the victim's behavior prior to the non-consensual act was declared formally void of legal significance. The emphasis shifted from the actions of the perpetrator to the victim's experience of having been violated (Snare 1985). The author of a recent dissertation interpreted young people's perceptions of rape in light of the cultural norms about gender and heterosexuality (Jeffner 1997). She found that what these young people perceive as rape depends on how they negotiate and reinterpret the encounter in question. Her findings indicate that distinctions made by these young people between rape and "good sex" seem to limit the action alternatives for young women while extending them for young men.

Until recently, there was no specific Swedish statute prohibiting "woman battering." Instead, such offenses have been prosecuted as assaults. However, in mid-1998, a new crime of gross violation of a woman's integrity was introduced to the Criminal Code, for the purpose of alleviating some of the difficulties in the encounter between abused women and the criminal justice system. The law is intended to establish a legal definition of woman abuse broad enough to include the entire complex of actions and processes reported by battered women. If a man repeatedly commits certain criminal acts (assault, unlawful threat or coercion, sexual or other molestation, etc.) against a woman who is a present or former spouse or cohabitant, he is to be sentenced for gross (collective) violation of the woman's integrity, instead of for the individual crimes that each act comprises. A necessary condition for sentencing under the new provision is that the acts be part of a repeated violation of the woman's integrity and aimed at seriously damaging her self-esteem. The punishment is imprisonment for at least six months and at most six years (sentences for aggravated assault range from one to ten years). One purpose of the new law is to allow prosecutors and the courts to take into account the entire situation of the abused woman.

How common is violence against women?

Over the past twenty years, an important question in the public debate has been just how widespread violence against women is, and there are no comprehensive sources to provide an accurate answer to this question. In this section, a look is taken at data on violence from cause-of-death and health-care statistics, police reports, and survey responses.

Violence resulting in death

Research is needed to determine how many women are killed by their male partners each year. Police statistics on homicide do not indicate the sex of the victim, a practice targeted for change by the Commission on Violence against Women (see above). However, statistics on causes of death do show the deceased's sex. In 1996, there were 110 deaths resulting from "murder, manslaughter or other injury willfully inflicted by one person on another." One-third of these were women (n = 36), six of whom were under 15 years old (Socialstyrelsen 1994). Over the 20-year period preceding 1996, the average total number of girls and women killed each year according to the cause-of-death statistics was slightly under 37 (Statistics Sweden).

Research from the 1970s and a more recent analysis of violent crimes ending in death during the 1990s have shown that 50 percent of all adult female homicide victims are killed by their present or former male partners (Somander 1979; Rying 1999). For 1996, this would be about 18 women. By comparison, less than 10 percent of male victims are killed by their female partners. Comparable Canadian statistics show that six in ten of women victims are killed by their male partners, compared with three in ten in the United States where murders committed by strangers are considerably more common (Stark & Flitcraft 1995).

Nonfatal violence

Of the more than 55,000 cases of assault that were reported to the police in 1997, 35 percent involved violence against women over the age of 14. Violence against men accounted for 56 percent of cases, while over one percent of cases involved children under the age of six and eight percent children between 7 and 14. This distribution roughly corresponds to the distribution of fatal violence. It was not until 1981 that statistics on assaults included the sex of the victim. The two largest sub-categories of assault reported to the police are assaults committed against men "outdoors by strangers" and those committed against women "indoors by persons known to the victim." The latter category corresponds most closely to what we term "woman battering," that is, abuse committed by a current or former husband or partner,[1] and accounts for roughly two-thirds of all assaults against woman victims (140 per 100,000 inhabitants in 1997), compared with only 20 percent of assaults against men. Table 1 shows the number of reported sex crimes and cases of woman battering committed in Sweden since 1987. During this period, the number of reported cases of woman abuse increased by 44 percent, while the number of rapes increased by 52 percent.

Table 6.1. Number of reported cases of "woman battering" and sex crimes in Sweden, selected years 1987–1997.

	1987	1989	1991	1993	1995	1997	Change 1987–1997
"Woman battering"	8 604	9 473	9 338	11 727	12 350	12 351	+44%
Of these, Aggravated	617	721	680	918	652	528	-14%
Sexual crimes	4 602	5 568	5 500	8 155	7 761	7 695	+67%
Of these, rape	1 114	1 462	1 482 2	153	1 707	1 692	+52%

Source: Tables on police-reported crimes from Statistics Sweden (SCB) up to and including 1993, Swedish National Council for Crime Prevention (BRÅ) after 1993.

In addition to rape, sex crimes also include other types of sexual coercion, exploitation and molestation. Statistics on reported rapes in Sweden have been available since 1950. The number of reported rapes per 100,000 has increased from five in 1950 to 19 in 1997. In 1997, 17 percent of rape victims were younger than 15—which is higher than the level in the mid-1980s, which was around 10 percent.

Criminal statistics show that other sex crimes, such as sexual coercion and sexual molestation, also increased substantially in the early 1990s. Examining the increase in reported crimes, Olsson (1994, p. 64) concludes that "the most likely interpretation is that the statistical increase in sex crimes against adults is due, first, to reduced tolerance for sex crimes in general and, second, to an actual increase in such crimes" (our translation). For a discussion of reported sex crimes against children, see Chapter 2.

The proportion of men is even higher among the perpetrators of violence than among victims. Statistics on police-reported crimes show that 89 percent of those suspected of homicide in 1997 were men, while 92 percent of assault suspects, 94 percent of robbery suspects, and 99 percent of sex-crime and rape suspects were men. For assaults, the gender of suspects is shown by the age and sex of the victims in Table 2.

Table 6.2. Gender distribution of assault suspects in Sweden in 1997 by victim's age and gender.

	Assaults against			
	Children 0–6	Children 7–14	Women >15	Men >15
By female suspect (8%)	28%	18%	12%	4%
By male suspect (92%)	72%	82%	88%	96%

Source: Swedish National Council for Crime Prevention (BRÅ), Tables 1997.

Surveys provide information on crimes not reported to the police

Researchers assume that the actual number of violent crimes committed is at least three times as high as the number of crimes reported to the police (Wikström 1992). The ratio of crimes that are not reported to the police to those that are is assumed to vary depending on the type of offense. The discrepancy is likely to be greater for crimes like woman abuse and rape, owing to the many factors that discourage women from going to the police (Ottoson Hindberg 1984).

Each year Statistics Sweden conducts nationwide surveys dealing with the conditions of people's lives and including questions on exposure to violence and threatening behavior. According to the 1992/93 surveys, 6 percent of women and about 9 percent of men between the ages of 16 and 84 had been exposed to violence or the threat of violence over a one-year period (Statistics Sweden 1995b). This represents an increase from the 1980s, and is due mainly to a rise in the number of threats. Surveys also indicate that violent behavior on the street and in other public places is usually directed against male victims, while women run a higher risk than men of being victims of violence or the threat of violence at home or on the job.

Based on the survey conducted by Statistics Sweden, we can estimate the number of violent crimes committed during one year in Sweden in several categories that are closely linked with woman abuse, which gives us some idea of how many crimes go unreported. Although even these surveys substantially underreport violence occurring at home, it is estimated that all together, women are exposed to about 161,000 incidents of violence or the threat of violence committed by someone they know well and to 145,000 incidents in their own homes. Women indicated that they failed to report 65,000 cases of violence or the threat of violence to the police for fear of reprisals or for family reasons. By comparison, some 11,000 cases of assault against women committed "indoors by a person known to the victim" were reported to the police during the same period. In addition, the survey shows that repeated violence (four or more incidents of violence or the threat of violence) is perpetrated against more female than male victims. The Statistics Sweden survey does not indicate how many women are victims of sexual abuse.

The same survey showed that in the course of one year, 17 percent of single mothers with small children were subjected to violence or the threat of violence in their homes, as compared with three percent of all young women and one percent of women and 1.7 percent of men in all age groups. The fact that women who live alone report experiencing violence in their homes more often than women who live with a partner may be due to the fact that it is easier, in both emotional and practical terms, for a woman to report such events if she is not living with the perpetrator. Moreover, violence and separation are frequently closely interlinked. Violence may lead to a separation, but a separation may also trigger violence. Research in other countries also shows a very high level of violence directed against women living alone (Stark & Flitcraft 1995; U.S. Dept. of Justice 1995).

Surveys conducted by specially trained interviewers and directed specifically at women appear to be the best way to estimate the extent of violence in the private and sexual spheres (Hanmer & Saunders 1984; Johnson & Sacco 1995; Russell 1984; Sorenson & Saftlas 1994; Statistics Canada 1993). A new Finnish mail questionnaire studying the prevalence of violence directed exclusively at women found that 40 percent of adult women have been victims of male physical or sexual violence or threats after their 15th birthday, 14 percent over the past twelve months. Further, the results show that 22 percent of all married and cohabiting women have been victims of physical or sexual violence or threats of violence by their present partner, 9 percent over the past year (Heiskanen & Piispa 1998). It was also shown that of those men who had been violent while the relationship lasted, more than one-third continued their violent behavior after separation. On the other hand, the violence stopped at separation in nearly 60 percent of the violent relationships.

The surveys conducted by Statistics Sweden show that violence and the threat of violence associated with the workplace increased between 1978 and 1993 among women of all age groups between 16 and 64. There has also been an increase in the number of reports submitted to the Swedish National Board of Occupation Safety and Health of work-related injuries associated with violence or threatening behavior. In the mid-1980s, such reports were quite evenly distributed between men and women, but the gender gap has widened since then, and the relative difference is especially great in the oldest age group (55–64 years of age). Men appear to have better career opportunities in the labor market that "provide them access to jobs with less risk of exposure to violence or threatening behavior" (Swedish National Board of Occupational Safety and Health 1998, p. 7–8, our translation). In addition, women are employed much more often than men in the health, care and service sectors, where work-related violence and threats commonly occur. Many women also find themselves in vulnerable positions as sales-clerks or cashiers at the post office, banks and retail stores. In the United States, murder and manslaughter are the most common reasons for work-related deaths among women, and represent between 39 and 57 percent of all women's deaths occurring on the job (Dannenberg et al., 1994).

Violence that is only temporarily visible

In concluding our discussion of how widespread violence is, we should note that some cases of violence that are reported to the police do not remain visible. Many reported cases of woman abuse and rape are dismissed or withdrawn before coming to trial (Leander 1989, 1992). This is certain to have a profound effect, not least psychologically, on women seeking protection and redress from the judicial system. There is a need for studies showing how the decision not to prosecute affects victims and perpetrators.

Women survivors of violence and the health system

> Violence against women may be an important, although often ignored confounding variable or effect modifier in studies of women's health… Studies that assess violence as a risk factor are likely to account better for women's health status. (Sorensson & Saftlas 1994, p. 144)

Many studies outside Sweden have shown that injuries caused by a male partner are one of the most common reasons why women seek emergency room treatment (Sorensson & Saftlas 1994), with some estimating that as many as 22 to 35 percent of all women who seek emergency care have been injured by a male partner, when we include secondary symptoms related to "the stress of living under abusive conditions" (Warshaw 1993, p. 134). Indeed, some experts claim that women in the United States seek medical treatment for injuries caused by violence approximately three times as often as for injuries resulting from automobile accidents (Dannenberg et al. 1994). According to estimates from the early 1990s in

Sweden, avowed violent injuries are responsible for one percent of all hospital-izations among women and three percent among men (Swedish National Institute of Public Health 1994b). Estimates of the prevalence of women experiencing violence during pregnancy in the U.S. have ranged between 1 and 20 percent (Ballard et al., 1998).

Systematic compilations of the reasons why people seek outpatient care, that is, treatment in emergency rooms or medical centers, are only available in certain counties in Sweden. An injury-surveillance system is currently being established for Stockholm County (Leander & Andersson 1995). In an experimental program that recorded all injuries treated at four emergency treatment centers in the Stockholm area (surgical and orthopedic centers), five percent of the women and more than 10 percent of the men treated in 1991 for injuries had been victims of violence (Karlsson et al. 1995). Nearly half of the violent injuries suffered by women were injuries to the head, while men's injuries tended to be more evenly distributed among various parts of the body. Health care statistics show that approximately 75 percent of those seeking treatment for violent injuries are men. This is only a rough estimate, since abused women also seek out facilities specializing in emergency treatment of gynecological, ears, nose and throat and psychiatric problems, and these cases are not captured in the records kept by the emergency treatment centers mentioned above.

In addition to the lack of statistical systems, there are other reasons why we do not know just how many abused women seek medical treatment. Medical personnel do not always "see" or document the violence that has led to injury (Landstingsförbundet 1991; Melinder 1994). The reluctance of medical personnel (especially physicians) to inquire as to whether injuries or other conditions are related to violence and to interpret signals accurately has been attributed to a lack of time, a perceived inability to change the situation, fear of violating a woman's integrity, and difficulty believing in the possibility of violence among certain socioeconomic groups (Risberg 1994a). Having a chance to tell someone and being treated with respect afterwards can be the first step toward a woman's rehabilitation. Silence from medical personnel may tend to reinforce a woman's feeling that she needs to deal with the problem on her own. Increased ability on the part of physicians to "dare to ask about and to see" violence, also among their long-term patients, is making such violence more apparent and leading to changes in the routines of health care workers (JAMA 1996).[2]

Much has been written about women's reluctance to talk about violence in their private spheres with others, and particularly with those in positions of authority (Risberg 1994a), such as members of the medical profession. This is thought to be due to abused women's feelings of shame and guilt, fear of reprisals, perceived lack of insight or understanding and even victim-blaming on the part of professionals, limited opportunities for redress, and ties to the abuser, as well as a failure on the part of those around them to condemn the perpetrator's behavior. These factors also account for the fact that violence against women is understated in criminal statistics and victim studies. Research has shown, though, that many of the barriers to disclosure of abuse within the health services can be overcome by, among other things, greater knowledge among physicians of the link between abuse and medical illness, improved sensitivity on the part of the physician, and the offer of a follow-up visit (McCauley et al. 1998).

Many women who have been abused seek treatment for other conditions and problems to which violence and sexual abuse may be contributing factors. In order to identify the impact of the abuse, one author has suggested two approaches to using medical records. First, she found a large percentage of sexually abused women in certain patient groups, such as patients with chronic pelvic pain, eating disorders, self-destructive behavior, chronic psychological and some personality disorders, as well as among patients in psychiatric care in general (Risberg 1994a). Second, she suggests studying the past and present medical records of women who are known to have been subjected to sexual abuse. For instance, among such women there is an increased incidence of sexual problems, chronic pain in the lower abdomen, infections of the reproductive organs, and psychological disorders such as depression, anxiety, insomnia and substance abuse. However, there are no specific symptoms manifested by all abused women (Risberg 1994a; for a discussion of rape as a health problem, see also Dahl 1993). When studying health consequences of physical, sexual, and psychological abuse, the chronology must be kept clear, that is, whether or not violence and abuse preceded these conditions.

Moreover, there are dangers in overemphasizing a medical model of violence against women, a model which can only "medicalize," reducing things to categories it can "handle and control" (Warshaw 1993, p 143). While it is crucial that health care responses be improved and rendered more sensitive, it is even more crucial to continue to stress the social roots of these phenomena. We should work to avoid stigmatization of those subjected to this violence and abuse, in part by recognizing that reactions to this treatment will differ from individual to individual. Assuming that physical and sexual abuse will inevitably lead to certain debilitating consequences and drawing conclusions about their duration, seriousness, or scope will not serve the interests of the victims. Indeed, we must avoid viewing them primarily as victims rather than as survivors of victimization with ensuing strengths, insights and resilience. An exclusively medical—or public health—model can never be sufficient for diminishing this violence or for enhancing women's empowerment. The health care sector must play a role, but we need to be sure that this role does not contribute to viewing abused women simply as objects to be cured.

Suicide attempts are much more common among women than men (see Chapters 2 and 5). Many women who have attempted suicide end up in hospital emergency rooms. Studies in Sweden and elsewhere have shown that domestic abuse is a factor in many suicide attempts by women (Bergman 1991; Stark & Flitcraft 1995). Both suicide attempts and substance abuse among abused women have been shown to be linked to the degree of control exerted by their partners, that is, how restricted these women are in their activities, access to money, contact to family and friends, and ability to control their sexual lives. This process of progressive infringement of women's freedom has been termed "entrapment" by American researchers (Stark & Flitcraft 1995). In many cases, violence is only one of several means used by an abuser to coerce, frighten and control a woman, and from her perspective it may, indeed, not always be the worst one. When violence goes unrecognized, for example by health care workers, this may contribute to increasing a woman's despair, isolation and sense of being trapped (Stark & Flitcraft 1995). This can lead to subsequent suicide attempts, which represent a desperate cry for help. The obstacles that continue to prevent women from·finding help are a social problem, not an individual one.

From chivalry to control

> Behavior by the man, adopted to control his victim, which results in physical, sexual and/or psychological damage, forced isolation, or economic deprivation or behavior which leaves a woman living in fear. (Definition of violence against women from Australia 1991, as quoted in Heise 1994:47)

What explains men's violent behavior toward women? There is no single universal theory. More than ten years ago, a researcher identified some twenty different theories of wife abuse and other types of violence within families (Okun 1986). According to a Swedish report on "violence against women in close relationships," there are two basic approaches researchers tend to take: ". . .the one focuses primarily on historical and social domination of women by men . . . and the other focuses on the question of why certain men, but not others, subject women to violence" (Swedish National Council for Crime Prevention 1994:4, p. 16, our translation). The former approach is primary and the latter secondary, since men who use violence against women are influenced by the patriarchal structure of society. The need to put violence in a larger social and cultural context is described as follows by another researcher: ". . . the priority is to understand why abuse is directed at women, not why each individual man abuses. . . The task is to discover what social conditions produce this target (i.e., women) generation after generation" (Schechter 1982:215–216).

A number of researchers invoke a gender-politics model to explain domestic violence against women (Stark & Flitcraft 1991). According to Stark and Flitcraft, this perspective is better able than one based on individual psychodynamics or a family dynamics model to explain why men abuse women. Violence within a family is seen as only one of many expressions of a man's control (over women, children or other men). The family dynamics model, for example, cannot explain why many women are abused even before a couple moves in together—courtship violence—or why men continue to exhibit violent behavior even after a divorce. Violence against women within the family or home setting should be seen against the backdrop of the existing power imbalance in society and the general discrimination directed against women. Resorting to violence is an alternative certain men choose when they see their privileged access to scarce resources (such as money or sex) threatened by women's independence (Stark & Flitcraft 1991). Typical conflicts that trigger violence include men's feelings of possessiveness and jealousy, their expectations regarding women's duties at home, their sense that they have the right to punish "their" women for perceived misdeeds—in other words, conflicts in which men's positions of authority are challenged (Dobash & Dobash 1992). Alcohol is also a significant factor in triggering violence. Finally, women are more likely to remain in violent situations for such reasons as fear, lack of support, criticism from their family and friends, and a lack of resources than because of their own psychological traits.

Turning to the issue of rape, one author has identified two broad theoretical explanations found in the literature for the "epidemic of rape" (O'Toole 1997). *Gender role socialization* theories focus on the ways the dominant culture indoctrinates males (through various media) to be sexual aggressors, to expect sex on demand, to believe aggression is a normative component of heterosexual relationships, and to embrace victim-blaming myths about rape. *Political-economic* theories of rape were developed based on women's historical powerlessness and their legal definition as the property of men. This perspective analyzes the commodification of women's sexuality—in advertising and the sex industry, for instance—which, in combination with the eroticization of dominance, contributes to escalating sexual violence.

How a situation of violence is perpetuated within a couple's relationship has been the focus of study by the Norwegian researcher Eva Lundgren, among others. Lundgren has interviewed both partners in relationships where violence has occurred. She describes the maintenance of violence in terms of a process of normalization:

> In an abusive relationship, we can view the development and continuance of violence as a process—a process of violence. Many mechanisms play a part in this process, mechanisms that both individually and in combination render abuse an active, dynamic process with profound consequences for the partners involved. The process of violence is characterized by a situation in which violence is normalized—in several different ways—by the abuser and the abused party. Borrowing an analytical concept, I use the term "normalization" for the process by which violence gradually becomes a normal part of everyday life and is both accepted and justified (Lundgren 1989, p. 114; our translation).

According to Lundgren, women and men in abusive relationships are similar to other couples in most respects other than violence. She believes that gradual transition takes place in these couples from a nonviolent to a violent relationship, "from a dominant male role to a violent male role and from a subordinate female role to a female role characterized by submission and abuse" (Lundgren 1989, p. 117, our translation).

The man's strategy in this process of normalization is goal-oriented and aimed at exerting control over the woman and seeking to define his own masculinity. Like other researchers (Hydén 1994; Skjørten 1995), Lundgren maintains that abusive men do not resort to violence in a state of frenzied rage. Skjørten shows that men's behavior is under their control in a number of respects: in their choice of a victim (in many cases, never anyone other than their wife), the time and place (when they are alone) and the instance of violence (how violently and in what way they strike out). Even if the man strikes out when he is in a state of affect, that state is associated with a high degree of control at the moment of abuse. Many of the men interviewed by Lundgren also described how the actual violence became an erotic experience for them. This may explain both why many physically abusive incidents end in rape and other sexual coercion and why men beat their wives. From being adopted as a strategy to achieve certain objectives, violence gradually develops its own dynamic.

Lundgren has also described what this process of normalization means for women. During the first phase, women begin to lose touch with their own sense of reality. Violence can no longer be explained by external factors (an accident, the fault of the man, etc.)—"it's just there." The line between what is acceptable and what is unacceptable behavior becomes hazy, and violence begins to be seen as normal. Gradually, women internalize violence and engage in self-blame,[3] in a process that affects their self-concept and sense of their own femininity. Violence comes to be a substantial part of these women's reality, which increases their emotional dependence on the abuser. At the beginning, their strategy is aimed at putting a stop to the violence. Gradually their efforts to adjust to the situation become a strategy aimed simply at survival. The woman begins to internalize the man's view of what a woman should be. In moving from a well-devised strategy to one of internalization, the woman shifts from being an active participant to being a victim. At this point, her control over the situation is greatly weakened.

The process is characterized by two important mechanisms. The first is the woman's isolation. In interviews, men have described their strategies for gradually cutting off the woman's contact with relatives, friends and others, and various ways for limiting her activities. Thus abused women are often isolated from other people who might be in a position to offer help or protect or validate their perceptions of what is happening. This process has also been termed "social battering" (Okun 1986, p. 116). Another control mechanism, according to Lundgren (1989, p. 122), is to alternate between violence and affection, between brutality and warmth, a tactic that is akin to torture: "The effects of violence are intensified when violence is alternated with affection and care. And it is the man who is in control of shifting from good to bad, from praise to punishment" (our translation).

The description provided by Lundgren and other researchers of couples in abusive relationships highlights the importance of outside support if women are to succeed in breaking off abusive relationships—which, indeed, many do.

Prevention in the spirit of public health

Although gender violence is a significant cause of female morbidity and mortality, it is almost never seen as a public health issue. Recent World Bank estimates of the global burden of disease indicate that in established market economies gender-based victimization is responsible for one out of every five healthy days of life lost to women of reproductive age (Heise et al. 1994, p. ix).

Violence constitutes a threat to women's health and well-being. Today violence against women is regarded as a criminal, social and political problem, and more recently also as an issue of human rights. Seen in historical terms, this is a breakthrough for a more comprehensive approach to the problem of violence against women, which was traditionally viewed as a problem confined to certain individuals. However, violence against women has rarely been seen as a public health issue (Sorensen & Saftlas 1994), perhaps because the problem is too complex to be addressed within the framework of public health measures. Sexism has also played a role in attaching a low priority to the issue of violence against women and its effects on women's health (Heise et al. 1994). It has been pointed out in numerous contexts that there is a clear connection between ideology and research on women's health (Larosa 1994).

Given the knowledge we have about the prevalence and deleteriousness of violence, it is certainly justified to speak of a public health issue (Leander 1995; Heiskanen & Piispa 1998). The consequences of violence are serious enough that we need to address this problem in every social arena. The topic of sexual abuse is increasingly being added to adolescent sexual health education agendas (Wood et al. 1998). Heise (1994) sees the plight of abused women as a hidden impediment to economic and social development. As women's vitality is eroded, their self-confidence undermined, and their health jeopardized, society loses the benefit of their contributions and full participation. Moreover, researchers who have studied women in extremely vulnerable social situations—drug abusers, prisoners and homeless women—have found that they report high levels of violence in their lives (Leander 1993; Järvinen 1995).

Fear of physical or sexual violence can also be viewed as a public-health problem. Studies from various parts of the world have shown that many women believe that "the worst parts of being a woman" are violence and the fear of violence at the hands of men (Heise 1994). Four to five times as many women as men interviewed in the Swedish surveys on living conditions report that at some point during a 12-month period they have refrained from going out in the evening for fear of violence (Statistics Sweden 1995b). The proportion of those expressing such fears is highest among the oldest women. To explain why more women (particularly among the elderly) are afraid, although they are victimized by far less street violence than men (particularly among the young), we might borrow Liz Kelly's term "the continuum of violence." Kelly (1987) interviewed 60 English women who provided information on men's threats and violence against them, and on how such behavior changed throughout childhood and into adulthood. The cumulative effect of violence during their lifetimes, including "hidden violence," that is, repeated experiences of vulnerability both at home and in public places, may help to trigger fear both among women who have experienced violence and among women who have not been directly affected (Pain 1995; Stanko 1987). Elisabeth Stanko sees women's lives as lived along a "continuum of insecurity" and provides examples of how women more or less constantly "negotiate" with men about their own safety (Stanko 1990).

Viewing violence against women from a public health perspective is appropriate because it emphasizes prevention, regarding violence as something that is not inevitable, but can be changed. In discussing measures to prevent violence, we should keep in mind the importance of counteracting the underlying causes of the problem as well as treating its symptoms. Every society has mechanisms that legitimize, hide, and deny—and thus perpetuate—violence, despite general condemnation of such behavior. This holds true particularly for violence against women. Every sector of society is called upon to identify and challenge such mechanisms.

The Swedish medical researcher Risberg concludes that measures on the structural level aimed at preventing violence against women are more appropriate and potentially effective than medical interventions. "We need to recognize the link between sexualized violence and the pattern of male dominance and female subordination that is found in our culture" (Risberg 1994b, p. 4773; our translation). Since the health care and medical sector is frequently alone in coming into contact with many types of violence against women, though, it is important to consider preventive efforts based in this sector. Flitcraft (1993) points out that health care and preventive efforts need to be linked, and uses a model that involves primary, secondary and tertiary levels of prevention.

Traditionally, *primary prevention* implies that the number of new cases declines as behavioral and environmental factors are changed. Preventing violence against women involves changing norms and calling for a comprehensive condemnation of violence and coercion in the private sphere as well as "an expansion of equality and an end to the existing power asymmetry" (Risberg 1994b, p. 4773; our translation).

Secondary prevention involves early detection and treatment of violence. Above all, woman abuse and other instances of violence within families need to be recognized as causing a host of medical problems, and it is important to give priority to prevention. Guidelines should be developed for diagnosis and treatment. Furthermore, changes need to be made in the structure of medical practice, with its hierarchical structure, male dominance and status orientation. A traditional relationship with an all-powerful, all-controlling physician can be directly harmful to an abused woman (Warshaw 1993).

Early intervention is critical, in part because violence is frequently repeated, and in part because many women seek out medical care before the process of "normalization" is fully underway (Risberg 1994b). Flitcraft (1993) emphasizes the need for new models of physician-patient interaction to increase "patient empowerment" and enhance a woman's ability to act independently. Effective prevention requires the involvement of a variety of groups within the health care system, such as nurses, medical social workers, and physiotherapists, who need to be able to provide advice on resources available to abused women.

In addition, Flitcraft (1993) points out that routine questions on domestic violence represent a type of health education. A physician's acknowledgment of this problem underscores the fact that wife abuse poses a threat to health. Just as questions about smoking may help a patient decide to quit smoking, questions about violence can be helpful in three ways: 1) by identifying an abused woman's problem; 2) by determining the current safety of a woman who has been abused in the past; and 3) by raising awareness of this problem among women who have not been abused. There should, of course, be some discussion to determine which patients should be asked such questions.

Tertiary prevention involves providing assistance to abused women to help put a stop to repeated abuse and alleviate the consequences of abuse. The health and medical care system needs to focus on crisis intervention, emergency interventions aimed at women's protection and security, counseling and other active measures; in other words, it should do more than simply identify the problem and refer women to other authorities. A model developed by the National Center for Battered and Raped Women is worthy of emulation by other parts of the health care system. At the Center, female physicians, psychologists, social workers, and physiotherapists provide various kinds of support and help to abused women, and it is also instrumental in generating further information about this issue. There are similar broad-based strategies, sometimes referred to as "postvention," for treating individuals who have attempted suicide or for dealing with child abuse (see Davidson 1996).

Protection and empowerment

In 1997, 23,732 contacts were made by women seeking help from women's shelters, according to the National Organization of Battered Women's Shelters in Sweden (ROKS, 1998). That year 1,239 women and 1,041 children stayed in women's shelters for a total of 50,646 nights. It is in large part thanks to these centers that violence against women and children has found a place on the public agenda. In the United States, women's shelters, together with other grass-roots organizations, have arrived at a consensus with decision-makers on three points (Flitcraft 1993):

First, violence within a family must be dealt with equally seriously as when perpetrated against someone outside the family; second, safety for victims of violence and their children is of primary importance; and finally, comprehensive changes in many social sectors are required if the needs of survivors are to be met. The World Bank has underscored the importance of this last point. Prevention will require tenacious and comprehensive efforts, and the World Bank's focus will be on "community-based organizations, public education, and women's empowerment" (Heise 1994, p. 43). Since the power imbalance between the sexes—on both a structural and an individual level—supports and perpetuates violence against women, societal measures should be devoted both to protecting women against violence and to strengthening their position. The World Bank report concludes by pointing out that some of the most effective short-term measures to combat violence against women can be taken within the framework of the health care system, not least because this is the only public institution that is likely to have contact with all adult women at some point in their lives.

Notes

1   Note that in certain cases assaults committed "indoors by persons known to the victim" may refer to violence at work or drinking parties, etc., or by a perpetrator other than the woman's partner. Conversely, certain cases of assault occurring outdoors may involve spouses. As of yet, there is no better way to estimate what portion of police statistics refer to woman battering other than to use the number of assaults against women committed "indoors by persons known to the victim."

2   An interesting example of medical practice leading to violence was pointed out by researchers in Baltimore, Maryland. Personnel working at various medical facilities for HIV-positive patients were required by new procedures to inform a patient's sexual partners if that patient tested positive for HIV. This led to considerable violence against female patients by their male partners. Results of this study lead to a change in these rules (North & Rothenburg 1993).

3   According to Stark and Flitcraft (1995), blaming oneself can be seen as a psychological mechanism for gaining some sense of control over the situation.

References

Ballard TJ, Saltzman, LE, Gazmararian JA, Spitz AM, Lazorick S, Marks, JS. *Violence during Pregnancy: Measurement Issues.* Am J Public Health 1998; 88 (2):274–6.

Bergman B, Brismar B. *Suicide attempts by battered wives.* Acta Psychiatr. Scand. 1991;83:380–4.

Blackman J. *Intimate Violence. A study of injustice.* New York, Oxford: Columbia University Press, 1989.

Dahl S. *Rape—A Hazard to Health.* Oslo: Scandinavian University Press, 1993.

Dahlberg A. *Misshandlade kvinnor och rätten [Battered women and the law].* In: Kvinnomisshandel [Woman Battering]. Stockholm: Delegationen för jämställdhetsforskning [Delegation for equality research] (JÄMFO), Report No. 14, 1989.

Dannenberg AL, Baker SP, Li G. *Intentional and Unintentional Injuries in Women: An Overview.* Ann Epidemiol 1994;4:133–9.

Davidson LL. Editorial: *Preventing Injuries from Violence towards Women.* Am J Public Health 1996;1:13.

Dobash RE, Dobash RP. *Women, Violence and Social Change.* London & New York: Routledge, 1992.

Edwards A. *Male Violence in Feminist Theory: An Analysis of the Changing Conceptions of Sex/Gender Violence and Male Dominance.* In: Hanmer J, Maynard M (Eds.): Women, Violence and Social Control. Houndmills etc.: MacMillan Press, Explorations in Sociology 23, 1987.

Federation of County Councils [Landstingsförbundet]. *Vården mot våld [Health care sector against violence].* Stockholm: Rapport till kongressen [Conference report], 1991.

Flitcraft A. *Physicians and Domestic Violence: Challenges for Prevention.* Health Affairs Winter 1993;154–61.

Hanmer J, Saunders S. *Well-Founded Fear: A Community Study of Violence to Women.* London: Hutchison & Co., 1984.

Heise LL, Pitanguy J, Germain A. V*iolence Against Women: The Hidden Health Burden.* Washington, D.C.: The World Bank, World Bank Discussion Papers 255, 1994.

Heiskanen M, Piispa M. *Faith, Hope, Battering. A Survey of Men's Violence against Women in Finland.* Helsinki: Statistics Finland, 1998.

Hydén M. *Women Battering as Marital Act. The Construction of a Violent Marriage.* Oslo: Scandinavian University Press, 1994.

JAMA. *When Physicians Ask, Women Tell About Domestic Abuse and Violence.* Medical News & Perspectives, JAMA 1996; 275(24):1863–4.

Jeffner K. *"Liksom våldtäkt, typ." Om betydelsen av kön och heterosexualitet för ungdomars förståelse av våldtäkt. ['Like, you know—rape.' On the importance of gender and heterosexuality to young people's perception of rape].* Uppsala: Dept of Sociology, Uppsala University, 1997.

Johnson H, Sacco VF. *Researching Violence Against Women: Statistics Canada's National Survey.* Canadian Journal of Criminology 1995;37(3):281–304.

Järvinen M. *De nye hjemløse. Kvinder, fattigdom, vold [The New Homeless: Women, poverty, violence].* Holte: Forlaget Socmed, 1993.

Karlsson A, Alberts KA, Andersson R. *Öppenvårdsregistrering av skador vid två akutsjukhus i Stockholms län: 1 års material för perioden februari 1991–januari 1992 [Outpatient injury registration at two emergency clinics in Stockholm County: One-year data for the period from February 1991–January 1992].* Sundbyberg: Landstingets hälsovård, Socialmedicin Kronan, 1995;258:93.

Kelly L. *The Continuum of Sexual Violence.* In: Hanmer J, Maynard M (Eds.): Women, Violence and Social Control. Houndmills etc.: MacMillan Press, Explorations in Sociology 23, 1987.

Larosa JH. *Women's Health: Science and Politics.* Ann Epidemiol 1994;4:84–88.

Leander K, Andersson R. *Utveckling av ett våldsförebyggande program i Stockholms län [Developing a violence prevention program in Stockholm County].* Sundbyberg: Landstingets hälsovård, Socialmedicin Kronan 1995;266.

Leander K. *Through the Looking Glass: A travel report on violence and violence prevention in the USA.* Sundbyberg: Landstingets hälsovård, Socialmedicin Kronan 1995;313.

Leander K. *Bortom kriminologin—En annan kunskap om kvinnor i fängelse [Beyond criminology: Another type of knowledge about women in prison].* Stockholm: Socialt Perspektiv 1993;4:23–28.

Leander K. *Kvinnomisshandel och våldtäkt i kriminalstatistiken [Woman battering and rape in criminal statistics].* In: Training materials for "Att möta våld mot kvinnor" [Confronting violence against women], Arlanda Hotel. Stockholm: Polishögskolan [Police Academy], October 12–13, 1992.

Leander K. *Misshandlade kvinnors möte med rättsapparaten [Battered women's encounters with the legal system].* In: Kvinnomisshandel [Battered women]. Stockholm: Delegationen för jämställdhetsforskning (JÄMFO) [Delegation for equality research], Report No. 14, 1989.

Lundgren E. *Våldets normaliseringsprocess. Två parter—två strategier [The normalization of violence: Two parties, two strategies].* In: Kvinnomisshandel [Battered women]. Stockholm: Delegationen för jämställdhetsforskning (JÄMFO) [Delegation for equality research], Report No. 14, 1989.

McCauley J, Yurk RA, Jenckes MW, Ford DE. *Inside "Pandora's Box." Abused Women's Experiences with Clinicians and Health Services.* J Gen Intern Med 1998;13:549–555.

Melinder K. *Registrering av våldsskador i landstingen [Registration of violent injuries by county councils].* Stockholm: Folkhälsoinstitutet [Swedish National Institute of Public Health], May 25, 1994.

North R, Rothenburg K. *Partner Notification and Domestic Violence.* New England J Medicine 1993;329:1194–6.

Okun L. *Woman Abuse: Facts replacing myths.* Albany: State University of New York Press, 1986.

Olsson M. *Sexualbrott. Sexuellt tvång och sexuellt ofredande mot vuxna [Sex crimes: Sexual coercion and sexual molestation against adults].* In: Ahlberg J (Ed.): Brottsutvecklingen 1992 och 1993 [Crime trends 1992 and 1993]. Stockholm: Brottsförebyggande rådet [Swedish National Council for Crime Prevention], BRÅ report 1994;3:34–73.

O'Toole LL. *Subcultural Theory of Rape Revisited.* In: O'Toole LL & Schiffman JR (Ed.): Gender Violence: Interdisciplinary Perspectives. New York and London: New York University Press, 1997.

Ottoson, Hindberg B. *Kvinnomisshandel [Woman battering].* Stockholm: Socialstyrelsen [Swedish National Board of Health and Welfare], Liber Förlag, 1984.

Pain RH. *Elderly women and fear of violent crime: The least likely victims?* A Reconsideration of the Extent and Nature of Risk. Brit J Criminol 1995;35:4.

Regeringskansliet. *Violence against Women.* Government Bill 1997/98:55. Fact Sheet from the Swedish Government Offices, February 1998.

Regeringskansliet. *Kvinnofrid [Women's Peace].* Stockholm: Arbetsmarknadsdepartementet, [Ministry of Labor], Regeringens proposition [Government Bill] 1997/98:55.

Risberg G. *Sexualiserat våld som hälsoproblem: Vårdgivarens motstånd att fråga försvårar rehabiliteringen för kvinnor [Sexualized violence as a health problem: Treatment providers' reluctance to ask questions makes women's rehabilitation more difficult].* Läkartidningen 1994a;50:4770–1.

Risberg G. *Varför går du inte? Fel fråga till offer: Sexualiserat våld i sociokulturellt perspektiv [Why don't you leave? The wrong question to ask the victim: Sexualized violence from a socio-cultural perspective].* Läkartidningen 1994b;50:4772.

ROKS [National Organization of Battered Women's Shelters in Sweden]. *ROKS Statistik 1997.* Stockholm: Riksorganisationen för kvinnojourer i Sverige (ROKS) 1998.

Russell D. *Sexual Exploitation.* Beverly Hills, CA: SAGE Publications, 1984.

Rying M. *Dödligt våld i Sverige: En deskriptiv studie. [Fatal violence in Sweden: A descriptive study].* Stockholm: Department of Criminology, Stockholm University. To be published 1999.

Schechter S. *Women and Male Violence: The Visions and Struggles of the Battered Women's Movement.* Boston: South End Press, 1992.

Skjørten K. *Voldsbilder i hverdagen: Om menns förståelse av kvinnemishandling [Violence in everyday life: Men's view of the abuse of women].* Oslo: Pax Forlag A/S, 1994.

Snare A. *The Crime of Rape and Criminal Policy.* In: Bishop N (Ed.): Scandinavian Criminal Policy and Criminology 1980–85. Stockholm: Scandinavian Research Council for Criminology (NSfK), 1985.

Somander L. *Dödsfall till följd av våldsbrott i Sverige 1976. Kvinnor i brottssituationen [Deaths resulting from violent crime in Sweden 1976: Women in crime situations]* (mimeo). Linköping: University of Linköping, 1979.

Sorenson SB, Saftlas AF. *Violence and Women's Health: The Role of Epidemiology.* Ann Epidemiol, March 1994;4:2:140–5.

SOU 1995:60. *Kvinnofrid: Slutbetänkande av Kvinnovåldskommissionen [Women's peace: Final report of the commission on violence against women].* Stockholm: Statens offentliga utredningar [Swedish Government Official Reports], Socialdepartementet, 1995.

Stanko E. *Everyday Violence: How Women and Men Experience Sexual and Physical Danger.* London, Sydney, Wellington: Pandora Press, 1990.

Stanko E. *Typical Violence, Normal Precaution: Men, Women and Interpersonal Violence in England, Wales, Scotland and the USA.* In: Hanmer J, Maynard M (Eds.): Women, Violence and Social Control. Houndmills etc.: MacMillan Press, Explorations in Sociology 23, 1987.

Stark E, Flitcraft A. *Killing the Beast Within: Woman Battering and Female Suicidality.* Intl J Health Services 1995;25;1:43–64.

Stark E, Flitcraft AH. *Spouse Abuse.* In: Rosenberg ML, Fenley MA (Eds.): Violence in America: A Public Health Approach. New York: Oxford University Press, 1991.

Statistics Canada. *Violence Against Women Survey: Survey Highlights.* Ottawa: Statistics Canada, 1993.

Statistics Sweden [Statistiska centralbyrån]. *Dödsorsaker [Causes of death].* Stockholm: Statistiska centralbyrån (SCB), relevant years up to and including 1993.

Statistics Sweden [Statistiska centralbyrån]. *Rättsstatistisk årsbok [Yearbook of Judicial Statistics].* Stockholm: Statistiska centralbyrån (SCB), relevant years.

Statistics Sweden [Statistiska centralbyrån]. *Offer för vålds—och egendomsbrott 1978–1993 [Victims of violent and property crime 1978–1993].* Stockholm: Statistiska centralbyrån (SCB), Levnadsförhållanden [Living conditions], Report 88, 1995b.

Swedish National Board of Health and Welfare [Socialstyrelsen]. *Dödsorsaker 1996 [Causes of death].* Stockholm: Socialstyrelsen (SOS), 1998.

Swedish National Board of Occupational Safety and Health [Arbetarskyddsstyrelsen]: *Våld och hot i arbetet: Statistik över anmälda arbetsskador, utsatthet och besvär. [Violence and threats at work. Statistics on reported work injuries, vulnerability and health complaints].* Stockholm: Arbetarskyddsstyrelsen, Rapport 1998:12.

Swedish National Council for Crime Prevention [Brottsförebyggande rådet]. *Våld mot kvinnor i nära relationer [Violence against women in intimate relationships].* Stockholm: BRÅ PM 1994:4.

Swedish National Council for Crime Prevention [Brottsförebyggande rådet]. *Kriminalstatistik [Criminal Statistics],* Stockholm: BRÅ Tables, 1997; BRÅ-rapport 1998:1.

Swedish National Institute of Public Health [Folkhälsoinstitutet]. *Kvinnojourskunskap—en översikt av kvinnojourernas kunskap om sexualiserat våld, speglad mot aktuell forskning [Information from women's shelters—an overview of what we have learned from women's shelters regarding sexualized violence, against the background of current research]* Stockholm: Folkhälsoinstitutet, 1994a:10.

Swedish National Institute of Public Health [Folkhälsoinstitutet]. *Svensk Skadeatlas. Baserad på dödsorsaks- och sjukvårdsregistren [Swedish Injury Atlas: Based on cause-of-death and health care registries].* Stockholm: Folkhälsoinstitutet, 1994b;28.

U.S. Department of Justice. *Violence against Women: Estimates from the Redesigned Survey.* Washington, D.C.: Bureau of Justice Statistics, Special Report. August 1995, NCJ-154348.

Warshaw C. *Limitations of the Medical Model in the Care of Battered Women.* In: Bart P & Geil Moran E (Eds.): Violence Against Women: The Bloody Footprints. London: SAGE Publications, 1993.

Wikström POH. *Våld: En kunskapsöversikt [Violence: A survey of what we know].* Stockholm: Brottsförebyggande rådet [Swedish National Council for Crime Prevention] (BRÅ), 1992.

7

Diseases of the musculoskeletal system and how they affect men and women

Eva Vingård, Åsa Kilbom

Introduction

THE MUSCULOSKELETAL SYSTEM IS made up of bones, muscles, tendons and ligaments, and accounts for approximately 50 percent of a person's body weight. Common musculoskeletal complaints include problems of the low back, like lumbago and sciatica; the neck and shoulders, like tendonitis and muscular pain; and the joints, like rheumatic diseases and arthrosis.

According to the Survey of Living Conditions (Statistics Sweden 94/95) the prevalence of musculoskeletal illnesses is higher among women than among men, in blue-collar as well as white-collar groups. Female blue-collar workers have the highest rate of all groups. The prevalence has increased somewhat over a five-year period, especially among lower-level white-collar workers (Statistics Sweden 1996).

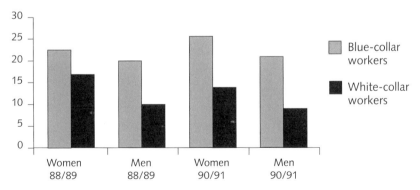

Source: Statistics Sweden's Surveys of Living Conditions (ULF 94/95)

Figure 7.1 Percentage of women and men aged 16–84 with illnesses of the musculoskeletal system, 1988–90 and 1993–95.

These figures refer to long-term illnesses of the musculoskeletal system. Rates are higher when respondents are asked whether they experienced a mus-

159

culoskeletal ailment at any time during the past year. A study in the Norrtälje region in Sweden is looking at potential risk and protective factors for ailments of the lower back and neck/shoulder area, and has found the incidence of such health problems to be remarkably high among people aged 20–59 who had not sought medical treatment for related complaints during the previous six months (Figure 7.2).

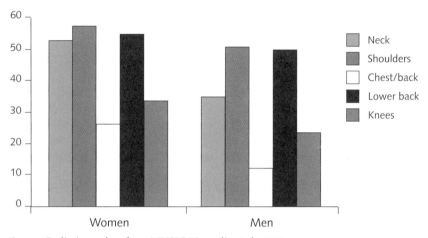

Source: Preliminary data from MUSIC-Norrtälje study 1995.

Figure 7.2. Percentage of self-reported health problems of the musculoskeletal system among a population aged 20–59 who had not sought related medical treatment in the previous six months.

All persons included in the study also undergo a clinical examination, which yields a substantially lower rate of illness as determined by an objective observer. When "healthy" individuals were examined, 14 percent of the women and 11 percent of the men were found to have low back trouble.

Illnesses of the musculoskeletal system seldom require hospitalization and do not directly cause death. However, they are the second leading cause of work absences and the leading cause of long-term work disability and early retirement in Sweden. No Swedish statistics are kept on the medical reasons accounting for missed work days. A study of 134,000 cases of illness conducted in 1983 and a similar study in 1990 showed that trends remained the same, with work absences and the length of illness distributed as shown in Table 7.1. Women are much more likely than men to miss work because of illnesses of the musculoskeletal system as well as to remain ill for longer periods with certain ailments, such as a slipped disc.

Table 7.1. Number of days absent from work and duration of certain health problems among all men and women in Sweden in 1990.

Primary diagnosis	ICD code	Women		Men	
		# of days in thousands	Average duration (in days) per year	# of days in thousands	Average duration (in days) per year
Arthrosis	715	1 448	254	1 399	171
Slipped disc	722	525	254	619	121
Neck/shoulders	723	4 087	40	1 860	25
Lower back	724	10 420	32	9 321	21
Rheumatism of soft tissues	726	4 780	54	3 477	41
Other illnesses of the soft tissues	729	8 016	48	3 444	26
Total of all musculo- skeletal diagnoses		35 164	43	24 189	29

Source: Swedish National Social Insurance Board (RFV). Diagnoses leading to work absences and ultimate causes, 1990.

A long-term work disability dramatically increases the risk of early retirement (see Table 7.2).

Table 7.2. New cases of early retirement approved in Sweden in 1998, resulting from certain groups of diseases and expressed as no. of cases and percentage (%) of the total number of retirements. A few selected subgroups of diseases are also presented (in italics).

	Women n %	Men n %
Psychiatric diseases	4116 (22)	4022 (25)
Cardiovascular diseases	996 (5)	2015 (13)
Pulmonary diseases	487 (3)	472 (3)
Illnesses of the musculoskeletal system	7976 (43)	4860 (30)
Rheumatoid arthritis	*397 (2)*	*161 (1)*
Arthrosis	*973 (5)*	*733 (5)*
Unspecified low-back disease	*1993 (11)*	*1587 (10)*
Tendinitis and related disease	*1804 (10)*	*340 (2)*
Accidents and poisoning	945 (5)	985 (6)
Other disease	4054 (22)	3555 (22)
Total	18 578 (100)	15 909 (100)

Source: Swedish National Social Insurance Board. Statistical information Is-1 1999:3.

Until July 1, 1993, when changes were made in the law on work-related injuries, health problems related to the musculoskeletal system were by far the most common reason for work-injury reports (Table 7.3a), and women are generally more affected by such health problems than men. The dramatic increase shown between 1992 and 1993 reflects the anticipated change in the law, since there was a rush to submit reports before the new provisions, which were much less generous. Thus the discrepancy between the figures for 1992 and 1993 is not indicative of a deterioration of the job environment during that period.

Table 7.3a. Officially reported work-related illnesses in Sweden between 1991 and 1997, expressed as number of reports per 1000 gainfully employed persons.

	Women:		*Men:*	
	Total	Due to illnesses of the musculoskeletal system	Total	Due to illnesses of the musculoskeletal system
1991	8.6	7.3	9.3	6.0
1992	7.1	6.3	8.3	5.5
1993	16.8	14.8	16.0	11.0
1994	4.4	3.4	4.0	2.6
1995	3.9	2.9	3.2	2.0
1996	3.4	2.5	2.8	1.7
1997	3.5	2.5	2.8	1.6

Source: National Board of Occupational Health and Safety, Sweden (ASS/ISA) and Statistics Sweden (SCB/AKU).

Table 7.3b. Officially reported work-related accidents in Sweden between 1991 and 1997, expressed as number of reports per 1000 gainfully employed persons.

	Women		Men	
	Total	Due to illnesses of part of the musculoskeletal system	Total	Due to illnesses of the musculoskeletal system
1991	9.2	2.8	22.5	4.0
1992	7.5	2.4	15.4	2.6
1993	6.6	2.1	13.1	2.1
1994	6.6	1.9	12.1	1.7
1995	6.1	1.7	10.7	1.4
1996	6.4	1.6	10.4	1.3
1997	6.6	1.7	9.7	1.2

Source: National Board of Occupational Health and Safety, Sweden (ASS/ISA) and Statistics Sweden (SCB/AKU).

To sum up, we note that women experience more health problems of the musculoskeletal system and report more related illnesses than men do. They take more sick days off from work, are more likely to retire early and submit more reports of work injuries. The situation in other countries is not entirely clear, nor is it clear how things have changed over time. In many countries today, as well as in Sweden in the past, other, more life-threatening problems have overshadowed these concerns. Access to medical care, the likelihood of a cure and the insurance system are also crucial factors influencing people's reporting of these kinds of health problems.

What accounts for the gender gap?

Biological factors

There are no clearly documented hereditary differences between men and women. Some unusual illnesses are passed on through the maternal or paternal line in certain families. These cases are so rare, however, that they are outside the scope of this anthology. Naturally, everything in existence has some linkage to hereditary factors. How well we do with what we are given, however, depends largely on the external influences with which we come in contact. By affecting these influences, we can damage, modify or improve the health of a group or an individual.

Muscles

As a rule, women are smaller and physically weaker than men because they have less muscle mass (Åstrand 1990). Various studies show a gender differential of between 20 and 50 percent. A study has found that women have 52 percent of a typical man's strength in the upper extremities and 66 percent in the lower extremities (Miller et al. 1993). However, muscular strength is affected not only by gender, but also by age, decreasing by some 25 percent between the ages of 25 and 65 (Åstrand 1990). At the same time, it should be kept in mind that these are statistics drawn from large groups and there is a wide range of individual differences. A well-trained younger woman may be stronger than a poorly-trained older man, while there may be an extremely large difference between the strength of a younger, well-trained man and a poorly-trained older woman.

Muscle fibers are divided into two main groups: slow (type I) and fast (type II). Slow muscle fibers are those that initiate a muscle contraction and are used during moderate activity. Fast muscle fibers are used during a vigorous activity of short duration. There are gender differences in the fibers found in the trapezius muscle (Lindman et al. 1990, 1991), with women having fewer slow and more fast fibers. It is difficult to assess how significant this is for the fact that ailments in the neck-shoulder region are disproportionately found among women.

The importance of differences in body dimensions and strength is well illus-trated by the following example (Mörck 1977). Cylinders containing gas, used for example in hospitals, are filled in factories by male workers who close the valve, a knob sized to fit a man's hand, with a clockwise twist of the wrist. In the hospital, a female nurse or assistant is usually the one to open the cylinder by twisting the valve counterclockwise. It is well known that a person's grip is significantly weaker when twisting in a counterclockwise than a clockwise direction. Furthermore, the knob is too large for the average woman's hand, so she has to extend her fingers to grip it, which again requires much more effort than gripping a knob made to fit her hand.

Edgren has proposed another explanation for gender differences in physical stress and patterns of health trouble (Edgren 1979). He takes as his point of depar-ture the positive and accelerating relationship between physical stress and per-ceived effort (Figure 7.3).

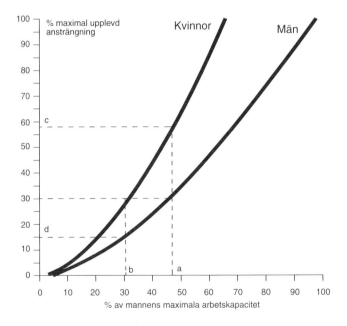

Figure 7.3 Model explaining gender differences in physical stress, perceived effort and health problems, adapted from Edgren (1979)

If we consider a "moderate" level of perceived effort on the job to be 30 per-cent, at that level the average man will achieve about 47 percent of his maximum performance (a in Figure 7.3). For the average woman, however, that same level of perceived effort would yield only about 30 percent of a man's maximum work capacity (b in the figure). In order for a woman to perform at the same level as a man, she would have to double her perceived effort, to about 60 percent (c in the figure). If those responsible for job requirements (production engineers, for example) are aware of gender differences in muscle strength and body size, one might expect them to be willing to adjust the job accordingly. For women to experience the same degree of effort as men, the stress level would have to be reduced to about 30 percent (b in the figure), which would reduce men's effort to a very low level—about 15 percent (d in the figure). A reduction in external stress by one-third corresponds to a 50-percent decline in perceived effort. A male production engineer would undoubtedly view this level as unrealistically low and likely to lead to monotony and understimulation.

Bones

Bone mass continues to increase up to the age of 25–30. During this period the increase in bone mass exceeds the breakdown of bone substance. A reversal occurs at about the age of thirty, when the body is no longer able to build bone mass as quickly as it is broken down. The bones become increasingly osteoporotic, and a fall, for instance, may result in a fracture. After reaching the age of fifty, one in three women and one in nine men are at risk of experiencing, at some time in their remaining years, a fracture related to osteoporosis. The female sex hormone estrogen also affects the development of bone mass. After menopause, a dramatic decline in estrogen production is accompanied by an equally dramatic decline in bone mass, and women have a higher risk of developing osteoporosis and experiencing complications such as aches and fractures (Gärdsell 1990 and Johnell 1995). Also of significance in maintaining bone mineral content are lifestyle factors such as physical activity, smoking and diet.

Living habits

Physical activity, smoking, diet and osteoporosis

Physical activity at a young age helps to build up bone mass. When the inevitable breakdown of bone substance begins to occur, those with stronger bones start out at an advantage. Moreover, the breakdown process can be slowed somewhat when people are physically active. Physical activity also has a positive effect on a person's sense of balance, flexibility and coordination, thus helping to prevent falls and their consequences. (Johnell 1995 and Gärdsell 1990).

Many studies have shown smoking to be a risk factor for osteoporosis. The bone density of women who smoke as adults is 5–10 percent lower than that of nonsmokers. Former smokers appear to be somewhere in between smokers and nonsmokers in terms of bone-mineral loss (Johnell 1995 and Nguyen et al. 1994). Young women who smoke do not achieve the same level of bone mass as female nonsmokers.

Vitamin D and calcium are important components in building bone mass. Swedes tend to have a high intake of calcium, since most of them consume large quantities of dairy products.

Physical exercise and health problems of the musculoskeletal system

Scientific studies have not been able to prove conclusively that physical exercise prevents musculoskeletal illnesses. However, it is certainly not harmful to have a flexible, well-functioning musculoskeletal system. People who are in good physical condition are more likely to recover quickly from illness. This holds true for athletes, and no doubt for others as well. A cross-sectional study of the exercise habits of the Swedish population, LIV 90 (Lifestyle-Performance-Health 1993), showed that women were somewhat less likely than men to engage in regular and frequent sports or other physical exercise, although the gender gap was not particularly large (Figure 7.4). The most prominent difference was that significantly more younger men were involved in comprehensive, intensive physical exercise, while younger women engaged in activities requiring a relatively low level of physical effort. Among middle-aged individuals, there was an equal share of men and women with high levels of activity, while the group of sedentary men was significantly larger than that of sedentary women.

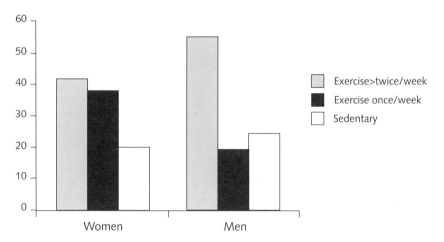

Figure 7.4 Exercise habits among persons aged 20–24.

Significance of the work environment

A Scandinavian study calculated that some 30 percent of illnesses of the musculoskeletal system were work-related, i.e., the work environment was seen as a contributing factor in triggering or exacerbating ailments of the muscles, joints

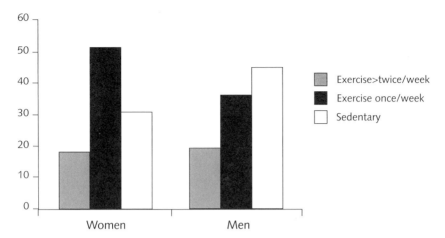

Figure 7.5 Exercise habits among persons aged 50–54.

or bones (Hansen 1993). Thus any gender differences in working conditions may be quite significant for differences in illness and other health problems. Accordingly, it is of interest to examine the distribution of men and women in various occupational groups and industries, as well as the stresses to which they are exposed.

Working conditions that may increase the risk of musculoskeletal illnesses include physical strains, in particular static working positions, repetitive movements and heavy manual labor, as well as psychosocial conditions, i.e., high performance requirements combined with a low level of influence, unclear roles and a lack of support from the work environment (Bongers et al. 1993). The quantitative significance of individual risk factors is not entirely clear, but it appears likely that physical stresses are most important early on, while psychosocial conditions are more liable to have a long-term effect on health problems and how people experience them, particularly as illnesses become chronic.

We see in Table 7.4 that women predominate in health care, administrative, office and service occupations. For most workers, health-care and service jobs involve regular heavy lifting and carrying as well as frequent conflict situations stemming from a high level of contact with patients and customers. Administrative jobs and office work often involve considerable static stress and repetitiveness. None of the typical "women's" occupations are physically demanding in the traditional sense, i.e., they do not require the exertion of a great deal of energy. However, relative to women's lower physical work capacity, particularly with advancing age, the physical demands of health-care, cleaning and restaurant jobs in particular are high.

Table 7.4. Averaged percentages of employed women and men in the population in various occupational branches in 1998. Total of 1 900 800 women and 2 078 600 men.

Branch of activity (SNI)	Women	Men
• Agriculture, hunting, forestry, and fishing	1.4	3.7
• Manufacturing, mining and quarrying, electricity, gas and water works	11.1	28.5
• Construction industry	1.0	9.7
• Wholesale and rental trade, transport, storage and communication companies	15.5	23.1
• Financial institutions and insurance companies, real estate, renting and business service companies	10.3	13.0
• Institutes for research and development, educational organizations	11.1	5.3
• Health and social work organizations	35.1	5.0
• Hotels and restaurants, recreational, cultural and sporting facilities, membership organizations, sewage and refuse disposal plants, sanitation facilities	9.1	6.6
• Public authorities and national defense, extra-territorial organizations and bodies	5.4	5.1

Source: Statistics Sweden labour force Survey 1998 (AKU).

It is noteworthy that older women make up a large proportion of women in service jobs. Many of the occupations within this group require a relatively low level of formal schooling, but place substantial physical demands on the employee. Similar findings have also been reported by Lannerheim, who followed a group of older women for a period of ten years (Lannerheim 1993). She showed that during that ten-year period, older women tended to gravitate toward occupations that required little training but a relatively high level of physical effort. At the same time, there was a decline in the percentage of women in occupations requiring advanced training. The Stockholm "MUSIC" study carried out some detailed measurements and interviews with a sample of employed people from Stockholm. Women and men were divided into older and younger groups, and the older men were consistently found to have a substantially lower level of physical stress in their jobs than younger men. In contrast, the physical stress on older women was only marginally lower than that experienced by younger women (Table 7.5).

Table 7.5. Various measurements of physical stress on younger and older women and men during a day's work, from the Stockholm "MUSIC" study (Kilbom et al. 1995).

	Women:		*Men:*	
	<40 years	>40 years	<40 years	>40 years
Number of steps per day	2,600	2,400	4,600	2,900
Lifting, times per day	164	136	154	39
Pushing/pulling, times per day	105	87	218	56
Percentage of the day spent with back bent >18°	35	30	29	20

These results probably reflect the fact that large numbers of women with little education were recruited into the labor market in the 1970s and 1980s. Unlike other groups, they were not targeted for further-training measures, so they remained stuck in low-level jobs with inferior working conditions. The combination of aging and years of performing low-level, hard work is probably one reason why older women have a high incidence of illness and early retirement due to illnesses of the musculoskeletal system.

Women, then, generally work in different occupations and follow a different career path than men. Yet even at the same workplace or within the same occupational group there are gender differences in working conditions that may explain why women often have more ailments of the musculoskeletal system than men. A Canadian study looked at male and female workers in poultry processing plants (Mergler et al. 1987). Comparing a sample of 580 male and female workers, the study found that women had a higher prevalence of complaints related to the musculoskeletal system. Where women and men were carrying out the same job responsibilities, however, these gender differences largely disappeared.

A study of female and male workers in the automobile industry looked at health problems of the forearm and hand, and asked participants to fill out questionnaires about their physical stress at work (Fransson-Hall et al. 1996). The female workers showed a higher prevalence of both perceived health problems and clinically diagnosed illness than the men did, and they also exhibited a different physical "exposure profile" (Table 7.6).

Table 7.6. Stress patterns of female and male automobile assembly workers (n=521).

	Women, %	Men, %
Repetitive finger work > 4 hrs per day	54	42
Repetitive hand movements > 4 hrs per day	68	54
Lifting of objects 1–5 kg > 4 hrs per day	48	40
Lifting of objects 6–15 kg > 4 hrs per day	34	16
Dorsal flexion of wrist	45	29
Palmar flexion of wrist	45	28

Gender differences were insignificant for reported use of muscle- or motor-driven tools. Both of these studies showed that despite the same job description and the same workplace, there may be hidden differences in physical stress patterns and work tasks between men and women.

So far, we have discussed gender differences in how jobs are distributed and in related physical requirements of the workplace. There are also important gender differences when it comes to psychosocial conditions on the job. As part of the work-environment statistics compiled by Statistics Sweden, questionnaires on working conditions are filled out every other year by ten to fifteen thousand Swedish workers. These interviews provide data on the perceived difficulty of people's jobs, the support they receive from their colleagues and superiors, the educational and training requirements for the job, and the opportunities workers have to determine how they do their jobs.

Results indicate that women have less opportunity to determine their own work pace and receive less help and support from their superiors and colleagues. Women are more likely to report that their work is stressful and that they are not involved in determining how it is structured. However, there are substantial differences depending on the type of work. It is particularly striking that far more women in manufacturing, transportation and communications jobs (some 60 percent, compared with 30–40 percent of comparable men) are given little opportunity to influence the structure of their jobs. It has always been assumed that unfavorable social conditions on the job have the same effect for women as for men in the development of illnesses of the musculoskeletal system, but the evidence is inconclusive. It is also possible that women's social networks outside the workplace play an important role with respect to work-related musculoskeletal ailments (see below). All of this would appear to indicate that large numbers of women experience worse physical and psychosocial conditions at work than men do.

How are the conditions described above reflected in society's laws and regulations? Women are not generally allowed to train as rescue workers for the fire department. It also used to be prohibited for women to work in the mines. Both of these jobs are exceedingly demanding physically, and require that the worker be in extremely good condition. So why are women permitted to perform hard physical labor in health-care and cleaning jobs? We have been willing for years to accept the risk that those kinds of jobs may result in injury to the worker or a third party. However, the risks associated with certain other kinds of hard physical labor have not been "sanctioned" by society to the same degree. This attitude of society is also reflected in recent legislative changes to make work-injury provisions more stringent. This does not benefit women.

Women's double role

Women continue to bear the main responsibility for household and children. The time-use studies conducted by Statistics Sweden show that women employed outside the home spend many more hours than men on housework. Although housework can usually be done at one's own pace and involves a greater variety of physical tasks than manual-labor jobs, it still commonly requires awkward physical positions and strenuous manual labor. Little study has been devoted to women's two-fold role as it relates to illnesses of the musculoskeletal system. A study carried out by the ABB company showed that women run a higher risk of shoulder and neck ailments, and that the risk increases further when they are caring for others in their household (small children, a sick husband) (Kvarnström 1983). Such activities as knitting and crocheting are also suspected of increasing women's overall stress and the risk of health problems, since they put strain on the same parts of the body as many industrial assembly jobs. A study of women working in the electronics industry provided some support for this hypothesis (Kilbom et al. 1986). A small amount of excess risk was confirmed, but only among individuals who engaged in needlework at least three times a week over a long period.

Women's double burden may also affect assessments of the association between musculoskeletal complaints and stresses at work that has been found in epidemiological studies. The above-mentioned study of automobile-industry workers showed a weaker link between job stress and the extent and severity of such health problems for female assembly workers than for comparable men (Hall 1995). One explanation may be that the women in the study group who were exposed to a low level of stress on the job encountered a relatively high level of stress in their households. Further study should be given to the interaction between work at home and on the job in the development of musculoskeletal illnesses.

The double role played by women may also mean that they are less committed to professional careers, and so they continue to work for years in low-level, physically demanding jobs (see above remarks on older women in service jobs). This two-fold role also means that women have less time for rest and recreation, which are believed to offer protection against musculoskeletal problems.

It has been suggested in recent years that social networks may play a different role for women than for men. In the case of cardiovascular disease, a social network has been shown to be a burden rather than an advantage for women. This is probably linked to the fact that women play a supportive, helping role among their friends and relatives, while men are more likely to be recipients of others' help and support. We do not know to what extent this applies to musculoskeletal illnesses as well, but a connection may well exist.

How women and men respond to ailments of the musculoskeletal system

A number of observations have indicated that there are differences between women and men in how they experience discomfort and pain of the musculoskeletal system. A series of studies have pointed out that women have a lower threshold for pain than men (Hall 1995). When pressure is slowly applied to the skin, the first perception is one of being touched. An increase in pressure will gradually change that perception to a feeling of pain, with the lowest level at which pain is experienced commonly referred to as the pressure pain threshold. It remains unclear to what extent gender differences in the pain threshold are biological or acquired. Women do not have more pain receptors than men per surface unit, but it is possible that gender differences in the functioning of the nervous system are present even at birth. However, pain thresholds are also influenced to some extent by the sex of the investigator, i.e., a male subject tends to receive higher threshold scores, meaning he shows less sensitivity to pain, if the investigator is female. These findings support the hypothesis that the pressure pain threshold is affected by the expectations that go along with reporting symptoms, and that gender differences are at least to some degree acquired. It is not certain to what extent these conditions also apply to pain experienced not on the skin but elsewhere in the body, or to non-laboratory conditions.

There are also differences between women and men with respect to aspects of perception other than pain. A study of 200 randomly selected individuals from Stockholm examined how people perceive their level of physical exertion during a working day and related these perceptions to their heart rate (Wigaeus Hjelm 1993). Findings showed consistently that there was a close association between these two variables for men, but only a weak link for women. One explanation might be that women's physical effort occurs in different circumstances than men's. Uncomfortable work positions and repetitive stresses are common among women but less frequent among men, and their effect on an individual's heart rate is insignificant. Men, in contrast, more frequently perform tasks that require a great deal of energy and have a substantial effect on their heart rate. One might also note that the study's design was based on years of experience of the stresses men encounter at work. Much less is known of the work women do and their responses to it. In this particular study, it may also be that wording the questions differently would have resulted in equally accurate estimates by both women and men. Furthermore, it is possible that women are influenced by their experiences at home and at leisure when they assess their fatigue, exertion and pain. Overall, they experience a higher level of physical load.

Most studies show that women have a higher incidence of musculoskeletal complaints and problems of the neck/shoulder area and the hand/forearm. While different studies produce somewhat contradictory findings on low back trouble, they frequently indicate a higher rate of such trouble among men. This holds true for subjective symptoms, clinical findings and diagnoses. Given the gender differences in types of job stress—strain on the upper extremities and neck is more common among women, while men are more likely to put stress on the low back—it is not surprising to find such differences in the types of illnesses affecting men and women. It is unclear how relevant the above-mentioned gender differences in pressure pain thresholds and subjective assessments are for clinical findings of illness. Those results were based on short-term studies of healthy individuals, which are quite different from a clinical setting.

We have already pointed out that women tend to have more long-term illnesses of the musculoskeletal system than men do. Women miss work for health reasons more than men do. This may be related to women's social situations and their responsibilities for caring for those around them.

Women appear to respond differently from men when health problems arise. While men frequently seek help from paramedical specialists, women are more likely to consult traditional health-care providers (Table 7.7).

Table 7.7. Percentage of individuals in the Norrtälje region seeking treatment from various specialists for lower-back or neck ailments.

Care provider	Neck pain		Low back pain	
	Women (n=174)	Men (n=71)	Women (N=364)	Men (n=305)
Physician, physical therapist	72%	44%	68%	45%
Chiropractor	9%	11%	13%	23%
Naprapath	14%	34%	14%	26%
Other	5%	11%	5%	6%

The reasons for this are unclear. Physicians, unlike osteopaths and chiropractors, have the authority to excuse an employee from work because of illness. Perhaps these gender differences are related to the difference in length of illness for men and women.

Conclusion

In conclusion, we note that women's physical constitution differs from that of men—they typically have 40–60 percent of the average man's muscular strength. At a level of 30 percent exertion, men utilize about 45 percent of their physical capacity, while the same perceived effort by a woman results in a performance equal to 30 percent of a man's typical physical capacity.

Women's and men's working lives also differ, with women staying in relatively monotonous jobs that involve substantial physical work. In terms of physical stress, women's career development tends to be negative. In addition, women are generally subject to greater physical demands in the household, and they are more likely to bear sole responsibility for household and family than men are. As for social support, which can be a modifying factor in the development of illness, women more frequently give support, while men receive it. Thus women have less time left for their own relaxation and recreation.

All of this doubtless contributes to the fact that women are absent from work for longer periods, experience longer episodes of illness, more frequently take early retirement and report more work injuries than men because of illnesses of the musculoskeletal system.

References

Åstrand I. *Arbetsfysiologi [Physiology of effort]*. Norstedts förlag, Stockholm 1990.

Bongers PM, de Winter CR, Kompier MAJ, Hildebrandt VH. *Psychosocial factors at work and musculoskeletal disease*. Scand J Work Environ & Health 1993;19:297–312.

Edgren B. *Forskning om sjukfrånvaro, medicinska och sociala faktorer [Research on work absences, medical and social factors]*. In: Cedermark M, Peterson G (Eds.): Kvinnans prestationsförmåga—psykiska, sociala och fysiologiska aspekter [Women's performance—psychological, social and physiological aspects]. FOA report, Stockholm: 1979;pp.49–54.

Fransson-Hall C, Byström S, Kilbom Å. *Characteristics of Forearm-Hand Exposure in Relation to Symptoms among Automobile Assembly Line Workers*. Am J Indust Med 1996;29:15–22.

Gärdsell P. *Osteoporosis prediction of fragility fractures*. Doctoral thesis, Lund University, 1990.

Hall C. *Hand function with special regard to work with tools*. Doctoral thesis, Karolinska Institutet, Arbete och Hälsa 1995:4.

Hansen S. *Arbejdsmiljø og samfundsøkonomi [Work environment and national economy]*. Nordiska Ministerrådet, 1993.

Johansson C (Ed.). *"Belasta Dig frisk" [Healthy through physical activity]*. Report from Arbetsmiljöfonden och Folksam, Stockholm 1992.

Johnell O. *Prevention of fractures in the elderly—A review*. Acta Orthop Scand 1995;66(1):90–98.

Kilbom Å, Persson J, Jonsson BG. *Disorders of the cervicobrachial region among female workers in the electronics industry*. Int. J. Ind. Ergonomics 1986;1:37–47.

Kilbom Å, Winkel J, Karlqvist L. *Is physical load at work reduced with increasing age? A pilot study*. In: Kuorinka I (Ed.): Proceedings of PREMUS II, Montreal 1995.

Kvarnström S. *Occurrence of musculoskeletal disorders in a manufacturing industry, with special attention to occupational shoulder disorders.* Doctoral thesis, Uppsala University 1983.

Lannerheim L. *Vinnare och förlorare.* En studie av medelålders och äldre kvinnors arbetsmiljö [*Winners and losers.* A study of middle-aged and older women's work environments]. Report No. 3, Gerontologiskt Centrum, Lund 1993.

Lindman R, Eriksson A, Thorell LE. *Fiber type composition of the human male trapezius muscle.* Am J Anat 1990;189:236–244.

Lindman R, Eriksson A, Thorell LE. *Fiber type composition of the human female trapezius muscle.* Am J Anat 1991;190:385–391.

Livsstil-Prestation-Hälsa [Lifestyle-Performance-Health]. Liv 90 Report 1. Folksam et al., Stockholm 1993.

Mergler D, Brabant C, Vézina N, Messing K. *The weaker sex?* Men in women's working conditions report similar health symptoms. J Occup Med 1987;29:417–421.

Miller AE, MacDougall JD, Tarnopolsky MA. *Sale DG Gender differences in strength and muscle fiber characteristics.* Eur J Appl Physiol 1993;66(3)254–62.

Mörck E. *Internrapport AGA* 1977.

Nguyen TV, Kelly PJ, Sambrock PN, Gilbert C, Pocock NA, Eisman JA. *Lifestyle factors and bone density in the elderly: Implications for osteoporosis prevention.* J Bone Miner Res 1994;9:1339–46.

Statistics Sweden [Statistiska Centralbyrån]. *Ohälsa och sjukvård 1980–1989 [Ill health and medical care 1980–1989].* Levnadsförhållanden [Life circumstances], Report No. 76, Stockholm 1992.

Wigaeus Hjelm E, Karlqvist L, Nygård CH, Selin K, Wiktorin C, Winkel J and Stockholm MUSIC 1 Study Group. *Validitet av enkätfrågor om upplevd fysisk ansträngning och fysisk aktivitet i Stockholmsundersökningen 1 [Validity of responses to self-enumerated questionnaires regarding perceived physical effort and physical activity in Stockholm study No. 1].* In: Hagberg M, Hogsted (Eds.): Stockholmsundersökningen 1, pp. 95–107. MUSIC Books, Stockholm 1993.

8

Work and cardiovascular disease among men and women

Töres Theorell

ALTHOUGH MEN STILL SPEND more time at paid employment than women do, women are more likely to experience conflicts between their work and their family lives. In addition, men's and women's working conditions are very different. Accordingly, it is important to determine just how working conditions affect the risk of cardiovascular disease for men and women. Since there are gender differences in the biological factors influencing the development of cardiovascular disease, it is difficult to draw conclusions about causal relationships. However, illuminating research is being carried out on work environments and the incidence of cardiovascular disease among men and women, and below we review some of the findings.

Historical developments: Survival and cardiovascular disease

Cardiovascular disease is a very significant cause of suffering and death for both men and women, and of major importance for life expectancy in the industrialized world today. Twentieth-century trends for longevity in the industrialized countries (21 countries in Northern, Western, Central and Southern Europe, North America, Australia, New Zealand and Japan; see Statistical Yearbook, Statistics Sweden 1995) have been less similar for men and women than might be expected. Figures 8.1 and 8.2 show life expectancy at birth for men and women at the turn of the century (Figure 8.1, 1900) and at the beginning of the 1990s (Figure 8.2, 1990) in these countries. Figure 8.1 shows a clear gender gap in life expectancy even at the beginning of this century (the average female advantage was 2.8 years, and certainly significant), while Figure 8.2 shows that the gap has grown over the course of the century. Life expectancy for both men and women has risen substantially in the industrialized countries, but the gap between men and women has grown to 6.4 years. The distributions are much narrower (with little variation across countries), and the distributions for men and women are almost entirely distinct. The reasons for this are unclear. Some conceivable explanations are the following:

a) Material conditions in general have improved considerably both for men and women in all of these 21 countries during the twentieth century, and the biological limits of life expectancy now seem clearer than at any time in human history;

177

b) Childbearing declined during this period. Particularly at the beginning of the century, childbearing was associated with substantial risks, and many women died of infections and other complications of pregnancy and delivery.

One might speculate that women's biological potential is to live longer than men. Perhaps they have evolved more tenacity relative to men to handle the risks of childbearing, and this has become more evident as other mortality risks have declined in highly civilized societies.

This tenacity-based explanation is consistent with the general observation in the epidemiology literature on men's and women's health in recent years showing that men die younger than women, but women experience more illness than men. A "male" interpretation might be that men are stoic, while women complain about insignificant aches and pains. An alternative interpretation, however, is that despite living under less favorable conditions and experiencing more symptoms than men, women still manage to live longer than men because they have a superior potential for survival. In certain respects, such as psychosocial working conditions of relevance to cardiovascular disease, women appear to be subject to worse conditions than men. These two interpretations have dramatically different implications for society's attitudes toward men and women, with the first dismissing women's complaints about their circumstances as "whining" and the second taking their complaints seriously.

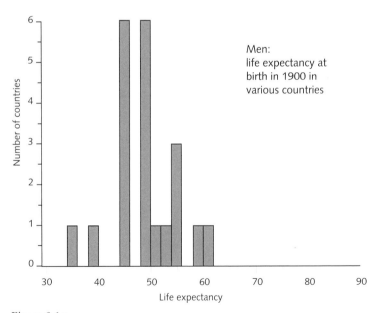

Figure 8.1a

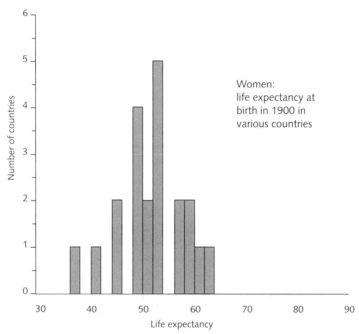

Figure 8.1b

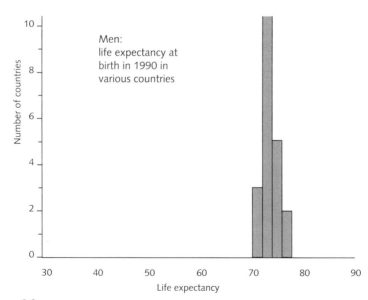

Figure 8.2a

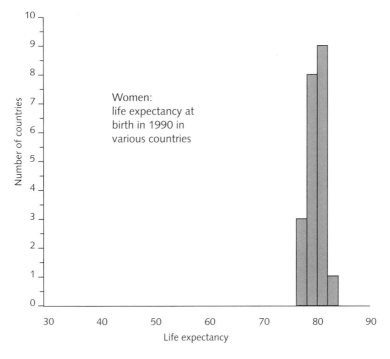

Figure 8.2b

Cardiovascular disease

Cardiovascular disease is a case in which it is possible to isolate underlying mechanisms. In the countries that have been industrialized for a long time cardiovascular disease is behind most of the differences in longevity. Since Sweden was one of the first countries to establish a social welfare state, it is particularly interesting to examine Swedish trends in cardiovascular disease. Both men and women in Sweden have long enjoyed good material living conditions, so we might expect the trends in cardiovascular disease that have been observed during this century in all industrialized countries to be particularly evident among Swedes. The underlying assumption is that it is mainly populations that survive up to middle and older age (and do not die because of infections and malnutrition) that "have the benefit of dying from cardiovascular disease." It has often been asserted that women's entry into the labor market would create a dual burden leading to an increased risk of cardiovascular disease, particularly for women in those age groups most likely to work outside the home. However, it is not clear that this has been the case.

Male and female trends in cardiovascular disease may be difficult to compare. As has been pointed out by McKinlay (1996) the incidence of myocardial infarction and other manifestations of coronary heart disease may have been underestimated in women simply because coronary heart disease before retirement has been regarded as a male phenomenon. There is, however, agreement that coronary heart disease is less common in women than in men (Wenger et al 1993) and that this difference is most likely partly biologically explained. Sex hormones such as oestrogen have been assumed to play a role. The difference is, however, also partly socially constructed (Wenger et al 1993).

In the industrialized world the incidence of myocardial infarction has been declining since the 1970s. It has been pointed out both in the US (Rosamond et al 1998) and in Sweden (Hammar 1997) that despite the persisting gender difference in coronary heart disease the decline in myocardial infarction risk is slower in women than in men. For instance between 1980 and 1995 the annual decrease in incidence was 1.8% in women and 2.2% in men in Sweden (Epidemiologiskt centrum, Stockholm 1997). For the same reason that McKinlay has addressed (see above), that the true incidence of myocardial infarction in women may have been underestimated, however, the small difference in myocardial infarction incidence between men and women may be a spurious phenomenon. With increasing awareness in the medical community regarding the possible underestimation of female coronary heart disease prevalence more female cases may be discovered.

The fact that even in recent years women have continued to have a lower risk of coronary infarction than men would appear to support the hypothesis that sex-linked genetic mechanisms are a major factor. Or could it be that the overall stress level for men and women has actually remained about the same? Or have women, throughout the twentieth century, managed to find ways of dealing with life's difficulties that are more favorable to their survival than men's strategies are to theirs?

If we apply to the question of cardiovascular disease among men and women the general model developed by Levi and Kagan for describing the interactions among stressors, heredity and experience in generating responses to environmental conditions (see Figure 8.3, modified by the author), we can use the same basic concepts used in psychosocial cardiovascular research. At the left are environmental conditions that can produce favorable or unfavorable responses that are relevant to cardiovascular disease. These interact with the individual's coping strategies. Coping behavior, in turn, is determined by two main factors: genetics and experience. Here we are referring to all kinds of experience throughout one's life, which means that coping patterns are constantly changing. Below we examine in more detail environmental factors, coping patterns and response patterns from a gender perspective, with particular attention to those that are relevant to cardiovascular disease.

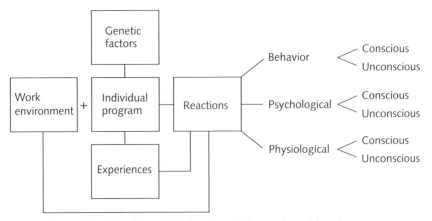

Source: Kagan, A. R. & Levi, L. 1971. Adaptation of the psychosocial environment to man's abilities and needs. In *Society, stress and disease. The psychosocial environment and psychosomatic diseases,* L. Levi (ed.). London: Oxford University Press.

Figure 8.3 Theoretical model of interactions among environment, individual and responses.

Environmental factors

The first question is whether men's and women's environments differ in some way that affects their risk of cardiovascular disease. Both physical and psychosocial factors in the environment can play a role in that risk. Men are exposed to more physical risks on the job than are women (Statistics Sweden 1991), including toxic substances like carbon disulphide, nitroglycerin, combustion exhaust and carbon monoxide (for an overview, see Kristensen 1989 and Gustavsson 1989). However, exposure to such risks is rare today, with the exception of carbon monoxide—which has not been clearly established as a risk factor for cardiovascular disease. Thus it seems unlikely that exposure to toxic substances can explain much of the gender gap in the risk of cardiovascular disease in Sweden. With regard to ergonomic risks, men are exposed to more static load than women are, which leads to an increase in pulse rate and diastolic blood pressure. This might, over time, heighten the risk of cardiovascular disease. However, severe static load is declining in importance (Statistics Sweden 1995).

It is important to analyze the psychosocial environment both on and off the job. Recent studies examining links between psychosocial factors and the risk of cardiovascular disease often use the "demand-control-support" model, in which psychological demands interact with an individual's control opportunities (Figure 8.4) and support. According to this theory, psychological demands do not substantially affect an individual's morbidity if he or she has a good deal of control. This kind of situation is referred to as *active* work. If, however, the individual has

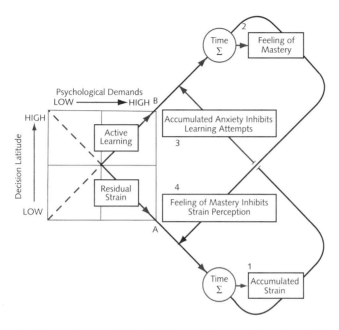

Figure 8.4 Dynamic associations linking environmental strain and learning to evolution of personality

little control, then such work is termed *strained*. The ideal work situation combines no excessive demands with a high degree of control (relaxed work). Many studies have examined the demand-control aspect of this model as it relates to men and cardiovascular disease, and for men there is a clear link between working in a situation marked by strain and an increase in coronary infarction (see overview by Schnall et al. 1994 and Kristensen 1989). Considerably fewer studies have looked at women, but those that have find corresponding links for women. For example, some studies link strained work and the risk of angina pectoris for women working at a computer. Orth-Gomér et al. (1995a) have recently shown that women who have experienced either a coronary infarction or angina pectoris are more likely than otherwise similar women to work at a job marked by strain. For both men and women, moreover, it has been shown that an individual's blood pressure level on the job is higher when the work is characterized by tension than when it is not (see, for example, Theorell & Karasek 1995 and Schnall & Landsbergis 1994).

In recent years, models have also taken into account support functions at work. In the case of men (see Johnson et al. 1989), a study showed that of people who eventually died of cardiovascular disease, those individuals who reported the favorable combination of low demands, high control and good support lived eight years longer than those who experienced high demands, little control and little support. However, there were differences both between men and women and across social groups, with the original demand-control model best able to predict the risk of early death from cardiovascular disease for men at the lowest social levels. For women and men in the upper social groups, the combination of inadequate control and inadequate support elevated the risk of dying of a cardiac infarction and the likelihood of angina pectoris more than the combination of high physical demands and inadequate control.

It has been more difficult to interpret the significance of work-related psychosocial factors for women than it has been for men (see, for example, Theorell & Karasek 1995). The Framingham study, for example, showed that men's risk of coronary-vessel disease was affected by different combinations of job-related psychosocial factors than women's (Haynes et al. 1980). One explanation may be that the home environment is of relatively greater importance to women than to men. Researchers have pointed out that women employed outside the home engage in substantially more housework than men. In the United States, employed women work a total of twenty hours more per week than men. Similar findings have been reported in Sweden as well (Lundberg 1989), but the fact that Swedish women frequently work part-time renders direct comparisons with the United States more difficult. Extremely long work hours are associated with an increased risk of coronary infarction (see Russek and Zohman 1958; Hinkle et al. 1968), but this, too, may differ for men and women (Alfredsson et al. 1985). For men, the risk of hospitalization for a coronary infarction is lower for men working in occupations where (at least moderate) overtime is common than for other men for whom overtime is less common. For women, working in occupations where moderate overtime (10 hours/week) is common is associated with excess risk of hospitalization for an infarction relative to other women who work in occupations with less overtime. This difference may perhaps be explained by the gender gap in the amount of unpaid work people do at home, although this gap appears to have narrowed somewhat in Sweden over the past decade (Nermo 1994). A more recent study (Hammar et al. 1994) of the risk of coronary infarction among individuals in various types of occupations also included deaths occurring outside the hospital, and did not find a similar gender gap. It may be, then, that such gender differences hold only for certain types of cardiovascular disease.

Many studies from countries like the United States, Sweden and Finland have shown that men and women have quite similar perceptions of the psychological demands of their jobs, but women view their opportunities to issue control over their job situations as much more limited than men do. Many studies in the United States and Sweden (see Karasek & Theorell 1990 and Theorell et al. 1993) have also found some correlation for men between psychological demands and control opportunities, while there is no similar correlation for women. Thus for men we find what one might expect—increased demands are generally associated with increased control—while this does not appear to be true for women. Similarly, for men, but not for women, there seems to be some correlation between age and control (see Theorell et al. 1993). In Western countries, the typical pattern is for men to have little control at the beginning of their careers, but control opportunities increase up to middle age, followed by a leveling off toward the end of their careers. In addition, a study in Stockholm has shown that men between the ages of 45 and 65 who experienced coronary infarctions were likely to have changed from higher- to lower-control jobs in the preceding three years. In contrast, the comparison group of men of the same age range in Stockholm, who did not change jobs, experienced a slight increase in control during the same period. The dynamics of change in control over a person's career may be significant—a man whose control decreases substantially when it might be expected to increase may run a particularly high risk of coronary infarction (Theorell 1994). This study did not show the same pattern for women suffering a coronary infarction, but instead a pattern of consistently low control, with no major changes during the period preceding the coronary infarction.

Control (see Karasek 1979), or *decision latitude,* involves two main components: the opportunity to develop competence and thus take control in unexpected and difficult situations *(intellectual discretion),* as well as the opportunity to affect decisions regarding one's own job *(authority over decisions).* Both components are affected by organizational conditions. It is well-known that male employees are promoted to higher positions more frequently than women are, and this can affect both components of control. It would appear from our studies that men and women who work in the same kinds of positions, grouped according to whether or not they have been promoted, have a similar perception of their control (see Theorell et al. 1993). In occupations we examined that permitted employees the least decision latitude—orchestral musicians and subway-train drivers—the point at which individuals are able to affect decisions is low for both men and women.

Also noteworthy is that men and women generally have quite different job responsibilities in the Swedish labor market. Far more women than men have jobs involving contact with the public (Statistics Sweden 1991). Thus women's low sense of control over their jobs may be linked to the fact that others' responses and relationships are difficult to control.

A study of Swedish employees (Hall 1990) showed that the group with the lowest sense of control over their work are women with few skills working in occupations dominated by men, indicating that control may involve factors other than the work itself—namely the gender culture that has been established at a particular workplace.

Research suggests that a well-developed network of social support at work is beneficial to men's health. These links are less clear for women. A major study of cardiovascular disease in women (Orth-Gomér et al. 1995) showed that social support on the job is not related to the likelihood of developing cardiovascular disease. Some have even raised the question of whether a large social network at work may mean additional stress for some women. Accordingly, the association between a social network and cardiovascular disease seems to be less clear for women than for men. A study of job-related stress factors affecting prison personnel in Sweden (Härenstam & Theorell 1990) showed that men who frequently felt isolated on their jobs and who also had high levels of liver enzymes (gamma GT concentrations in the blood), i.e., men who probably consumed large amounts of alcohol, also had the highest concentrations of plasma cortisol (a measure of dissatisfaction). This is one of a number of indications that men who feel isolated on the job show more signs of physiologically harmful stress reactions than other men. Among female employees, in contrast, those who never felt isolated at work and who had normal or low liver enzyme levels showed the highest concentrations of plasma cortisol. Of course, this may also have something to do with the complex interaction between social support and other conditions on the job. For example, a study conducted by Johnson and Hall (1988) showed that for women, symptoms of cardiovascular disease occurred most frequently when little control at work was coupled with little social support from coworkers.

A more complete look at how cardiovascular disease affects men and women should consider the presence of social support in people's life situations as a whole. Many studies of men have shown a lack of social support to be associated with an increased risk of coronary infarction (see, for example, Orth-Gomér et al. 1993). The picture is less clear for women. Indeed, a Swedish population study (Orth-Gomér & Johnson 1987) indicated that older women with an extensive network of social contacts had a higher risk of dying of cardiovascular disease than other women of the same age. It may be that for certain women, a large network of contacts causes psychosocial stress.

Another psychosocial factor that has been discussed in the context of cardiovascular disease is the occurrence of negative life events. A longitudinal study of risk factors for cardiovascular disease showed a deterioration after individuals experienced important negative life events, while an improvement occurred following significant positive events (Theorell & Emlund 1993). Here, too, more study has been devoted to men than to women (see, for example, the summary in Theorell 1992). A Stockholm study of women and cardiovascular disease (Orth-Gomér et al. 1995) showed that more negative life events, many of them family-related, occurred in the group suffering from diseases of the coronary vessels than the comparison group.

To sum up, we note that life circumstances as they relate to cardiovascular disease have been studied much more thoroughly for men than for women. However, some parallel observations have been made for men and women. Thus, for example, a lack of control at work, particularly when combined with high psychological demands, has been shown to be a risk factor for cardiovascular disease for both men and women, while the effects of social support may differ by gender.

In general, research shows that women experience more stress than men in their psychosocial living environments. Women probably work more total hours than men and perceive their control to be more limited. The picture of the role of social support in people's lives is unclear. At any rate, however, differences in psychosocial stresses cannot entirely explain the fact that men have a higher risk of coronary infarction than women do. The gender gap undoubtedly stems from other factors as well. Differences in coping patterns (which, in turn, result to some degree from earlier experiences of life stresses) and biological factors should also be studied.

Coping patterns

We find systematic gender differences in responses to unfair treatment by bosses or coworkers (Theorell et al. 1999). "Hidden coping"—when an individual does not say or show what he or she is thinking—is clearly more common among female than male employees in Stockholm. "Open coping," in which the individual speaks his mind, either immediately or after some thought, tends to be more common among men. The origins of this gender difference are uncertain, but it seems quite clear that socialization into the different gender roles is significant. Links between coping patterns and cardiovascular disease have not been the subject of comprehensive studies, although some related studies are currently underway in such countries as Sweden. There is some indication that less open coping strategies are associated with an increased risk of cardiovascular disease, and preliminary observations of men and women in the Swedish prison population have lent support to that hypothesis (Härenstam & Theorell 1990). The less open the coping method, the higher the likelihood of ischemic ECG changes, which are indicative of coronary vessel disease. A Swedish study of women with coronary vessel disease (Orth-Gomér et al. 1995) found that coping, defined as the ability to deal with difficulties in life, was less effective among patients with diseases of the coronary vessels than the women in the comparison group. Various aspects of coping behavior and personality patterns as they relate to cardiovascular disease have been studied for both men and women.

Several studies have indicated that for men, Type-A patterns, particularly hostility, are associated with increased risk of an early coronary infarction (see, for example, Matthews & Haynes 1986). In a Swedish study of women who were followed for 12 years to assess their risk of cardiovascular disease, Hällström et al (1986) showed that for women it was other aspects of personality that were significant for the risk of coronary infarction. Hostility and Type-A personality showed no link with cardiovascular disease. Moreover, different personality aspects led to different manifestations of cardiovascular disease among women. In a study of characteristics of men and women who had experienced a myocardial infarction, Welin et al. (1994) also showed that personality patterns among such men and women differed in various ways from their respective comparison groups. Male coronary patients differed from healthy men in reporting more irritability and depression, while this was not a distinguishing factor for women. The Swedish case control studies of women with cardiovascular disease showed no connection between Type-A personality and cardiovascular disease, but did link such health problems and optimism, with less optimism found among the ill women. A study conducted by Hällström et al. (1986) revealed that women with little self-confidence had an increased risk of angina pectoris—which contrasts sharply with the male risk pattern for myocardial infarction. Research in this area has not yet been able to present clear conclusions, but it appears that the picture of coronary infarction is quite different for men and women.

Physiological response patterns

Might one explanation for the gender difference in the risk of cardiovascular disease be that men's and women's coronary-vessel systems respond differently to situations of stress? Many authors have suggested this, and a number of experiments have been conducted to determine whether men and women have different response patterns. However, the empirical findings are difficult to interpret, since the situations that men find most stressful may not be perceived in the same way by women, and vice versa. For instance, Lundberg and Palm (1989) showed that mothers secreted more stress hormones (catecholamines) in situations involving children than fathers did. Otherwise, a considerable amount of research has indicated that men generally respond with a slightly larger increase in catecholamine secretion in pressure situations than women do (Frankenhaeuser 1988). Some research more directly related to the cardiovascular system has been published in recent years.

Laboratory experiments have focused on situations of high versus low psychological demands and good versus poor decision latitude. Diastolic blood pressure rose least among individuals (both men and women) with Type-B personality (opposite of Type-A) in situations with low demands and good decision latitude. However, men and women differed in that hostility was significant for men's blood pressure responses in these situations, but insignificant for cardiovascular responses of women (Burns, Hutt & Weidner 1993).

In another experiment, researchers observed the cardiovascular responses of children between the ages of 10 and 14 to anger expressed by adults (Ballard, Cummings & Larkin 1993). Sons of parents with high blood pressure showed a stronger reaction in terms of systolic blood pressure when they observed adults quarreling than did sons of parents with normal blood pressure. A similar difference was not observed for girls.

A third study examined how the degree of hostility (measured, as in the other studies, using a questionnaire completed by the individual) related to lack of oxygen, ischemia, in the heart muscle in connection with physical exertion. For both middle-aged men and middle-aged women, a high level of hostility was found to be associated with a substantial lack of oxygen in the heart muscle when physical exertion was present. In this case, there did not appear to be a difference between men and women (Helmers et al. 1993).

The third study differed from the first two in that the stress situation to which individuals were exposed was gender-neutral—the experience of physical effort may be similar for men and women. In the other studies, it is conceivable that men and women interpret a given situation differently, and thus have a different physiological response to it.

One interpretation of psychophysiological research may be that men and women respond somewhat differently to different situations (e.g., family or work situations), but that the basic mechanisms are really the same and hence the observed differences may reflect difference in degree rather than nature of response.

Biological factors

An extensive body of literature has been published on biological risk factors for cardiovascular disease, for both men and women. This literature shows that here, too, there are systematic differences between the sexes. Serum cholesterol, for example, appears to be a much better predictor of the risk of coronary infarction for men than for women, while other blood fat fractions seem to be more important in determining women's risk of a coronary infarction. Apparently there are similar differences with respect to coagulation factors. Thus biological risk factor patterns appear to be different for men and women, and this, of course, may help explain the remaining gender differences in the risk of cardiovascular disease.

A recent study showed that various indicators of socioeconomic status were strongly related—independently of a number of biological confounders—to HDL cholesterol in women. A particularly strong relationship was found between low decision latitude at work and low HDL cholesterol (Wamala et al 1997). Plasma fibrinogen concentration has been studied both in men and women in two different studies (Brunner et al 1996 and Tsutsumi et al 1999) in relation to psychosocial factors. In particular more objective measures (expert ratings in the first study and indirect population measures in the second study) of job control were associated with fibrinogen, the lower the control the higher the fibrinogen. These findings were more significant in women than in men. Thus there is evidence that both fibrinogen and lipids are more closely related with job control in women than in men.

While smoking was always more common among men in the past, this pattern has changed. Among younger people it is women who smoke the most today, and women also seem to have a harder time quitting than men do. For both men and women, there is a striking difference in smoking habits between social classes —the lower the social status, the higher the prevalence of smoking. Smoking is particularly common in Sweden today among younger women with little education (see, for example, the 1994 Public Health Report for Stockholm county). These gradual changes in health-related behavior naturally have long-term consequences for cardiovascular disease. The reasons behind the increase in women's smoking have been discussed extensively by Chesney (see Franken-haeuser et al. 1991). One question is to what extent increased smoking among women may be a result of changed social roles for men and women. Cohen et al. (1991), for example, conducted a study of randomly selected men and women in an American population. For men, the only indisputable link was that prior depression increased the risk of cigarette smoking. For women, on the other hand, there were four significant psychological or social factors: prior depression, marital conflict, the occurrence of unwanted life events and full-time work. A Swedish study of women and cardiovascular disease (Orth-Gomér et al. 1995b) showed cigarette smoking to be significantly more common among women with low levels of education relative to highly educated women. As for the work environment, high psychological demands coupled with low levels of control increased the risk of smoking among men (but not women). This may indicate that the overall life situation is of greater significance for women's smoking habits, while work is of great importance for men's smoking habits—which is yet another illustration of the fact that the pattern of interactions between life situation and living habits is different for men and women.

Another question that psychophysiological research has attempted to answer is whether or not men and women show different patterns of psychophysiological response in connection with smoking. Here there is some disagreement, but a recent study has shown that cigarette smoking has a more pronounced effect on the heart rate of women than of men (Stone et al. 1990).

Consequences of myocardial infarctions for men and women

In recent years, there has been some discussion in the literature on whether men and women receive equivalent care in the hospital following a coronary infarction. At present, the consensus seems to be that a good portion of the observed difference results from the fact that women are usually older than men when they are treated for a coronary infarction. It has also been pointed out, however, that women have more difficulty participating in rehabilitation activities than men do. For several years I observed this myself, while I was working in rehabilitation for coronary patients and organizing group meetings for patients and their families. Female patients were frequently absent from the late-afternoon meetings, and the reason, as it turned out, was that they were expected to be cooking dinner for their husbands—the husband's dinner was perceived as more important than the patient's rehabilitation. It appears that rehabilitation departments have every reason to provide a little extra help for women!

General conclusions

It is unlikely that gender differences in the risk of cardiovascular disease are due solely to either hereditary or environmental factors. Women have a somewhat different endocrinological makeup than men, and this is reflected in gender-specific differences in blood fats and coagulation factors. Might women have a biologically-determined potential for longevity that is greater than men's? This could certainly be part of the explanation. However, men's and women's life situations are different as well. Furthermore, there are differences in how men and women deal with stress, and these differences are reflected in differing interactions between psychosocial factors and the risk of cardiovascular disease. As for lifestyle factors, women have caught up with men when it comes to cigarette smoking, and it is the women who are most at risk psychosocially who are most likely to smoke.

References

Alfredsson L, Spetz CL, Theorell T. *Type of occupation and near-future hospitalization for myocardial infarction and some other diagnoses.* It J Epidemiol 1985;14:378–388.

Ballard ME, Cummings EM, Larkin K. *Emotional and cardiovascular responses to adults' angry behavior and to challenging tasks in children of hypertensive and normotensive parents.* Child Dev 1993;64:500–515.

Brunner, E., Davey Smith, G. Marmot, M, Canner, R., Beksinska M. and O'Brien, J: *Childhood social circumstances and psychological and behavioural factors as determinants of plasma fibrinogen.* Lancet 1996; 347:1008–1013.

Burns JW, Hutt J, Weidner G. *Effects of demand and decision latitude on cardiovascular reactivity among coronary-prone women and men.* Behav Med 1993;19:122–128.

Cohen S, Schwartz JE, Bromet EJ, Parkinson DK. *Mental health, stress and poor health behaviors in two community samples.* Preventive Medicine 1991;20(2):306–15.

Folkhälsorapport om hälsoutvecklingen i Stockholms län [Public health report on health trends in Stockholm county]. Stockholms läns landsting. Hälso- och sjulvårdsnämnden, 1994.

Frankenhaeuser M. *Stress and reactivity patterns at different stages of the life cycle.* In: Pancheri P, Zichella L (Eds.): Biorhythms and Stress in Physiopathology of Reproduction. Washington, D.C.: Hemisphere, 1988.

Frankenhaeuser M, Lundberg U, Chesney M (Eds.). *Women, Work and Health.* Chicago: Plenum Publishing Corporation, 1991.

Gustavsson P. *Cancer and ischemic heart disease in occupational groups exposed to combustion products.* Arbete och hälsa 1:21. National Institute of Occupational Health, Solna, 1989.

Hall EM. *Women's Work: An Inquiry into the Health Effects of Invisible and Visible Labor.* Ph.D. dissertation, The Karolinska Institute, Stockholm, 1990.

Hammar N, Alfredsson L, Theorell T. *Job characteristics and the incidence of myocardial infarction.* Int J Epidemiol 1994;23:277–284.

Haynes SG, Feinleib M, Kannel W. *The relationship of psychosocial factors to coronary heart disease in the Framingham study. III. Eight-year incidence of coronary heart disease.* Am J Epidemiol 1980;111:37–58.

Helmers KF, Krantz DS, Howell RH, Klein J, Bairey CN, Rozanski A. *Hostility and myocardial ischemia in coronary artery disease patients: Evaluation by gender and ischemic index.* Psychosom Med 1993;55:29–36.

Hinkle LE, Jr., Whitney LH, Lehman EW, Dunn J, Benjamin B, King R, Plakun A, Flehinger B. *Occupation, education and coronary heart disease.* Science 1968;161:238–248.

Hällström T, Lapidus L, Bengtsson C, Edström K. *Psychosocial factors and risk of ischaemic heart disease and death in women: A twelve-year follow-up of participants in the population study of women in Gothenburg, Sweden.* J of Psychosomatic Research 1986;30:4:451–459.

Härenstam A, Theorell T. *Cortisol elevation and serum gammaglutamyl transpeptidase in response to adverse job conditions: How are they interrelated?* Biological Psychology 1990;331:157–171.

Härenstam A, Theorell T, Kaijser L, Köster M. *Psychosocial working conditions and signs of CHD on ECG recordings.* Manuscript, 1996.

Johnson JV, Hall EM. *Job strain, workplace social support and cardiovascular disease: A cross-sectional study of a random sample of the Swedish working population..* Am J Public Health 1988;78:1336–1342.

Johnson JV, Hall EM, Theorell T. *Combined effects of job strain and social isolation on cardiovascular disease morbidity and mortality in a random sample of the Swedish male working population.* Scand J Work Environ Health 1989;15:271–279.

Karasek RA. *Job demands, job decision latitude, and mental strain: Implications for job redesign.* Admin Sci Q 1979;24:285–307.

Karasek RA, Theorell T. *Healthy Work.* New York: Basic Books, 1990.

Kristensen TS. *Cardiovascular diseases and the work environment. A critical review of the epidemiologic literature on chemical factors.* Scand J Work Environ Health 1989;15:245–264.

La Croix AZ. *Occupational exposure to high demand/low control work and coronary heart disease incidence in the Framingham cohort.* Ph.D. dissertation, Department of Epidemiology, University of North Carolina, 1984.

Lundberg U, Palm K. *Workload and catecholamine excretion in parents of preschool children.* Work & Stress 1989;3:255–260.

McKinlay JB. *Some contributions from the social system to gender inequalities in heart disease.* J Health and Social Behavior 1996;37:1–26.

Mathews KA, Haynes SG. *Type A behavior pattern and coronary disease risk: Update and critical evaluation.* Am J Eidemiol 1986;123:923–960.

Nermo M. *Den fullbordade jämställdheten [Completed equality].* In: Fritzell J, Lundberg O (Eds.): Vardagens villkor. Levnadsförhållanden i Sverige under tre decennier [Everyday conditions: Life circumstances in Sweden over three decades]. Stockholm: Brombergs, 1994.

Orth-Gomér K, Johnson JV. *Social network interaction and mortality: A six year follow-up study of a random sample of the Swedish population.* J Chron Dis 1987;40:949–957.

Orth-Gomér K, Rosengren A, Wilhelmsen L. *Lack of social support and incidene of coronary heart disease in middle-aged Swedish men.* Psychosom Med 1993;55:37–43.

Orth-Gomér K, Eriksson I, Högbom M, Wamala S, Blom M, Moser V, Belkic K, Schenk-Gustafsson K, et al. *Psykosociala riskfaktorer för kranskärlssjukdom hos kvinnor [Psychosocial risk factors for diseases of the coronary vessels among women].* Stressforskningsrapporter no. 255, Statens Institut för Psykosocial Miljömedicin, 1995a.

Orth-Gomér K, Schenk-Gustafsson K, Wamala S, Blom M, Högbom M, Moser V, Rosenberg U. *Socialklass och hjärtkärlsjukdom hos kvinnor i Stor-Stockholm [Social class and diseases of the coronary vessels among women in the greater Stockholm region].* Medicinska Riksstämman, Sammanfattningar (P. 370), 1995b.

Russek HI, Zohman BL. *Relative significance of heredity, diet and occupational stress in coronary heart disease of young adults; based on an analysis of 100 patients between the ages of 25 and 40 years and a similar group of 100 normal control subjects.* Amer J Med Sci 1958;235:266.

SCB [Statistics Sweden]. *Kvinnors och mäns arbetsmiljö [Women's and men's work environments].* Information om arbetsmarknaden 1991: 1. Stockholm: Statistiska Centralbyrån, 1991.

SCB [Statistics Sweden]. *Statistisk Årsbok [Statistical yearbook]* (Table 495). Stockholm: Statistiska Centralbyrån, 1995.

Schnall PL, Pieper C, Schwartz JE, Karasek RA, Schlussel Y, Devereux RB, Ganau A, Alderman M, Warren K, Pickering T. *The relationship between "job strain," workplace diastolic blood pressure, and left ventricular mass index.* JAMA 1990;263:1929–1935.

Schnall PL, Landsbergis PA. *Job strain and cardiovascular disease.* Annual Review of Public Health 1994;15:381–411.

Schnorr TM, Thun MJ, Halperin WE. *Chest pain in users of video display terminals.* JAMA 1987;257:627–640.

Stockholms läns landsting [Stockholm county council]. *Hjärtinfarkt i Stockholms län under 1980-talet [Coronary infarctions in Stockholm county during the 1980s].* A report from the county council office of epidemiology, Stockholm county council, 1992.

Stone SV, Dembroski TM, Costa PT, Jr., MacDougall JM. *Gender differences in cardiovascular reactivity.* Journal of Behavioral Medicine 1990;13(2):137–56.

Szulkin R, Tåhlin M (Eds.). *Sveriges arbetsplatser—Organisation, personalutveckling, styrning [Sweden's jobs: Organization, personnel trends, management].* Stockholm: SNS förlag, 1994.

Theorell T. *Health promotion in the workplace.* In: Badura B, Kickbusch (Eds.): Health promotion research. WHO Regional Publications, European series No. 37, pp. 251–266, 1991.

Theorell T. *Critical Life Changes. A review of research.* Psychother Psychosom 1992;57:108–117.

Theorell T, Emllund N. *On physiological effects of positive and negative life changes—A longitudinal study.* J Psychosom Res 1993;37:653–659.

Theorell T, Karasek RA. *Current issues relating to psychosocial job strain and cardiovascular disease research.* J Occ Health Psychology 1995, in press.

Theorell T, Olsson A, Engholm G. *Concrete work and myocardial infarction.* Scand J Work Environ Health 1977;3:144–153.

Theorell T, Perski A, Åkerstedt T, Sigala F, Ahlberg-Hultén G, Svensson J, Eneroth P. *Changes in job strain in relation to changes in physiological state.* Scand J Work Environ Health 1988;14:1889–196.

Theorell T, Michélsen H, Nordemar R, Stockholm MUSIC 1 Study Group. *Levnadshändelser och copingmönster i Stockholmsundersökningen 1 [Life events and coping patterns in Stockholm study 1].* In: Hagberg M, Hogstedt C (Eds.): Stockholmsundersökningen 1. Data från en tvärsnittsundersökning av ergonomisk och psykosocial exponering samt sjuklighet och funktion i rörelseorganen [Data from a cross-sectional study of ergonomic and psychosocial exposure as well as of illness and functioning of the musculoskeletal system]. Stockholm: MUSIC Books, 1991.

Theorell T, Michélsen H, Nordemar R, Stockholm MUSIC 1 Study Group. *Validitetsprövning av psykosociala indexbildningar [Validation study of psychosocial indices].* In: Hagberg M, Hogstedt C (Eds.): Stockholmsundersökningen 1. Utvärdering av metoder för att mäta hälsa och exponeringar i epidemiologiska studier av rörelseorganens sjukdomar [Evaluation of methods of measuring health and exposure in epidemiological studies of illnesses of the musculoskeletal system]. Stockholm: MUSIC Books, 1993.

Theorell T, Reuterwall C, Hallqvist J, Emlund N, Ahlbom A, Hogstedt C. *Metodstudier kring psykosociala faktorer i SHEEP [Methodological studies of psychosocial factors in SHEEP].* ONYX 1994, No. 1.

Wamala SP, Wolk A, Schenck-Gustafsson K, and Orth-Gomér K: *Lipid profile ans socioeconomic status in healthy women in Sweden.* J Epidemiology and Community Medicine. 1997; 51: 400–407.

Welin C, Rosengren A, Wedel H, Wiklund I, Wilhelmsen L. *Psychological characteristics in patients with myocardial infarction—A case-control study.* Cardiovascular Risk Factors 1994;4:154–161.

9

Biological and social conditions: Hypotheses regarding mortality differentials between men and women[1]

Örjan Hemström

Introduction

IT IS A PARADOX THAT WOMEN tend to have poorer health but longer lives than men. Statistics presented in Chapter 2 documented the discrepancy between the life expectancy of men and women. In virtually all industrialized countries, there has been an increase in this gender gap over the last century (Hart 1989). In a period when the life expectancy of both men and women has increased, gains for men have lagged behind those for women.

Some social scientists have asked whether it is women's relatively low mortality that should be studied, or rather men's relatively high mortality (Erikson 1987; Gee & Veevers 1983). There might be different kinds of explanations for low female mortality, for high male mortality, and for the differentially rapid decline in mortality for men and women. In short, certain factors affect men's and women's mortality equally, while other factors affect one sex more than the other.

However, views differ with respect to the additional years of life enjoyed by women. Comparing the number of active years after the age of 65, Silman (1987) concludes that there is no gender gap. In Finland, a country with relatively high excess male mortality, disability-free life expectancy was only slightly higher for women both at age 25 (1.5 years) and 65 (1.3 years) (Valkonen et al. 1994). The 1994 Swedish Public Health Report clearly shows that women experience more years of life than men do between the ages of 65 and 84. However, if we look instead at the number of years of full health in this age group, there is no gender difference (National Public Health Report 1994: 44). These estimates may depend on what one considers to be ill health. The relationship between ill health and mortality was discussed at the end of Chapter 2. Here we focus on the fact that men have a higher mortality rate over the entire life cycle, even in utero (Stillion 1984).

The primary purpose of this chapter is to examine why the observed mortality differential between men and women exists. In this analysis we do not focus on age; differences found for various ages are given only peripheral attention. We first present the difference in life expectancy in a number of countries, recent changes in a few of them, and the differential mortality of Swedish men and women for an extended time period. This is followed by an overview of various hypotheses and presumptions that might explain men's higher mortality rate. We offer some critical comments on the conclusions drawn from these hypotheses. It should be noted that the discussion is not exhaustive, but limited to some of the most common hypotheses. The chapter ends with a general discussion.

Changes in mortality among men and women

A list of 52 countries from all continents and representing most types of society, with gender-specific life expectancy (LE) at birth and the differences between men's and women's life expectancy, is presented in Table 9.1. This table shows a range of differentials, from the country with the largest negative gender difference (shorter LE for women) to the country with the largest positive gender difference (shorter LE for men). It has been noted that a few countries (such as India and Pakistan) used to have excess female mortality (Nathanson, 1984). Similarly, our data show that in other South Asian countries (Nepal, Bangladesh and the Maldives) men could expect to live longer than women do. However, India is perhaps not a suitable example due to large regional variation. In the state of Kerala, for instance, the common finding of higher male mortality has been observed for decades (Ram, 1993). India, Algeria and Iran also had very small gender differences (one year or less). In general, the global trend indicates that life expectancy is shorter for men than for women by between 3.1 years (Kenya) and 13.5 years (Russia), with a mean of 6.0 years. One should note the predominance of Eastern European countries among those having the largest gender differences.

Over the last two decades or so, a narrowing of the gender differences has been observed for many countries (Waldron, 1993). Figure 9.1 shows the change in gender differences in LE for 15 developed countries from around 1980 (1977/82) until 1992/94. A narrowing of the gender differences can be observed for most of these countries during this period. The largest decrease was observed for Iceland, while the clearest increases were found in Hungary, Japan and Israel. By comparison, France, Germany and Switzerland experienced only small changes.

Among the selected countries Sweden occupies a 'middle position,' both with regard to the size of the gender gap in survival and to recent changes. Figure 9.2 shows trends in mortality rates for men and women in post-war Sweden. We see that the decline in women's mortality rates has been virtually uninterrupted throughout this period. For men, there was a decline in the 1940s and 1950s, followed by a period of stagnation in the 1960s and 1970s. One can observe a marked decline in men's mortality rates, exceeding those for women, from the early 1980s onwards. 1980 was a turning point in the post-war trend; it was here that the gender gap began to narrow (in absolute numbers).[2] The general view is that it was

Table 9.1: Gender Differences in Life Expectancy at Birth for 52 Countries

Countries (year)	Life Expectancy at Birth (Years)		
	Men	Women	Women-Men
Nepal (1981)*	50.9	48.1	-2.8
Bangladesh (1988)*	56.9	56.0	-0.9
The Maldives (1992)*	67.2	66.6	-0.6
India (1986-90)*	57.7	58.1	0.4
Algeria (1987)*	65.8	66.3	0.5
Iran (1990-95)*	67.0	68.0	1.0
Kenya (1990-95)*	54.2	57.3	3.1
China (1990-95)*	66.7	70.5	3.8
Iceland (1993)	77.1	80.9	3.8
Israel (1992)	74.7	78.5	3.8
Sri Lanka (1981)*	67.8	71.7	3.9
Egypt (1991)*	62.9	66.4	4.0
Brazil (1990-95)*	64.0	68.7	4.7
Costa Rica (1990-95)*	72.9	77.6	4.7
Argentina (1990-91)*	68.2	73.1	4.9
Turkmenistan (1994)	61.5	66.5	5.0
Denmark (1993)	72.7	77.9	5.2
Ecuador (1995)*	67.3	72.5	5.2
Greece (1993)	75.0	80.4	5.4
Ireland (1992)	72.6	78.2	5.6
Sweden (1992)	75.5	81.1	5.6
United Kingdom (1992)	73.6	79.2	5.6
New Zealand (1990-92)*	72.9	78.7	5.8
Australia (1992)*	75.0	80.9	5.9
South Africa (1990-95)*	60.0	66.0	6.0
The Netherlands (1993)	74.0	80.1	6.1
Japan (1993)*	76.3	82.5	6.2
Norway (1992)	74.2	80.5	6.3
Austria (1994)	73.4	79.9	6.5
Germany (1994)	73.1	79.7	6.6
Switzerland (1993)	75.0	81.7	6.7
Belgium (1989)	72.3	79.1	6.8
Canada (1985-87)*	73.0	79.8	6.8
Italy (1991)	73.7	80.5	6.8
USA (1991)*	72.0	78.9	6.9
Albania (1993)	70.3	77.3	7.0
Czech republic (1993)	69.3	76.5	7.2
Portugal (1993)	70.6	77.9	7.3
Romania (1993)	65.9	73.3	7.4
Bulgaria (1993)	67.5	75.0	7.5
Finland (1993)	72.1	79.6	7.5
Spain (1992)	73.8	81.3	7.5
France (1992)	73.8	82.3	8.5
Poland (1993)	67.4	76.0	8.6
Slovakia (1991)	66.5	75.3	8.8
Hungary (1994)	64.8	74.3	9.5
Ukraine (1992)	63.9	74.0	10.1
Belarus (1993)	63.8	74.6	10.8
Estonia (1994)	61.2	73.2	12.0
Lituania (1994)	62.8	74.9	12.1
Latvia (1994)	58.9	72.3	13.4
Russia (1994)	57.7	71.2	13.5
Mean	*68.2*	*74.2*	*6.0*

Sources: WHO statistical data base (Health for all 2000);
* *Demographic Yearbook 1994.* New York: United Nations, 1996, Table 22.

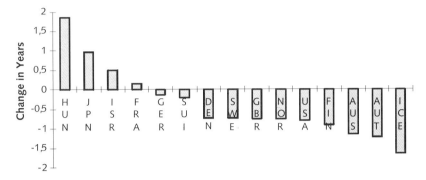

Sources: 1977/82: *Demographic Yearbook 1983*. New York: United Nations, 1985, Table 22.
          1992/94: *Demographic Yearbook 1995*. New York: United Nations, 1997, Table 22.

Figure 9.1: Change in Gender Differential in Life Expectancy at Birth for 15 Selected Countries, 1977/82–1992/94.

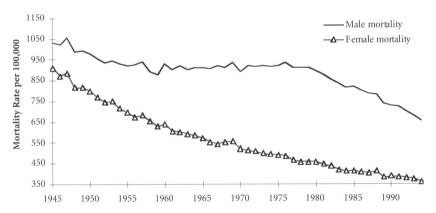

Figure 9.2: Male and Female Mortality Trends 20–74 Years, 1945–94. Age Standardized by the Mean Swedish Population in 1965 as the Standard Population (5-Year Age Weights). Calculated from Annual Causes of Death Reports ("Dödsorsaker"). Published by Statistics Sweden.

the relatively constant male mortality in the period 1960–80 that led to the rise in excess male mortality in Sweden. Consequently, it is the rapid fall in male mortality after 1980 that contributes to the narrowing of the gender-gap in mortality in the most recent period.

Another way to view the changes that have taken place during this period is to look at the various causes of death that have contributed to a higher mortality rate among men. Particularly significant in industrialized countries are external causes[3] among younger adults and circulatory diseases among older people (see Hart 1989; Nathanson 1984). For the latter group, ischemic heart disease (IHD)[4] is especially prominent. With this in mind, we have divided causes of death roughly into three groups: external causes, IHD and other causes. As Figure 9.3 makes clear, there were changes in the distribution of excess male mortality between 1952 and 1992 across these groups. In 1952 there was substantial excess male mortality from external causes and IHD, but the gender differential was slight for other causes of death. However, the period in question saw a decline in the differential for external causes. Fourteen percent of total excess male mortality was accounted for by external causes in 1992, compared with 37 percent in 1952. At the same time, the category "other causes of death" has gained in importance. In 1992, these 'other causes' contributed as many deaths as ischemic heart disease to total excess male mortality.

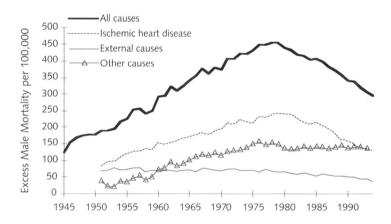

Figure 9.3: Excess Male Mortality in Absolute Numbers 1945–1994 for Ischemic Heart Disease (IHD), External Causes (Accidents, Poisonings, Suicide, Homicide), Other Causes and All Causes. Difference in Men's and Women's Mortality Rates Ages 20–74. Age Standardized by the Mean Swedish Population in 1965. Calculated from Statistics Sweden's Annual Causes of Death Reports (Dödsorsaker")
1945–1994.

The increasing importance of 'other causes of death' raises certain questions. Does this category contain certain causes of death that have affected men disproportionately? When comparisons are made over time, various classification problems can arise as a result of changed coding guidelines.[5] Since a lack of space here restricts further detail, we shall limit ourselves to a comparison of various causes of death in the first and last years (1952 and 1992) under study. By breaking down overall mortality into twelve different causes of death, we arrive at a more detailed picture of the changes that have occurred (Figure 9.4).

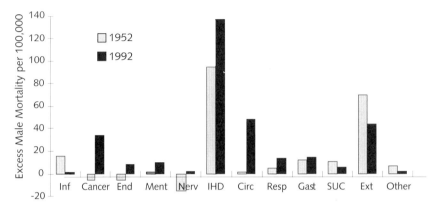

Note abbreviations: *Inf* = Infectious and parasitic diseases; *End* = Endocrine and metabolic diseases; *Ment* = Mental disorders; *Nerv* = Diseases of the nervous system and sense organs; *IHD* = Ischemic heart disaese; *Circ* = Other diseases of the circulatory system (excluding IHD); *Resp* = Respiratory diseases; *Gast* = Gastrointestinal diseases; *SUC* = Symptoms and unknown causes; *Ext* = All external causes (accidents, poisonings, suicide, homicide); *Other* = All other causes not specified elsewhere (diseases of the blood organs, uro-genital diseases, diseases of pregnancy, childbirth & puerperalism, diseases of the skin, musculoskeletal diseases, and conditions from the perinatal period & congenital malformations).

Figure 9.4: Excess Male Mortality in Absolute Numbers 1952 and 1992 for Twelve Selected Causes of Death. Age 20–74. Age Standardized by the Mean Swedish Population in 1965. Calculated from Statistics Sweden's Causes of Death Reports *("Dödsorsaker") 1952 and 1992. The Total Excess Male Mortality per 100,000 Persons was 188.6 in 1952 and 319.3 in 1992.*

In 1952, some causes of death, including cancer, had female excess mortality. In contrast, in 1992 men had a higher mortality rate for all types of deaths listed. During this forty-year period, male mortality increased relative to female mortality, particularly for cancer and diseases of the circulatory organs (including ischemic heart disease). However, cancer accounts for a large proportion of men's higher mortality (10.6 percent) because cancer is a common cause of death, not because the gender gap is particularly large in relative terms (see also Chapter 2). The proportion of those dying from cancer is in fact larger among women than among men. For a few other causes of death, male mortality did in fact decline relative to female mortality. However, these causes of death, with the exception of violent deaths, were uncommon in 1992 (such as infectious diseases).

In summary, the factors which account for the increase in excess male mortality in Sweden appear to have been particularly significant during the 1960s and 1970s. They primarily affected increases in excess male mortality from cancer and various diseases of the circulatory organs (but also from other diseases).

Causes of the mortality gender gap

Earlier studies of excess male mortality in industrialized countries have focused particularly on the following question: Do women enjoy a natural (biological) advantage, or do men live in an unfavorable environment (Ortmeyer 1979)? The fact that the relationship between men's and women's mortality varies considerably over time, from country to country and between different social groups, has often been seen as an indication that the gender gap is due primarily to the social environment (Macintyre 1994; Retherford 1975). Seeking social explanations for this gap, epidemiologists have concentrated on individual risk factors, while sociologists have focused on roles, socialization and structural aspects of society (Nathanson 1984). Before addressing social factors, however, we shall begin by examining some of the biological factors assumed to favor the life expectancy of women.

Biological and genetic factors

Sex hormones.
The group of biological factors that has received the most attention in this context is probably sex hormones. Female sex hormones, primarily estrogen, are believed to protect women from cardiovascular disease, particularly during a woman's fertile years (Kalin & Zumoff 1990; Waldron 1983a). There is, however, another side to the protection afforded by female sex hormones; they may cause disease or death for certain women through breast cancer, for example. Moreover, both prior to puberty and after menopause men's mortality is higher than women's (Östberg 1996; Silman 1987). One reason why research results are not clear-cut is that it is difficult to isolate a pure effect of sex hormones. It has been shown that women, who experience early menopause, whether spontaneously or for medical reasons, have a higher risk of heart disease than other women. However, women's 'protective' hormones decrease only gradually after menopause (Kalin & Zumoff 1990), and there is no sudden increase in disease or mortality among elderly women (McKinlay 1996). Furthermore, while post-menopausal treatment with estrogen reduces risk for these women, estrogen treatment does not appear similarly to lower the risk of cardiovascular disease for men (there are endogenic hormones, according to Kalin and Zumoff, that are associated with a lower risk of heart disease).

It may even be the case that male sex hormones facilitate the development of heart disease. This view is supported, for example, by the fact that men with low levels of testosterone have a lower risk of heart disease, while women with higher levels of testosterone have an increased risk (Kalin & Zumoff 1990). Such findings, however, have not been obtained on 'healthy' individuals. Furthermore, male testosterone and other sex hormones may affect men's tendency toward aggressive behavior (Parsons 1982), which may contribute to the excess male mortality from accidental deaths (Waldron 1983a). This effect might be expected to be strongest during puberty, but there is no conclusive evidence that the increased rate of accidents among teenage boys is caused by an upsurge of male sex hormones or is due to socialization (Parsons 1982). Parsons, as well as Fausto-Sterling (1992:126–32), points out that the level of testosterone can be affected by social factors. The fact that the gender gap in mortality shows up today at an earlier age than forty years ago may reflect changed social conditions, as well as a change in the onset of (biological) puberty, in itself a result of improved nutrition and other social circumstances. If sex hormones contribute to changes in the male/female mortality gap, it must be through interactions with other factors.

Cholesterol levels and body fat distribution.

When examining a number of biomedical risk factors for cardiovascular disease in the United States, Janghorbani et al. (1993) observed that serum cholesterol was the only risk factor to increase the mortality risk for men but not for women.[6] One reason is that the ratio of ('the healthy') HDL cholesterol to ('the unhealthy') LDL cholesterol[7] differs for men and women. Women have approximately 25 percent higher levels of the more desirable HDL cholesterol than men, and this difference has been viewed as explaining about half of excess male mortality from ischemic heart disease (Waldron 1995). Women's higher HDL cholesterol levels are due to sex hormones, according to Waldron. However, triglycerides can pose considerable risk to women (Orth-Gomér 1992), so Waldron's estimate of the total influence of cholesterol could be somewhat exaggerated (see also Chapter 8).

Gender differences in body fat distribution may also play a role in causing higher male mortality from certain heart diseases. One research group found that the waist/hip ratio was the only known risk factor to markedly change the gender difference in myocardial infarction in multivariate analyses (Larsson et al. 1992). Excess abdominal fat, which is more common among men, seems to raise cholesterol levels, showing that there is a close link between such levels, body fat distribution and excess male mortality from heart disease.

Iron levels.

A possible biological explanation for men's higher mortality rates from ischemic heart disease lies in the higher levels of iron stored in men (Waldron 1995). Stored iron can heighten risk by increasing the oxidation of LDL cholesterol, a process that tends to accelerate the artherosclerotic process. High levels of stored iron are associated with myocardial infarction. In the case of hemoglobin, men's average levels are about 10 percent higher.

Genetic factors.

Perinatal deaths[8] and congenital defects are more common among boys. This may indicate that females enjoy some sort of genetic protection, possibly linked to natural selection and the survival of the species (Stillion 1984). Stillion suggests that the stresses of pregnancy and the immediate postnatal period imply a certain genetic protection for women, to ensure that the species will survive, a situation that is not unique to human beings. The X chromosome contains genes that affect the functioning of the immune system. Since women have two sets of these chromosomes (XX), while men have only one (XY), they may have greater resistance to infectious diseases (Waldron 1983a). This may also explain women's generally greater resilience to external stress and greater recovery during periods of growth (Ferembach 1978). Ferembach believes that girls' growth and maturation are less affected than boys' by external environmental conditions. This may help explain the gender gap in infant mortality,[9] as well as the fact that class differences in adult height are larger for men than for women (Nyström-Peck & Vågerö 1987).

One can also observe differences in biological development as children grow up. Girls develop earlier than boys, on average; they are at birth more neurologically advanced (although boys are physically larger); they reach certain developmental milestones (such as walking and speaking) at an earlier age; and they reach sexual maturity earlier than boys do (Parsons 1982). Boys' achievements in school may also be more dependent on 'favorable' social conditions, such as having a married mother, than those of girls (Modin 1998).

However, it is unclear what significance this has for the higher mortality rate of adult men, and it would appear difficult to prove that boys' 'susceptibility' stems from the fact that they have a Y rather than an additional X chromosome. Moreover, purely genetic factors are difficult to distinguish from social factors as children grow up. Nathanson (1984) holds that genes are of little significance for the gender gap in adult mortality, since there is a gendered socialization in modern society regarding what is appropriate behavior for 'men' and 'women' in adult life. The observations above would tend to indicate that genes and sex hormones are, if anything, significant in particular circumstances, such as in combination with environmental factors.

Social factors

Social factors (including behaviors) that may affect the gender gap in mortality are divided here into three groups: individual, group-related and societal (macrosocial) factors. These categories should not be seen as completely distinct from one another. In practice it is nearly impossible to isolate the pure effect of any such risk factors. People's choices are partly determined by conditions in their environment, and a health outcome of such choice (in this case death) depends also on various protective social factors that vary from group to group. Susceptibility to various diseases is influenced by social circumstances (Cassel 1976). These three categories are nonetheless useful in shedding light on some of the conditions in the social environment that may be responsible for the fact that men's lives, on average, are shorter than women's.

Individual behavior

Differences in smoking between men and women have been a predominant explanation for the gender difference in mortality rates in the industrialized countries (see, for example, Hart 1989; Retherford 1975; Waldron 1976, 1983b). This is particularly because it has been estimated that a heavy smoker can expect to live a 25-percent shorter life than a person who has never smoked (Rogers & Powell 1991). Retherford calculated that 47 percent of the gender gap in mean longevity can be attributed to smoking. In a recent study of five Northern European countries, smoking was estimated to contribute on average 40 percent to men's higher mortality in the period 1970–74 and around 30 percent in 1985–89 (Valkonen & van Poppel 1997). It was also found that smoking probably contributed somewhat less to excess male mortality in Sweden than in some other countries (14 percent in 1985–89), for example, because of smaller gender differences in smoking in Sweden than in the other countries. In a Swedish time-series analysis, changes in cigarette consumption were found to be associated with changes in excess male mortality (Hemström 1999a). However, the relationship was clearly significant only for changes in excess male mortality from ischemic heart disease.

In the 1960s, a comprehensive study was made of smoking habits in Sweden, in which 49 percent of men and 23 percent of women indicated that they smoked every day (Statistics Sweden 1965). The proportion of heavy smokers[10] and smokers who inhaled deeply was also considerably higher among men. Since the 1960s, the proportion of men smoking has decreased by more than one-half. This led to the situation in 1990s, when the traditional gender gap in smoking prevalence had disappeared (see Chapter 2). Similar observations have been made in other countries, although in Japan, Greece and Portugal, for instance, smoking continues to be primarily a part of the male lifestyle (Nathanson 1995). More similar smoking habits have led to a narrowing of lung-cancer mortality rates between men and women (Nathanson 1995; Qvist 1993), but any corresponding narrowing of differences in circulatory diseases has not been observed (Waldron 1993). This may be an effect of biological interaction.

In countries where there is no longer a substantial gender difference in smoking behavior, the significance of smoking as an explanation for the gender gap in mortality has undoubtedly declined. Nevertheless, reduced male smoking is certainly an important factor in the declining mortality rate for men since 1980. Smoking may have been one reason why life expectancy did not improve, or improved only little, among Swedish men in the 1960s and 1970s. The substantial difference between men's and women's smoking habits observed in the Statistics Sweden study of smoking behavior in the 1960s offers the strongest support for this hypothesis. Men smoked substantially more in the sixties and seventies than women do today, so smoking is not likely to have the same consequences for women's health (and mortality) as it had for men in the past, unless women are more vulnerable than men. Nathanson (1984) observes that smoking tends to increase the risk of mortality for men more than for women.

However, arguing against smoking as a general explanation for the gender gap in mortality lies in the fact that a mortality differential also exists between male and female non-smokers (Nathanson 1984). We should also examine which factors influence the probability of someone being a smoker. There is evidence that work-related stress and weak social support increase a person's likelihood of smoking, both in Sweden (Brännström 1993) and in the United States (Sorensen et al. 1985).

Higher *alcohol consumption* by men manifests itself primarily in deaths that can be directly linked to alcohol use, such as from cirrhosis of the liver.[11] There is significant excess mortality among men in the case of such deaths. Some accidents can also be linked to alcohol consumption (Skog 1986). Mortality from mental illnesses ('mental' column in Figure 9.4) is approximately three times as high for men as for women. This excess mortality is largely due to alcohol-related psychoses, alcoholism and alcohol abuse. Based on survey data, men in Sweden are about 2.5 times as likely as women to be heavy consumers of alcohol (FHI & CAN 1996:72). Alcohol probably continues to be of substantial significance, since countries with a high level of alcohol consumption (such as France) have a large gender gap in mortality (Pampel & Zimmer 1989; see Table 9.1).

Along with the level of consumption, drinking patterns are also important. Women's more moderate drinking may be beneficial, while immoderate ('male') drinking is probably harmful. What is moderate for men may differ from what is moderate for women, owing among other things to the sex difference in average body weight. For the period 1945–92 changes in alcohol consumption in Sweden were related to changes in excess male mortality, and the contribution of alcohol consumption to Swedish men's excess mortality was estimated to be even larger than the contribution from smoking in the most recent period, namely 15–20 percent (Hemström 1999a). The relationship was significant for changes in the excess male mortality from external causes and from 'other causes' (excluding ischemic heart disease). Thus, even though Sweden has relatively low levels of alcohol consumption, it seems nevertheless to be an important contributor to excess male mortality, and it certainly could help explain the absence of a drop in male mortality between 1960 and 1980.

In the United States it has been observed that women have somewhat healthier *eating habits* than men (Posner et al. 1993). The gender gap for being *overweight* appears to be small in Sweden (Kuskowska-Wolk and Bergström 1993a, 1993b). However, obesity[12] was more common among women than men in the late 1980s (9.1 percent for women versus 5.3 percent for men). On the other hand, it has been suggested that diets high in saturated fats may contribute more to health risks for men than for women due to interactive effects with sex hormones

(Waldron 1995). Retherford concluded in his 1975 study that diet and over-weight had no substantial significance for the gender differential in mortality. However, in view of more recent research it seems that diet generally, as a risk factor for ill health, may be particularly complex and difficult to evaluate from a gender perspective.

Retherford (1975) believed that men had reduced their *physical activity* levels more than women during this century, primarily due to changes in the work environment (towards more sedentary work). Unfortunately, he could not verify this hypothesis with available data. The Swedish study "Liv 90" showed the proportion of physically inactive individuals (20 percent of men and 10 percent of women) to be relatively constant throughout all age groups (Engström et al. 1993:157). This contradicts the assumption of some researchers that a higher percentage of women than men are physically inactive (see Verbrugge 1989).

How one interprets such research findings may depend on the level of activity being measured. Both going for walks and everyday kinds of exercise[13] were included as physical activity by Engström et al. in "Liv 90," which contained a thorough discussion of various types of activities. In her study of the United States, Verbrugge included only exercise requiring a quite high level of effort. "Liv 90" also showed exercise requiring considerable exertion[14] to be more common among men. This type of exercise is relatively uncommon among the population, nor is it necessarily the most beneficial exercise for one's health (Shaper & Wannamethee 1991). Women are more likely to pursue such activities as going for walks, a kind of exercise that is important from a health standpoint but which is frequently ignored when activity is studied. The fact that it is common for those men who do take exercise to exert themselves more than women do carries with it certain risks, such as sudden unexpected death (Drory et al. 1991).

Further problems arise with the measurement and definition of physical activity. When activity is defined, as it usually is, in terms of (planned) leisure-time exercise, this results in such a high prevalence of physical inactivity that the explanatory power of the 'risk factor' disappears. Regardless of these problems, the results of "Liv 90" indicate that physical inactivity may have been paid too little attention in past research on gender differences in mortality. In conclusion, it is possible that women's 'activity behavior' is, in fact, more beneficial for health than that of men.

It is generally well known that women seek medical care more frequently than men. It may be that women value health more highly than men do, and women may pay greater *attention to health issues.* Verbrugge (1989) observed that it was primarily for mild health problems that women sought medical treatment more often than men did. She points out that health attitudes are more alike than different for both men and women, and in the case of chronic and serious illnesses[15] there is no gender differential in the inclination to seek medical care. Results from a Scottish study on common cold symptoms found that women tended to underreport disease symptoms (Macintyre 1993). Some researchers argue that differences in seeking professional help for illness could contribute to corresponding differentials in mortality, for instance between men and women (Gove 1973; Vallin 1995). Others contend that medical science in general makes only a minor contribution to changes in population mortality rates (e.g. McKeown 1979). There seems thus to be contradictory evidence and ideas about the role of gender differences in the willingness or reluctance to seek medical attention and its impact on the gender gap in mortality.

However, it is assumed that women are more ready than men to accept advice on lifestyle changes to help prevent certain kinds of heart disease (Baker et al. 1993). Observations from a large-scale Swedish public-health project indicate that this is not true for all types of health-related preventive measures. Between 1985/86 and 1989/90 more women than men took up smoking (Brännström 1993). Nonetheless, Brännström demonstrates that women generally changed their health-related behavior (for example by improving their eating habits) more than men did during the study period. This observation gives some support to Baker and co-workers' hypothesis, but it remains unclear just how important such lack of compliance with positive behavior change may be for men's excess mortality overall.

When Sorensen et al. (1985), using an American sample, studied gender differences in certain kinds of behaviors and attitudes thought to be associated with cardiovascular disease, they found that men were more caught up in their work, impatient and overly competitive than women, while women reported more work-related stress than men. The behavior analyzed by Sorensen et al. can be classified as *Type-A behavior,* which is believed to facilitate the development of cardiovascular disease. Since Type-A behavior is more common among men, this may affect the gender differential in mortality (Waldron 1976, 1983b, 1991). However, it has been observed that Type-A personality may result in an even larger increase in mortality for women than for men (Wingard 1982), and excess male mortality has also been found among Type-B (opposite of Type-A) personalities. Type-A behavior is also linked to a person's labor-market position and social class. It is unusual among housewives but extremely common among women in managerial positions (Frankenhaeuser 1991; Nathanson 1984). The overall picture, then, is somewhat unclear with regard to Type-A behavior (see also Chapter 8).

Family and group-related factors

The hypotheses in this section focus on protective social factors rather than on direct causes of illness or death. Here an individual's family circumstances are important, but other sources of social support (relatives, friends and colleagues) may be more significant for the gender gap in mortality. American researchers, among others, have found that unmarried men have a relatively higher mortality rate than unmarried women (Gove 1973; Retherford 1975). The higher mortality of unmarried people in general has been explained primarily in terms of various selection mechanisms and protective factors provided by marriage. These selection mechanisms mean that people in poor health are more likely to be unmarried. Social integration and social support are seen as protective factors that are presumed to encourage a healthy lifestyle (Anson 1989; Umberson 1987). Men, to a greater extent than women, may be dependent on marriage as a source of social support. It can be argued that one of the reasons for single women's lower mortality (compared with that of single men) is their more extensive social networks, including more contacts with friends and relatives (Gove 1973; Nathanson 1984; Retherford 1975). This is hardly a controversial observation, but it is not certain that there is a substantially higher mortality risk for men than women among those who have never married or those who are no longer married.[16]

A large-scale longitudinal study analyzing the effect of changes in marital status, taking into account age and social circumstances, found small differences in the effect of such changes on men's and women's mortality (Hemström 1996). Widowers had a somewhat higher increase in mortality than widows, but the high mortality rate among divorced men was largely explained by the fact that they belonged to socio-economic groups with high mortality rates, were unemployed and/or rarely had children in their households. Moreover, men who were divorced (and remained divorced) had a mortality rate 76 percent higher than men who did not experience the breakup of their marriage, while divorced women (who remained divorced) had 70 percent higher mortality than women who remained married to the same person. Thus the remaining association between divorce and mortality does not diverge greatly between the sexes.

The social protection provided by children may have been underestimated in the past. Backet and Davison (1995) found that parenthood leads to certain changes in attitudes toward health. The 'health gains' of parenthood appear to be similar for men and women (Hemström 1996), but since relatively few men receive (or seek) custody of their children following a divorce or separation, and since single fathers are still unusual and atypical, certain gender differences still arise.

Therefore, it does not appear that gender-specific effects of marital status constitute the crucial factor in men's total excess mortality. First of all, a majority of both men and women are already married or living with a partner, and a hypothetical introduction of obligatory marriage would lead only to a marginal improvement in men's life expectancy relative to that of women (Retherford 1975). Moreover, the high mortality rate of divorced men is due to other factors, one of which is that women are more likely to have children in their household following divorce. Divorced fathers would likely live longer if they had more contact with their children.

Societal factors

Some social scientists have found links between certain general social changes and gender-specific mortality trends in Europe. There seems to have been a trend shift in gender-specific mortality along with the transition from an agricultural to an industrial society, and along with growing urbanization (Hart 1989). In Sweden, where industrialization was accompanied by a less dramatic urbanization process, the increasing gender differential appeared later than in such countries as England and Wales. Hart demonstrated that male and female mortality rates are more similar in rural than in urban areas. This seems to be true as well after the industrialization process was well under way. The author's own analyses of Swedish data from the 1980s show that the gender gap for mortality was greatest in large urban areas (Stockholm and Gothenburg).[17]

It is unclear what aspects of urbanization have had an adverse effect on men. It has been suggested that, in pace with modernization, men have adopted a lifestyle posing greater danger to their health (Nathanson 1984). Might migrating involve men in greater risks? We know that in modern Swedish society, young women are more likely than men to move to urban areas, while men are more likely to stay put (see, for example, Brännström 1993:10). There is also evidence that men who move from one place to another are more liable to have psychological difficulties than are women (Dryler 1993). Dryler suggests that moves are more stressful for men, particularly if they have weak social support. This may in turn affect their mortality risk. However, it does not seem likely that changes in urbanization were determining factors in men's relatively high mortality in the 1960s and 1970s, although there may be a link between urbanization and male consumer behaviors that could cause changes in excess male mortality (Hemström 1999a).

A common explanation for the increase in the gender gap in mortality in the recent century is *falling fertility* rates (Erikson 1987; Hart 1989). Over a long period this may be a significant factor. Countries with high fertility rates tend to have smaller gender differences in mortality than countries with low fertility rates (Ram 1993). However, lower birth rates and a reduction in maternal mortality are only marginal explanations for the striking improvement in women's longevity that has occurred in Sweden during the second half of the twentieth century. In 1952, for instance, there were only sixty-five deaths in Sweden from "pregnancy, childbirth or puerperalism" (Causes of Death 1952). However, there are other long-term consequences of bearing children. Beral (1985) found that among women in England and Wales who reached the age of forty-five, those who had not borne children had a longer average lifespan. If the decline in fertility does have an effect, then it is probably in the form of long-term consequences for women's health, affecting, for example, diseases of the circulatory organs. A significant relationship was found between changes in crude birth rate and changes in female mortality, but there was no corresponding association with changes in excess male mortality in Sweden (Hemström 1999a). Lower birth rates may have contributed to women's emancipation, since pregnancy and childbirth have been the foremost obstacle to women's labor force participation and economic independence.

Some researchers have looked to the *increase in female labor force participation* to explain the gender differential in mortality. One large-scale study conducted by Pampel and Zimmer (1989) found that the gender gap was larger in countries with a high level of education and employment for women than in countries where women were less likely to be employed. They viewed this as support for the so-called discrimination hypothesis: improvements in women's education, employment and professional status have a more favorable effect on their longevity than such improvements would have for men, since women have been subjected to various kinds of social discrimination in the past.

Researchers comparing the longevity of women employed outside the home and housewives have found that employed women have a lower mortality rate. This is true for Finland (Martikainen 1995), England and Wales (Weatherall et al. 1994) and Sweden (Vågerö & Lahelma 1998). But employment is not necessarily the reason for this striking result. Martikainen (1995), among others, argues for health-related selection—that the healthiest and most enterprising women move into the labor market. Vågerö and Lahelma (1998) concur, but they believe that not even a very extreme self-selection of healthy women can fully explain why employed women live longer, on average, than housewives. Since housewives have a higher mortality rate than women employed outside the home, some researchers view housework as a risk factor for poor health and premature death (Smith & Waitzman 1994). Housework may indeed be comparable to unemployment in this respect. It is suggested that labor-force participation offers greater opportunity for social support (Hibbard & Pope 1992). Housewives are more likely to be socially isolated.

Despite the findings of these studies, there are those, according to Waldron (1991), who link the recent narrowing of the gender gap in mortality with women's increased employment. These researchers believe that homemaking offers protection against mortality because it avoids risks posed by the workplace (the so-called protection hypothesis). In a period when the increase in Swedish women's employment was rapid (1970s), it was observed that the type of work that increased most among women was associated with low mortality (Hemström 1999b). When Nathanson (1995) analyzed the links between women's social position in various industrialized countries and their life expectancy in the 1970s and 1980s, she suggested that the association between women's social position and their life expectancy was largely determined by the rate of smoking among women in these countries. According to Nathanson, countries in which large numbers of women had long been in the labor force, and in which women were quite likely to be active in political life, also had a larger share of women smokers than countries in which the status of women had not improved to the same degree. Consequently, smoking has worked against the improvement in women's life expectancy in countries with a high level of gender equality (such as Sweden, Norway and Denmark) compared with those that have seen less progress toward equality (e.g., Japan and southern European countries). However, in Sweden lung cancer deaths are as common among women in full-time employment as among housewives (Vågerö & Lahelma 1998).

In conclusion, there is in general little support for the so-called protection hypothesis, which posits that women are protected by not taking part in gainful employment. In spite of the possibility that women might be expected to emulate a male risk-taking lifestyle as their participation in the labor market increases, increased employment may have considerably improved their life expectancy. However, there does not seem to be any strong association between changes in female labor-force participation and changes in excess male mortality, although perhaps changes in the wage gap between men and women have had some influence on excess male mortality (Hemström 1999a).

Occupation, work environment and class. Do men and women experience different kinds of social support at work? A Swedish study has found that unemployment leads to higher mortality rates for men than for women (Stefansson 1991). Stefansson's interpretation is that work status has a stronger effect on the social and psychological identity of men than of women. However, suicide and alcohol-related deaths among the unemployed did not completely explain excess mortality among long-term unemployed men. A number of other factors also provide more protection for women than for men against ill health and early death. Social support from friends may be such a factor, while men seem to be more dependent on work as a source of social support. Like the effect of marital status, the effect of unemployment on the overall gender gap in mortality is quite small, since most people in Sweden are already employed.

Some major demographic studies have shown that the longevity difference between social classes is larger for men than for women (Vallin 1995; Vågerö & Lundberg 1995). In the latter Swedish study, it was particularly striking that the mortality rate of nonmanual workers, both men and women, began a sharp decline in the beginning of the 1960s. In contrast, male manual workers experienced hardly any decline in their mortality rate. Male manual workers, particularly between the ages of 40 and 54, experienced only a very small improvement in life expectancy between the early 1960s and the mid-1980s, (Vågerö & Lundberg 1995).

An ecological analysis of the mortality differential between men and women in the United States showed socio-economic status to be the most significant factor (Park & Clifford 1989). Park and Clifford concluded that improved working conditions for certain groups of workers would result in a substantial reduction in deaths from cardiovascular disease for men but not for women. This might also hold for other causes of death. Men are much more exposed to physically risky work environments than women (Waldron 1991). In Sweden the occupational groups with the highest mortality rate are certain heavy-industry jobs usually held by men (Swedish Commission on Working Conditions 1990). The Swedish

Commission on Working Conditions estimated that 10 percent of coronary infarctions and a maximum of 5 percent of cancer cases were work-related. Waldron (1991) estimated that 5–10 percent of the mortality differential between men and women in the United States was accounted for by gender differences in the work environment.

The report from the Swedish Commission on Working Conditions (1990) indicates that blue-collar occupations with high mortality rates were found primarily in stagnant and outdated manufacturing industries. Certain male laborers may have slipped behind the rest of the working population (Vågerö & Lundberg 1995). However, it is unclear if it is solely due to work environment factors that social class differences are generally larger among men than among women. Most working conditions have improved across time, and the development has generally been towards fewer health risks at work (Theorell 1991).

An analysis of the role of some work-related factors for excess male mortality shows a clear picture: Swedish men's common experience of traditional male manufacturing work, and high levels of physical work hazards, did not contribute to men's excess in all-cause mortality or to their excess in ischemic heart disease mortality (Hemström 1999b). Given that women are more likely to have jobs with low status and low levels of work control and workplace social support (as compared with men) one should indeed be cautious in concluding that excess male mortality is due to the work environment (or to gender-specific relationships between social class and mortality). Generally, the increase in excess male mortality has been observed during a period when physical job hazards have been reduced (probably more so for men than for women). In sum, it seems clear that only a very small proportion of the gender gap is due to occupational or class differences between men and women (Vallin 1995). Furthermore, it is women who are disadvantaged on the labor market. We will provide some evidence for the latter proposition below.

For women, overall stress is less related to work itself than it is for men. It is rather the pressures of combining employment with home and family responsibilities, which generate more stress for women. Among individuals who work only a modest amount of overtime, women have a relatively higher risk of cardiovascular disease than men (Alfredsson & Theorell 1983). In general, women—particularly highly educated women—tend to experience more stress than men (Frankenhaeuser 1991; Koskinen & Martelin 1994). The social environment of the job can also be an important factor. Frankenhaeuser observed that low-level female white-collar employees received more social support from colleagues than did women in higher-level white-collar jobs. Theorell and Karasek (1989) suggest that women experience a higher proportion of work-related coronary infarctions than men do, perhaps because women have less control over their work (Hall 1989). Swedish women, too, have been experiencing increasing job stress. The number of women in high-strain occupations increased significantly between

1981 and 1991 (Szulkin & Tåhlin 1994). It is difficult to sort out the net effects of the larger increase in stress that women have experienced relative to men, especially when one considers the greater biological protection that women may have. It is not clear that these factors have resulted in a reduction in the advantage enjoyed by women when it comes to mortality from cardiovascular disease. We need to know more about the interactions of biological and social factors.

Socialization and roles are important for understanding the difference between men's and women's longevity, particularly when it is clear which underlying roles and behaviors lead to a given cause of death, such as accidents, suicide, cirrhosis of the liver and emphysema, all of which show higher mortality rates for men than for women (particularly among younger adults). According to Waldron (1976, 1991) this excess mortality stems from behaviors that are more readily accepted among men: use of weapons, alcohol consumption, smoking, acceptance of dangerous jobs, adventurous behavior and general risk-taking.

Recent decades have seen some changes in the social roles of men and women. Employment for women has become the norm in Sweden. Today there is a small difference in the labor-market participation of men and women. Swedish official statistics (Labor Force Survey 1999) show that in 1999, 70.9 percent of women and 74.8 percent of men (aged 16–64) were gainfully employed. Changes have also taken place in methods of coping with stress. Men are traditionally thought to handle psychosocial stress by consuming socially acceptable (for men) drugs such as alcohol or tobacco, while women have more frequently resorted to medication (Hart 1989; Waldron 1983b). The traditional male strategies seem more unhealthy. Men are more likely to choose these 'problem-solving strategies' because they are brought up to be independent, according to Stillion (1984). A need to be independent is one characteristic of the traditional male role. However, it has become more acceptable for women to use various stimulants like tobacco and (to a much lesser extent) alcohol as well, which is an important factor in the increase in rates of smoking and lung cancer among women in recent decades (Hart 1989; Qvist 1993). Thus, what is appropriate gender behavior changes over time.

The protection hypothesis, mentioned briefly above, assumes that gender roles will converge and that the risk of accidents, for example, will increase for women as their employment rate rises. Statistics presented above indicate that accidents and other violent deaths have declined in importance for men's overall mortality as well as for excess male mortality. Thus we can reject the hypothesis that men's lifestyles have become less healthy as urbanization has progressed. On the contrary, the male role in the industrialized countries has been marked by less risk-taking in the last decades, while violent deaths have increased somewhat among women. In Sweden, violent deaths fell by 23 percent for men and rose by 16 percent for women between 1952 and 1992. This period, then, has probably seen a certain convergence of roles and behaviors. There have been similar findings from Canada (Maxim & Keane 1992). Nevertheless, large gender differences remain. As Maxim and Keane have pointed out, gender roles have not so far converged to any great degree. Any such convergence seems to be most visible in mortality from motor-vehicle accidents and has had no noticeable effect on total mortality rates.

Discussion

What supports the view that biological and genetic factors cause the gender gap in mortality? The fact that today there is no excess female mortality in any industrialized country, nor has there been in Sweden or France, in the past 200 years (see Chapter 2; Pressat 1973), lends some weight to biological or genetic explanations. In countries where women do have a higher mortality rate than men, it is usually because women have fewer resources, less food and worse medical care than men. Such conditions have been observed where cultural traditions consistently favor men (Nathanson 1984). It appears that when social discrimination against women has become less pervasive, women have increased their life expectancy beyond that of men, indicating that women have a biological advantage in such societies. Certain researchers who have carefully studied social factors as well support the hypothesis that women have better biological protection than men (Gee & Veevers 1983; Wingard 1982). The question is how this accounts for the changes in the gender gap over the last half century. In the case of Sweden, it is difficult to explain the stagnation of men's life expectancy during the 1960s and 1970s solely to biological factors. A change in male lifestyle factors provides a better explanation. Such changes may affect certain biological conditions as well. Eating habits, for example, may affect body fat distribution and cholesterol levels, which influence men's mortality more than women's.

Neither biology nor the social environment need to be singled out as the primary factor in men's excess mortality. It is widely recognized that behavior and environmental factors interact with various biological components (e.g., Macintyre 1994; Waldron 1983a). A social scientist may find it tempting to dismiss biological factors, since mortality differences vary so much over time. But biological conditions also change in the short term, although not genetic factors. While it is difficult to determine just which biological factors protect women more than men, there seems to be agreement on certain ones—primarily female sex hormones and the ratio of HDL to LDL cholesterol. Since these affect the risk of cardiovascular disease, which is the most common cause of death among men over 45,[18] their effect on the gender gap could be quite substantial.

This does not mean, however, that men's higher mortality rates are due exclusively to biological conditions. Women's biological protection means that it takes more unhealthy behavior by women or worse social conditions for women's mortality rates to equal those of men's. Thus if conditions affecting women were to improve, this would probably increase the mortality gender gap rather than equalizing men's and women's mortality rates.

It should also be noted that some social conditions are unfavorable to female survival. This is true, for example, of the prognosis for certain diseases. Despite protective biological factors, cardiovascular diseases are also common among women and the risk of death after being hospitalized for ischemic heart disease is somewhat higher for women. Furthermore, in the 1980s the lethality[19] of these diseases during hospitalization declined in the United States more for men than for women (Demirovic et al. 1993). Men may receive better hospital care, perhaps because women with heart disease show different symptoms than men, so the disease may not be diagnosed as early in women.

Looking at possible social explanations for the gender gap, we see that certain behaviors and social conditions do indeed have an unfavorable effect on men's lifespan; furthermore, many of the social factors interact with one another (for instance, the likelihood of being a smoker and also physically inactive is greater for men than for women).

We will give three examples of the types of mechanisms stemming from the interactions of social and biological factors: (1) Poor eating habits, as well as smoking, carry with them a greater increase in risk of cardiovascular disease for men, since women are afforded some protection by their endogenic hormones and are less likely than men to gain excessive abdominal weight. (2) Gender-specific stressresponses are sometimes reported. Stress researchers have observed that men tend to secrete larger amounts of adrenaline in response to stress than women do (Frankenhaeuser 1991). (3) Gender-specific reactions have also been observed for competitive behavior and its effect on serum cholesterol levels: serum cholesterol levels rise for men but not for women (Sorensen et al. 1985). However, the type of effect given in the second example is not determined exclusively by biological factors. Female engineers, for example, showed the same level of adrenaline secretion as men (Frankenhaeuser 1991). Thus, particular social circumstances and socialization seem to play a role in at least some biophysical outcomes.

We observed at the beginning of this chapter that there were gender differences for all listed causes of death. Most studies have concentrated on men's higher mortality from accidents and ischemic heart disease. Smoking and men's 'risk-taking role' clearly dominate as primary explanations. These are powerful risk factors for poor health and mortality, and may offer some explanation for past gender differences in mortality. Statistics presented above, as well as an examination of how these two risk factors have changed over time, indicate that smoking may be an important reason for the lack of improvement in men's mortality rates in the 1960s and 1970s, as well as central in the decline in men's mortality that began in 1980. However, recent findings indicate that in Sweden at present, alcohol consumption probably contributes more to excess male mortality than smoking (Hemström 1999a). Male risk-taking in general has become less prevalent. Risk-taking can be viewed as a biological, hormone-related male characteristic, but it is also thought to be an effect of socialization (Parsons 1982). In fact, we can postulate that culture mediates and even (to some degree) controls the effect of hormones. Thus socialization towards the traditional male role, and corresponding lifestyle factors, appear to be important in men's higher mortality rates.

We pointed out that the life expectancy of male manual workers was stagnant in the 1960s and 70s, just when gender differentials in mortality increased most rapidly. The most obvious explanations for the lack of a decline in this group's mortality would seem to be smoking and alcohol consumption. However, the truth is probably more complicated, as risky behavior has underlying causes associated with a person's choices and social position. Material and social factors affect lifestyle and health (Whitehead 1992:336). Traditional male lifestyle features, such as drinking alcohol, in combination with increased material resources, may have been accentuated among male manual workers. It has been suggested that lifestyle factors may explain something of manual workers' excess mortality over nonmanual workers, as well as excess male mortality (Vallin, 1995). A rise in men's wages seems to have been accompanied by increased cigarette and alcohol consumption, which has been less common among women (until recently for cigarettes in some countries), even though women's wages have increased relatively more than men's. Thus, in the second half of the 20th century, economic growth has been more beneficial to women's survival than to men's survival (Hemström 1999a).

Some of these examples show how certain social conditions and behaviors interact with biological processes to cause excess male mortality. We can probably go on to discuss the fact that men have a higher mortality rate than women for almost all causes of death. It should be noted that men and women do not react in the same way to a given set of conditions and environmental risks. Men appear to be more vulnerable than women to social stresses affecting such things as biological resilience, growth during childhood and adolescence and mortality over the entire life cycle—despite the fact that women are still socially disadvantaged in a number of ways (such as in wages and work control). There may be changes in social factors over time, which interact with biological conditions. Biological characteristics can also be changed by social influences; this holds for such things as the onset of puberty, body height and weight, blood-pressure levels and physical condition. All of these result from a combination of social and genetic factors. This makes it difficult to draw conclusions as to the precise proportions of excess male mortality that is attributed to social, biological and genetic factors. We can conclude that, even if accepting that biogenetic factors are of significance for men's excess mortality, there are 'social ways' to affect this situation, for example by addressing traditional 'male' role patterns that involve risk-taking, coping with stress, physical inactivity, limited contact with children, consumer behavior and 'male lifestyles' in general. Positive social changes in Sweden with regard to such behaviors as smoking and risk-taking have led to a decline in the mortality gender gap. Since social improvements for women came to a partial halt in the 1980s, owing for example to increased work-related stress, we may expect further convergence of men's and women's mortality rates over the next few years.

Notes

1 The author would like to thank the participants in a seminar held on June 15, 1995 for valuable comments on an earlier version of this chapter, in particular Helen Dryler and Magnus Nermo. Denny Vågerö and the editors of this book have also contributed helpful suggestions. This paper was financed in part by the Bank of Sweden Tercentenary Foundation (Grant No. 92-0315:03) and the Swedish Council for Work Life Research (Grant No. 95-0419).

2 In relative terms (rate ratios by gender) the gap does not begin to narrow until 1987.

3 Accidents, poisonings, suicide and homicide. Last main section in the ICD (International Classification of Diseases) listing of causes of death (E800-E999).

4 This includes heart trouble in which the flow of blood to portions of the heart tissue is impeded by thrombosis (constriction of blood vessel/blood clot), causing an interruption in the supply of blood and oxygen to the affected portion of the heart. A cardiac infarction is the most common result in such cases.

5 There are three versions of ICD for the period under study, 1952–1992: ICD-7 1952–1968, ICD-8 1969–1986 and ICD-9 1987–1992. The most substantial change occurred between the 7th and 8th versions. Note that while the 7th version coded diseases in the cerebral blood vessels as diseases of the central nervous system, these diseases are found in the 8th and subsequent versions in a section on diseases of the circulatory organs.

6 Other factors, such as high blood pressure, involved approximately the same amount of risk for both men and women.

7 LDL=Low Density Lipoproteins: the type of cholesterol most closely associated with heart disease. HDL=High Density Lipoproteins: the "good" cholesterol that offers some protection against heart disease.

8 Stillborn babies as well as deaths within the first weeks of life.

9 Mortality of live births within the first year of life.

10 More than 25 cigarettes per day.

11 Cirrhosis of the liver, alcohol poisoning, alcohol-related psychoses, alcoholism and alcohol abuse.

12 Obesity was determined using the conventional measure of body weight composition, the Body Mass Index (BMI), which is calculated by weight/height squared. The Swedish study defined obesity as BMI>28.6 kg/m^2 for women and >30 kg/m^2 for men.

13 "Inactive" people in this context are those who "do not pursue a voluntarily selected type of exercise, nor carry out everyday exercise amounting to one hour per day" (Engström et al. 1993: 157). Everyday exercise might, for example, include taking the dog for a walk, cleaning house, walking to work, walking to the bus, etc.

14 A high level of exertion was subjectively determined by the individuals involved in the study, using criteria such as high pulse rate, sweating or shortness of breath while involved in a given type of exercise.

15 Illnesses more likely to be life-threatening, such as coronary infarction and cancer.

16 Through the death of a spouse or divorce. Divorce is the more common case.

17 The analyses were done using 1960, 1970 and 1980 population and housing data linked to the death registry for 1980–86. Cumulative deaths among people aged 20–84 were standardized using five-year age groups and the mean population in 1983. Population density was divided into ten equal groups according to the population within a thirty-kilometer radius from the home parish church.

18 According to Statistics Sweden's Causes of Death for 1992.

19 Mortality after diagnosis/discovery of a disease.

References

Alfredson L, Theorell T: *Job characteristics of occupations and myocardial infarction risk: Effect of possible confounding factors.* Social Science and Medicine 1983; 17: 1497–1503.

Anson O: *Marital status and women´s health revisited: The importance of a proximate adult.* Journal of Marriage and the Family 1989; 51: 185–94.

Backett KC, Davison C: *Lifecourse and lifestyle: The social and cultural location of health behaviours.* Social Science and Medicine 1995; 40: 629–38.

Baker D, Illsley R, Vågerö D: *Today or in the past? The origins of ischaemic heart disease.* Journal of Public Health Medicine 1993; 15: 243–8.

Beral V: *Long term effects of childbearing on health.* Journal of Epidemiology and Community Health 1985; 39: 343–6.

Brännström I: *Community participation and social patterning in cardiovascular disease intervention.* Umeå: Umeå University, Department of Epidemiology and Public Health, 1993. [Dissertation]

Cassel J: *The contribution of the social environment to host resistence.* American Journal of Epidemiology 1976; 104: 107–23.

[Causes of Death] *Dödsorsaker*: Stockholm: Statistics Sweden, annual reports 1945–92.

Demirovic J, Blackburn H, McGovern P, Sprafka JM, Doliszny K: *Sex differences in coronary heart disease mortality trends: The Minnesota Heart Survey, 1970–1988.* Epidemiology 1993; 4: 79–82.

Drory Y, Turetz Y, Hiss Y, Lev B, Fisman EZ, Pines A, Kramer MR: *Sudden unexpected death in persons <40 years of age.* The American Journal of Cardiology 1991; 68: 1388–92.

Dryler H: *Flyttningar, socialt stöd och psykisk ohälsa* [Moves, social support and psychological distress]. Sociologisk Forskning 1993; (4) 46–58. (Available in Swedish only).

Engström L-M, Ekblom B, Forsberg A, v Koch M, Seger J: *Liv 90. Rapport 1: Motionsvanor, fysisk prestationsförmåga och hälsotillstånd bland svenska kvinnor och män i åldrarna 20–65 år* [Liv 90. Report 1: Exercise habits, physical performance and health among Swedish women and men aged 20–65]. Stockholm: Folksam, Högskolan för lärarutbildning, Idrottshögskolan, Karolinska Institutet, Korpen, Riksidrottsförbundet, 1993. (Available in Swedish only).

Erikson R: *Disparities in mortality.* In Erikson R, Åberg R (Eds.): Welfare in transition: A survey of living conditions in Sweden 1968–1981. Oxford: Clarendon Press, 1987, pp. 43–58.

Fausto-Sterling A: *Myths of gender: Biological theories about women and men.* New York: Basic Books (second edition), 1992.

Ferembach D: *Sexe et adaptation au milieu* [Sex and environmental adaptation]. Recherche 1978; 9: 14–9. (Available in French only).

FHI, CAN: *Alkohol- och narkotikautvecklingen i Sverige* [Alcohol and drug trends in Sweden]. Stockholm: Folkhälsoinstitutet (FHI) and Centralförbundet för alkohol och narkotikaupplysning (CAN), Report No 4, 1996.

Frankenhaeuser M: *The psychobiology of sex differences as related to occupational status.* In Frankenhaeuser M, Lundberg U, Chesney M (Eds.): Women, work, and health. New York/London: Plenum Press, 1991, pp. 39–61.

Gee EM, Veevers JE: *Accelerating sex differentials in mortality: An analysis of contributing factors.* Social Biology 1983; 30: 75–85.

Gove WR: *Sex, marital status and mortality.* American Journal of Sociology 1973; 79: 45–67.

Hall EM: *Gender, work control, and stress: A theoretical discussion and an empirical test.* International Journal of Health Services 1989; 19: 725–45.

Hart N: *Sex gender and survival inequalities of life chances between European men and women.* In Fox J (Ed.): Health inequalities in European countries. Aldershot: Gower, 1989, pp. 109–41.

Hemström Ö: *Is marriage dissolution linked to differences in mortality risks for men and women?* Journal of Marriage and the Family 1996; 58: 366–78.

Hemström Ö: *Explaining differential rates of mortality decline for Swedish men and women: A time-series analysis, 1945–1992.* Social Science and Medicine, 1999a; 48: 1759–77.

Hemström Ö: *Does the work environment contribute to excess male mortality?* Social Science and Medicine, 1999b; 49: 879–94.

Hibbard JH, Pope CR: *Women's employment, social support, and mortality.* Women and Health 1992; 18: 119–33.

Janghorbani M, Hedley AJ, Jones RB, Zhianpour M, Gilmour WH: *Gender differentials in all-cause and cardiovascular disease mortality.* International Journal of Epidemiology 1993; 22: 1056–63.

Kalin MF, Zumoff B: *Sex hormones and coronary disease: A review of the clinical studies.* Steroids 1990; 55: 330–52.

Koskinen S, Martelin T: *Why are socioeconomic mortality differentials smaller among women than among men?* Social Science and Medicine 1994; 38: 1385–96.

Kuskowska-Wolk A, Bergström R: *Trends in body mass index and prevalence of obesity in Swedish men 1980–89.* Journal of Epidemiology and Community Health 1993a; 47: 103–8.

Kuskowska-Wolk A, Bergström R: *Trends in body mass index and prevalence of obesity in Swedish women 1980–89.* Journal of Epidemiology and Community Health 1993b; 47: 195–9.

[Labor Force Survey 1999] *Arbetskraftsundersökningen 1999.* Stockholm: Statistics Sweden, 2000. (English summary).

Larsson B, Bengtsson C, Björntorp P, Lapidus L, Sjöström L, Svärdsudd K, Tibblin G, Wedel H, Welin L, Wilhelmsen L: *Is abdominal body fat distribution a major explanation for the sex differences in the incidence of myocardial infarction?* American Journal of Epidemiology 1992; 135: 266–73.

Macintyre S: *Gender differences in the perceptions of common cold symptoms.* Social Science and Medicine 1993; 36: 15–20.

Macintyre S: *Understanding the social patterning of health: the role of the social sciences.* Journal of Public Health Medicine 1994; 16: 53–9.

Martikainen P: *Women's employment, marriage, motherhood and mortality: A test of the multiple role and role accumulation hypotheses.* Social Science and Medicine 1995; 40: 199–212.

Maxim PS, Keane C: *Gender, age, and the risk of violent death in Canada 1950–1986.* Canadian Review of Sociology and Anthropology 1992; 29: 329–45.

McKeown T: *The role of medicine.* Oxford: Basil Blackwell, 1979.

McKinlay JB: *Some contributions from the social system to gender inequalities in heart disease.* Journal of Health and Social Behavior 1996; 37: 1–26.

Modin B: *Uppväxt och skolbetyg: En uppföljning av barn födda på Akademiska sjukhuset 1915–1929* [Growing up and school reports: A follow-up on children born at Akademiska Hospital 1915–1929]. Socialmedicinsk Tidskrift 1998; (4): 190–7. (Available in Swedish only).

Nathanson CA: *Sex differences in mortality.* Annual Review of Sociology 1984; 10: 191–213.

Nathanson CA: *Mortality and the position of women in developed countries.* In: Lopez A, Caselli G, Valkonen T (Eds.): Adult mortality in developed countries. Oxford: Oxford University Press, 1995, pp. 135–57.

[National Public Health Report 1994] *Folkhälsorapport 1994.* Stockholm: Social-styrelsen, SoS Report 1994: 9.

Nystöm-Peck M, Vågerö D: *Adult body height and childhood socioeconomic group in the Swedish population.* Journal of Epidemiology and Community Health 1987; 41: 333–7.

Orth-Gomér K: *Varför ökar ischemisk hjärtsjukdom hos yngre svenska kvinnor?* [Why is ischemic heart disease increasing among younger Swedish women?] Läkartidningen 1992; 89 (21): 1861–2, 1867. (Available in Swedish only).

Ortmeyer LE: *Female's natural advantage? Or the unhealthy environment of males? The status of sex mortality differentials.* Women and Health 1979; 4: 121–33.

Östberg V: *Social structure and children's life chances: An analysis of child mortality in Sweden.* Stockholm: Swedish Institute for Social Research, 1996. [Dissertation]

Pampel FC, Zimmer C: *Female labour force activity and the sex differential in mortality: Comparisons across developed nations, 1950–1980.* European Journal of Population 1989; 5: 281–304.

Park KE, Clifford WB: *Sex differentials in cardiovascular mortality: An ecological analysis.* Social Science and Medicine 1989; 29: 869–76.

Parsons JE: *Biology, experience, and sex-dimorphic behaviors.* In Gove WR, Carpenter GR (Eds.): The fundamental connection between nature and nurture. Lexington, Massachusetts/Toronto: Lexington Books, 1982, pp. 137–70.

Posner BM, Cupples LA, Franz MM, Gagnon DR: *Diet and heart disease risk factors in adult men and women: The Framingham offspring-spouse nutrition studies.* International Journal of Epidemiology 1993; 22: 1014–25.

Pressat R: *Surmortalité biologique et surmortalité sociale* [Biological excess mortality and social excess mortality] Revue Francaise de Sociologie 1973; 14: 103–10. (Available in French only).

Qvist J: *Dödsorsak: Rökning* [Cause of death: Smoking]. Välfärdsbulletinen 1993; (2), 4–7. (Available in Swedish only).

Ram B: *Sex differences in mortality as a social indicator.* Social Indicators Research 1993; 29: 83–108.

Retherford RD: *The changing sex differential in mortality.* Westport, Connecticut: Greenwood Press, 1975.

Rogers RG, Powell GE: *Life expectancies of cigarette smokers and nonsmokers in the United States.* Social Science and Medicine 1991; 32: 1151–9.

Shaper AG, Wannamethee G: *Physical activity and ischemic heart disease in middle-aged British men.* British Heart Journal 1991; 66: 384–94.

Silman JS: *Why do women live longer and is it worth it?* British Medical Journal 1987; 294: 1311–2.

Skog O-J: *Trends in alcohol consumption and violent deaths.* British Journal of Addiction 1986; 81: 365–79.

Smith KR, Waitzman NJ: *Women, work and whether occupation matters: Differences in mortality by occupation in the U.S. 1971–1987.* Paper presented at the XIIIth Congress of Sociology, Research Committee 19, Session 10 (Health Inequalities, Class and Gender). Bielefeld, Germany, July 18–23, 1994.

Sorensen G, Pirie P, Folsom A, Luepker R, Jacobs D, Gillum R: *Sex differences in the relationship between work and health: The Minnesota Heart Survey.* Journal of Health and Social Behavior 1985; 26: 379–94.

Statistics Sweden: *Rökvanor i Sverige. En postenkätundersökning våren 1963* [Smoking habits in Sweden: A postal questionaire in spring 1963]. Stockholm: Statistics Sweden, 1965. (Available in Swedish only).

Stefansson C-G: *Long-term unemployment and mortality in Sweden 1980–1986.* Social Science and Medicine 1991; 32: 419–23.

Stillion JM: *Perspectives on the sex differential in death.* Death Education 1984; 8: 237–56.

Swedish Commission on Working Conditions: *A survey of jobs posing special risks to health.* Stockholm: Ministry of Labor, The Report of the Health Risks Study Group to the Swedish Commision on Working Conditions, 1990.

Szulkin R, Tåhlin M: *Arbetets utveckling* [The evolution of work]. In Fritzell J, Lundberg O (Eds.): Vardagens villkor. Levnadsförhållanden i Sverige under tre decennier. Stockholm: Brombergs, 1994, pp. 87–116. (Available in Swedish only).

Theorell T: *On cardiovascular health in women: Results from epidemiological and psychological studies in Sweden.* In Frankenhaeuser M, Lundberg U, Chesney M (Eds.): Women, work, and health. New York/London: Plenum Press, 1991, pp. 187–204.

Theorell T, Karasek R: *Kan vi minska antalet hjärtinfarkter genom att förbättra den psykosociala arbetsmiljön?* [Can we decrease the number of coronary infarctions by improving the psychosocial work environment?] Läkartidningen 1989; 86: 1455–6. (Available in Swedish only).

Umberson D: *Family status and health behaviors: Social control as a dimension of social integration.* Journal of Health and Social Behavior 1987; 28: 306–19.

Vågerö D, Lahelma E: *Women, work and mortality: An analysis of female labor participation.* In K. Orth-Gomér, M. Chesney and N. K. Wenger (Eds.), Women, stress and heart disease. Hillsdale, N. J.: Lawrence Erlbaum, 1998, pp. 73–85.

Vågerö D, Lundberg O: *Socio-economic mortality differentials among adults in Sweden.* In Lopez A, Caselli G, Valkonen T (Eds.): Adult mortality in developed countries. Oxford: Oxford University Press, 1995, pp. 223–42.

Valkonen T, Sihvonen A-P, Lahelma E: *Disability-free life expectancy by level of education in Finland.* In Mathers C, McCallum J, Robine J-M (Eds.): Advances in health expectancies: Proceedings of the 7th meeting of the international network on health expectancy (REVES), Canberra, February 1994. Canberra: Australian Institute of Health and Welfare, 1994, pp. 160–8.

Valkonen T, van Poppel F: *The contribution of smoking to sex differences in life expectancy: Four Nordic countries and The Netherlands 1970–89.* European Journal of Public Health 1997; 7: 302–10.

Vallin J: *Can sex differentials in mortality be explained by socio-economic mortality differentials?* In Lopez A, Caselli G, Valkonen T (Eds.): Adult mortality in developed countries. Oxford: Oxford University Press, 1995, pp. 179–200.

Verbrugge LM: *The twain meet: Empirical explanations of sex differences in health and mortality.* Journal of Health and Social Behavior 1989; 30: 282–304.

Waldron I: *Why do women live longer than men?* Social Science and Medicine 1976; 10: 349–62.

Waldron I: *Sex differences in human mortality: The role of genetic factors.* Social Science and Medicine 1983a; 17: 321–33.

Waldron I: *Sex differences in illness incidence, prognosis and mortality: Issues and evidence.* Social Science and Medicine 1983b; 17: 1107–23.

Waldron I: *Effects of labor force participation on sex differences in mortality and morbidity.* In Frankenhaeuser M, Lundberg U, Chesney M (Eds.): Women, work, and health. New York/London: Plenum Press, 1991, pp. 17–38.

Waldron I: *Recent trends in sex mortality ratios for adults in developed countries.* Social Science and Medicine 1993; 36: 451–62.

Waldron I: *Contributions of biological and behavioural factors to changing sex differences in ischaemic heart disease mortality.* In: Lopez A, Caselli G, Valkonen T (Eds.): Adult mortality in developed countries. Oxford: Oxford University Press, 1995, pp. 161–78.

Weatherall R, Joshi H, Macran S: *Double burden or double blessing? Employment, motherhood and mortality in the longitudinal study of England and Wales.* Social Science and Medicine 1994; 38: 285–97.

Whitehead, M: *The health divide.* In: Inequalities in health: The Black report and the health divide. England: Penguin Books, 1992, pp. 215–400.

Wingard D: *The sex differential in mortality rates: Demographic and behavioral factors.* American Journal of Epidemiology 1982; 115: 205–16.

10

Two sets of responsibilities: Weaknesses and strengths in women's history

Ann-Sofie Ohlander

On Tuesday, July 29, 1934, three women, Catrina Andersdotter, Catrina Lars-dotter and Anna Andersdotter, were drilling a hole in the Nya Kärrgruvan mine in Striberg, to be used for explosives. One of them held and turned the drill, while the other two took turns pounding on it. When the drill bits had become dull and were in need of sharpening, the women sent them to the surface, but the con-tainer broke, fell 22 meters to the bottom of the mine and struck Catrina Ander-sdotter in the spine, below the shoulders. The two other women splashed water on her to revive her, but soon blood was coming out of her nose, mouth and ears. When they loosened her clothing, they found bluish-red marks where she had been struck. There was nothing more they could do, and her lifeless body was hoisted up out of the shaft.

"Women have long been accustomed to working in the forestry and mining industries," wrote a mine foreman in the 1820s. According to his report, there were 628 miners in the Nora mining district in 1826, at least two-thirds of whom were women. There are reports from as far back as the seventeenth century of women who were injured or killed working in the mines. It was common until the mid-nineteenth century for women to work as miners.

According to a study of one particular mine, female miners were usually mar-ried and working with their husbands. But what about their children? Pregnancy was no obstacle to working in the mines. A report from a country doctor in 1835 observed that "female miners continue to work in the mine until their labor pains begin, then they climb up 50, 60, 90 fathoms on ladders, give birth to the child at the entrance to the mine, and then carry the child home, a distance of perhaps two or three miles, where they remain, more for the sake of custom than neces-sity, until they are readmitted into the social community of the church. For these women, a midwife would just mean unnecessary expense."

But how could these women care for their children and work in the mines at the same time? Sometimes they could take their children along. Older children could work alongside their parents, but what about the younger ones? Employers did not want infants in the mines. According to the Pershyttе mining law, female miners were not permitted to take "babes in arms" or other children who required supervision along with them to work, and were fined for doing so. These children had to be left without supervision while their mothers were working, or perhaps left in the care of an older relative. Fathers, at any rate, do not seem to have assumed any responsibility for their children.

After work, female miners had to tend to their household responsibilities. In 1825, a mine foreman wrote: "Weary from working hard at a job that is utterly inappropriate for a woman, she returns home, dejected at the thought of the unfinished work that awaits her there. . . Instead of coming home to a comfortable, warm dwelling and a frugal but healthy meal, her husband finds that he has exchanged the damp chill of the mine for the stuffy air of a closed-up hut and is served a meal that his wife has prepared with no thought other than to satisfy their hunger and, finally, to rest."

The mine foreman's sympathy is with the husband, although he is not the one burdened with the responsibilities of both work and household. His wife, in contrast, is expected to work in the mine as well as to bear sole responsibility for her children and household.

The myth of the housewife

But didn't female mining workers have an exceptionally hard lot? Was it really common in earlier times for women to have production jobs as well as to assume all responsibility for household and children?

We may have the impression that it was not until the 1960s that large numbers of women entered the labor market. Before that time, it seems, they were housewives, perhaps working outside the home for a few years before marrying. At any rate, many people think that was the way it was.

This view, however, is false. As far back as we can follow Swedish history, women have worked in production jobs. They have worked hard and long hours, and made a major contribution to the country's economy. The overwhelming majority of women worked on farms.

Women's work in farming

In 1850 there were three-and-a-half million people living in Sweden. Nearly all of them, ninety percent, lived in rural areas, and before then the percentage was even higher. Agriculture was by far the major industry. Accordingly, nearly all women were involved in farming, whether as farmers' wives, tenant farmers or farmhands. Unmarried women worked as maids. There was a clear delineation between the work of men and women, and it is a simple matter to identify what was women's work.

Women were responsible for all aspects of dairy production. They tended the grain and took care of the barns, while men were in charge of the stables and horses. The women also took care of smaller animals, such as sheep, pigs, goats and hens. They milked the cows, churned the butter and made the cheese. In many parts of the country the women spent the entire summer in the mountains, taking care of the animals.

The dairy industry was a central part of the country's economy, with butter long one of Sweden's most important exports. Starting in the mid-nineteenth century, dairy production began to undergo industrialization. It was almost exclusively women who worked in the dairies. At the end of the nineteenth century, dairy products made up the third largest group of export goods in Sweden, after lumber and iron. It was not until the 1930s that men entered the dairy industry in a serious way.

Women also worked in other aspects of agriculture. They raked hay and bound the sheaves at harvest time. Before scythes came into use in the nineteenth century, workers used a sickle for harvesting grain, and it was common for women to cut as well as bundle the grain. Women weeded the beets and turnips, and planted and harvested potatoes.

In an interview shortly after the turn of the twentieth century, a maid described the constant work expected of her. First she helped with the harvest in the fields. Then she had to help cook dinner and wash the dishes, as well as tending to the animals in the barn and doing the midday milking. Men could take a break at noon and were not expected to do indoor chores in the evenings, she said, but women were never off duty.

"Gored by an animal" is one cause of death listed in long-ago Swedish statistics. However, owing to a lack of related research we know little about other types of accidents and work injuries related to farming. We can assume that injuries related to overwork must have been common. Such cases were probably included under the heading "gout and podagra, joint pain or rheumatism," among the causes of death listed for the years 1811–1820. There was little security for people who were old and worn out. Children were required to provide for their parents, who were often granted certain privileges, called "undantag," in their old age. This meant that they had the right to a place to live, some land and a portion of the farm harvest. Disputes regarding these privileges were common.

Maids were dependent on the generosity of their employers; otherwise the relief services for the poor had to assume responsibility for them. Each parish was divided into districts, and each district was required to take care of its poor people, which sometimes meant that these people had to move from farm to farm. Poorhouses were built later on, which were characterized by a lack of human warmth or even the bare necessities of life. The great majority of paupers were women, both in the cities and in rural areas—in part because women lived longer than men did, but also because they lacked the opportunities men had to make a living and provide for their own security in sickness and old age. As a rule, a maid earned only half as much as a farmhand did.

Working with fabric and clothing

Women were also responsible for the manufacture of yarn, fabric and clothing, from tending the sheep to producing the finished cloth and sewing the clothing.

Every girl had to learn how to spin. All of the yarn in Sweden was spun by women on a spinning wheel. Women were supposed to use every free moment to work on their spinning. In addition, they wove all the fabrics.

An example from Iceland shows just how important the manufacture of cloth used to be. Long ago, in the twelfth and thirteenth centuries, there was no money in Iceland. Instead, people measured value in terms of their most valuable possession—homespun cloth. This was the only standard of value, or "currency," and all of it was produced by women. Indeed, the sails of the Viking ships were woven by women.

In addition, flax production and the weaving of linen cloth were largely women's work. Women sewed clothing for their families, and when fabrics wore out and turned to rags, they were used to make paper. Without the introduction of the spinning wheel in Europe in the tenth century, women would not have been able to produce as much cloth as they did, and perhaps the art of printing would not have been invented at the end of the fifteenth century. Rags were the most important raw material for making paper up to the nineteenth century, when wood pulp began to be used instead. Women worked in paper mills as well.

Housewives helped with their husbands' work, and widows assumed responsibility after their husbands died

Until 1846, women were officially excluded from trades, commerce and citizenship, which were reserved exclusively for men. Nor were women allowed to hold government or other public offices.

Nevertheless, women were involved in these matters. When women were widowed, they frequently carried on their husbands' work. Widows in earlier times were allowed to become citizens and continue their husbands' businesses, since most women had been already quite involved in their husbands' trade or business. It was not until their husbands died that the work that women had already been doing was recognized.

Women worked side by side with their husbands in the mines, and this was true in the ironworks as well. In the seventeenth and eighteenth centuries, forges were run by a blacksmith with the help of his family, with the blacksmith and his wife working together at the anvil. Women also performed other demanding jobs, such as hauling pig iron, and they often helped their husbands to sell the iron. When a blacksmith died, his widow—and sometimes his daughters as well—were capable of continuing the work of the smithy.

Strong women

Visitors from the upper classes who came to the ironworks perceived the women who worked there as big and coarse. Indeed, this was the feminine ideal in farming and other kinds of physical labor. A woman was supposed to be big, strong and capable of working hard. Dairymaids and midwives had long been known for such characteristics.

A researcher on women's issues has contrasted that robust feminine ideal with the "white-collar ideal" of a thin woman mincing along on high heels, an upper-class ideal that gradually took hold in other parts of society as well.

Women as postmistresses, blacksmiths and constables

In other cases, too, widows were allowed to take over after the death of their husbands. When the Swedish post office was established in the 1630s, its jobs were reserved for men only. However, many widows succeeded their husbands in their capacity as postmasters, and in two cases—national postmistresses Gese Wechel and Margareta Beijer—women even headed the Swedish postal service.

Starting in 1722, however, widows were no longer permitted to succeed their deceased husbands. It was viewed as inappropriate for women to ride the horses of the postal service, and women were not considered strong enough to handle the exhausting transport work. This limited widows' opportunities to earn a living even more. It was not until the 1860s that women were again permitted to work for the post office, as postal clerks. Even then, however, there was opposition from those who claimed women lacked the necessary strength—that they were too weak to stamp several copies at a time.

In earlier times, Swedish women were denied certain rights. For example, they were not permitted to represent themselves in a court of law, and their testimony as witnesses was generally disregarded. So it is surprising to learn that two women served as constables in Finland in the seventeenth century. One of them, Karin Thomasdotter of Pargas, was the head of the constabulary for forty years. It is said that her appearances at court showed a remarkable degree of authority.

Teachers of Christian doctrine

It may also seem surprising that women not only were able to read as well as men, but also that they had significantly greater knowledge than men of the main tenets of the Christian faith, according to priests' records. This has been shown by researchers studying literacy and knowledge of Christianity among the Dalarna population of the seventeenth century. This apparently stems from the fact that women were the ones who taught children to read and instructed them in the basic Christian texts in preparation for the priests' home visits during which household members were questioned about church teachings.

Female entrepreneurs

Women were not officially authorized to conduct business, although an exception was made for widows. A few other exceptions were made as well: Women in cities were frequently allowed to run an inn, and very poor women were granted permission to support themselves by selling brandy.

Other women obtained permission to sell goods from a stand or cart, or at the market. They were allowed to sell odds and ends like kerchiefs or buttons as well as to make and sell sweets. Women from Dalarna went to Stockholm to work in stearin factories or as assistants in construction. They also made and sold intricate jewelry out of human hair.

After laws establishing greater freedom of trades were passed in 1846 and 1864, women were allowed to start their own businesses, often small enterprises like dairies, haberdasheries, bakeries and women's beauty shops. The 1940s saw the largest number of female entrepreneurs.

Women and the industrial revolution

Early on, women were involved in industrial work at ironworks, paper mills and glassworks. The textile industry was largely built on the efforts of women and children, both at home and in factories. In the 1840s, more than half of the workers in the textile industry were women and children. Women also worked in the lumber industry and in match factories, they rolled cigars for the tobacco industry, and they threw pots and glazed china for the porcelain industry.

Industrial work was hard and hazardous to workers' health, and the hours were long. Dust was a problem in the textile industry. In addition, the threat of tuberculosis was spread through work routines, particularly among weavers. "Shuttle kissing" was the term used to describe a weaver sucking the thread through the weaving reed, which helped to spread tuberculosis. In 1911 a female textile worker wrote to her foreman requesting her own loom, because she did not want other workers to touch her shuttle: "Lotta is the only one who wants to teach (others how to do it), but she needs new shuttles, since the boy she was teaching has already died of consumption. . ."

There was no provision for child care, so women had no choice but to take their children with them and expose them to the dangerous environment of the factory, or else to leave them home alone or in the care of relatives. Older children often had to watch their younger siblings. Women generally bore sole responsibility for their household and children. Here, too, men were not involved: "It would be almost embarrassing for a man to go to the well to fetch water. That was something his wife was supposed to do . . . It would never occur to a man to go and shake out the rugs. It would be beneath his dignity." However, men could tend to the potato patch and cut wood for the household.

Women and children also worked with hazardous materials in tobacco and match factories. The phosphorus used for dipping matches was dangerous, and not only at the factory. At the turn of the century, there was a dramatic increase in the number of women's suicides by phosphorus poisoning. Gradually these figures have been corrected—these women were not trying to take their own lives, but to induce an abortion.

Responsibility for food

Throughout the centuries, women have also been responsible for all aspects of food storage and preparation. It was up to women to make sure that their families were fed when there was a shortage of grain for flour. When the price of bread went up or when the potatoes ran out, women took action. They held protest meetings, started hunger riots and even fomented revolution. During the French Revolution of 1789, protesting women left Paris for the king's palace in Versailles and forced the royal family to return with them to Paris. Female textile workers, protesting the high price of bread, started the Russian Revolution in 1917. That same year, Swedish women took part in riots triggered by a potato shortage in Stockholm.

Women did the washing, cleaning and housekeeping. They washed their laundry in lakes or streams, even in the cold of winter. Scrubbing laundry on a bridge over ice-covered water cannot have been beneficial to women's health.

In addition to all these responsibilities, women had to care for their children. Families were large, and deliveries were dangerous, resulting in many women's deaths. Danger to the child was great as well. In 1800, twenty percent of Swedish children died before reaching their first birthday. Average life expectancy at birth was low—in 1800 it was 36 years for women and 34 for men. This was largely because of the high rate of infant mortality, but deaths of young adults were also more common at that time than they are now, meaning heightened insecurity for everyone. It was common for a child to lose one or both parents before reaching adulthood.

Because of high mortality rates among adults, remarriage was common. Low average life expectancy and late marriage made it uncommon for grandparents to be involved in the upbringing of their grandchildren, or, indeed, for children to know their grandparents at all.

Women took on men's work

Thus even under normal circumstances, women's production work played an essential and indispensable role in European and Swedish history. Under abnormal circumstances, for example during the frequent wars that were waged, their contributions were even greater, as large numbers of women stepped in and took over men's responsibilities.

In the seventeenth century, when the young, able-bodied men were called up to serve as soldiers in the Thirty Years' War, women assumed the jobs they left behind. A study of the consequences of conscription in the Norrland parish of Bygdeå shows that these women managed to keep agricultural production going, although nearly all able-bodied men had gone off to fight in the war. Per-capita productivity increased while women were in charge.

During other wars as well, women assumed men's work responsibilities. This was a widespread phenomenon during World Wars I and II, particularly in the countries actively engaged in hostilities. One result of women's contributions during wartime was that universal suffrage was established in the European countries—in most of Northern Europe following World War I, and in Southern Europe at the end of World War II.

The first European countries to introduce universal suffrage were in Scandinavia: Finland in 1906 and Norway in 1913. In Finland, women had been active in the early years of the twentieth century in the fight against Russian influence. In Norway, women had called for the dissolution of Norway's union with Sweden in a nationwide petition drive undertaken in 1905. Some women obtained the right to vote in Norway in 1907, and suffrage was granted to all Norwegian women in 1913.

There were other circumstances, too, in which women took over the occupations formerly held by men. Men were absent for reasons other than war. Particularly in the nineteenth century, work-related migration was common. Men went to work in sawmills in Norrland, while their families stayed home. During the great migration waves to America in the nineteenth century, men frequently emigrated by themselves or ahead of their families. In some years, 20,000 more married men than married women emigrated from Sweden. In such cases as well, married women were the sole provider for their families, and in addition they frequently took over their husbands' work duties.

A study from Österbotten, in Finland, at the end of the nineteenth century showed a very high infant-mortality rate, with nearly one in two infants dying during the first year of life. This was because women were not breastfeeding their babies, which, in turn, was due to the fact that women had taken on men's work on the farms. In Österbotten, men were engaged in tar production, seal hunting and sailing, occupations that required them to be away from home for long periods. So women took care of all the farming responsibilities themselves—they plowed, sowed, harvested, dug ditches and burned woodland. They could not take their children along while they were working, so babies were not breastfed, which increased their vulnerability to infectious diseases. Since breastfeeding has a certain contraceptive effect, fewer women nursing their children also meant a higher birth rate. The strain on women's health must have been substantial.

However, they evidently did well at their jobs. Then, during the twentieth century, men stopped pursuing second jobs and stayed home again. Nevertheless, women continued for some time to be involved in all types of work related to both agriculture and forestry.

It has already been pointed out that widows frequently entered occupations otherwise reserved for men. The picture is clear: When men were unable to carry out their jobs, for whatever reasons, women stepped in. Women's areas of social activity and their competence throughout history stand out as extremely wide-ranging, encompassing practically every conceivable type of work or occupation.

. . . but men did not take on women's work

What about men? Did they, in turn, start doing women's work?

The answer seems to be no. It was considered shameful for a man to do a woman's work, such as taking care of the cattle or working in milk production. They preferred not to set foot in the barn. Perhaps a tramp or vagabond could be asked to milk the cows or churn the butter.

Writing home, a farmhand who emigrated from Sweden to America in the nineteenth century described the strange conditions he found in his new home: "In this country, it is men who tend to the barns and do the milking," he wrote, adding, "but don't tell anyone at home, or people will talk!"

It was not until milking machines were introduced and milk production was taken over by dairies that work in the dairy industry was considered acceptable for men.

Nor were taking care of the household and preparing meals considered suitable for men. In Icelandic sagas, for instance, men who did such work were held up to ridicule. Moreover, it was not only women's production work that men could not see themselves doing. They did not feed or care for young children, so women were responsible for child care until children were old enough to start working on their own.

There were grave consequences to this "one-parent system," as is distressingly clear when we look at a study of 226 prisoners in Västernorrland during the nineteenth century. The study followed these prisoners from an early age, and shows quite persuasively how the impoverished and miserable circumstances of their childhood put them on a path of criminal activity. No fewer than 40 percent of the men and 60 percent of the women had lost one or both parents before turning sixteen. If it was the father who had died, the mother nearly always managed to keep the family together and provide for her children, even in conditions of extreme poverty and hardship. However, if the mother died, the family usually broke up immediately, with the children cared for by the parish or left in some other less than satisfactory situation. This was true even though fathers were generally in a better financial and legal position than mothers.

The mother's life and that of her child were virtually inextricable from each other. This is borne out by a study of maternal deaths in childbirth in Sweden between 1750 and 1950, which also looked at what happened to the children of a mother who died in childbirth, both the newborn and older siblings. In the past, children under five who lost their mother were at great risk of dying themselves. In other words, a mother was absolutely essential to the lives of small children. If she died, her children died as well. Only quite recently has it become common and acceptable for fathers to care for their small children.

Women, then, assumed men's jobs and responsibilities in society when their help was needed. *But men did not take over women's responsibilities.* Thus women's areas of responsibility and competence were considerably more extensive than men's.

From powerlessness to influence

Throughout history, women's double burden and women's responsibility for all aspects of life have been the rule rather than the exception, and surely this is a familiar picture today as well. How have women's work and women's position in society changed up to the present?

Women have always worked extremely hard, but they have had little control over basic conditions in their lives. Children were always dependent primarily on their mothers, and as long as women were powerless, the position of children, too, was a vulnerable one. There are clear indications that women's position gradually deteriorated between the seventeenth century and the beginning of the nineteenth century. Since that time, however, trends have been more favorable.

Improved conditions: Single women

Equal inheritance rights for women and men were established in 1845. Up to that time, women in rural areas inherited only half of what men received. Compulsory guild membership was abolished the following year. Working at a trade or business was now possible also for women, as well as for men who were not guild members. In 1864, a liberal law on trade freedom was passed, making it easier for women to start their own businesses. In 1858, single women had also been given full legal rights as of the age of 25.

These developments primarily benefited unmarried women, whose plight had also triggered many of these improvements. The percentage of single women had increased so much by the mid-nineteenth century that supporting them posed a problem for their male relatives. Accordingly, men began to demand from parliament more rights and better support for their unmarried female relatives. At the same time, feminists like Fredrika Bremer stepped forward to demand civil rights for women.

The newly-established freedom to pursue a trade gave women the opportunity to start their own small businesses, such as shops or dressmaking businesses. Some women established larger-scale enterprises. The industrialization that began in Sweden in earnest in the 1870s offered many women the opportunity to make a living, even if their wages were generally lower than men's.

There were also improved opportunities for education and training. New kinds of jobs were introduced, for both men and women. In 1842, primary schools were established throughout the country for all boys and girls.

Not long after the primary schools were opened, women were allowed to become teachers. In 1859 the first teachers' college for women was founded, and by the end of the century, nearly half of all primary school teachers were women.

By that time women had also gained admission to higher education, either at a newly-established women's teachers' college or at the universities, which had opened their doors to women in 1873. However, women were not permitted to hold high-level government positions until 1923.

Since women did not gain access to public secondary schools until 1927, only a small number of women were actually able to pursue a college education. Many of those who did go to college became teachers at private schools or physicians in private practice. Some also opened their own schools and clinics.

Midwifery has been a women's occupation for centuries. As early as the beginning of the eighteenth century, formal training was offered for midwives. The first nurses were trained in the mid-nineteenth century, and nursing became an important female-dominated occupation. Starting in the 1920s, advanced training for district nurses was made available. These nurses had a great deal of autonomy and were important pioneers in the field of preventive health care in Sweden. Women also worked as assistant nurses, for a long time without receiving any formal training.

Other service jobs also began to accept women. Women were allowed to work as post-office clerks and as telephone and telegraph operators, and they were hired by banks and as office workers.

While women with advanced training and high-level positions were rare, such individuals played an important role in establishing feminist groups and calling for political influence and other progress for women.

The overwhelming majority of middle-class employed women were unmarried. Except for primary-school teachers, district nurses and midwives, marriage still, for a long time, meant leaving the job world. Many women made a conscious decision not to marry so that they would be able to pursue a career. In 1938, a law was passed prohibiting employers from firing women who chose to marry.

Unmarried women, however, were often given equal treatment relative to men, although they were usually assigned lower-level jobs and paid less.

Improved conditions: Married women

Married women had to wait longer to achieve official equality with men. However, all women were covered by the new law governing inheritances, and women at all levels of society attended the new schools that had been established.

Toward the end of the nineteenth century, some working-class people in Stockholm were living together without benefit of marriage. These "Stockholm marriages" may have resulted from the fact that marriage meant the loss of women's legal rights and control over their income and their children.

The plebiscite held in 1922 on the issue of banning alcohol highlighted the conflicts that sometimes arose over how family income should be spent. As many as 60 percent of women, compared with only 40 percent of men, voted in favor of prohibiting the dispensing and sale of alcohol. In the working-class neighborhoods of Gävle, 90 percent of women voted for prohibition. Far more women than men joined the new temperance movement that was founded in the late nineteenth century.

The relative lack of rights permitted to married women became more apparent as the position of single women improved. In 1874, married women were given the authority to make decisions regarding their income, and ten years later they were given control of their property as well. Full legal rights were granted to married women in 1920.

Married women's work outside the home

Long before then, however, many married women had begun to gain new visibility and recognition as a result of their work outside the home. While middle- and upper-class women did not generally work outside the home after marriage, working-class women did, and their work in the factories was essential to their family income. Indeed, many of these women brought home their family's only paycheck.

Married female blue-collar workers had jobs that were recognized outside the home and were listed independently in the wage lists, so their production work was an indisputable fact that was included in the new labor statistics that were being kept. Here they differed from farmers' wives, for example, whose vital contribution to the economy was not reflected in Swedish labor statistics until 1965.

With women working away from home, the unacceptable aspects of their circumstances and those of their children gradually became more obvious. Finally, there was some recognition of the conflict in society between production and reproduction, between making a living and parental responsibilities, a conflict that had hitherto been an unspoken part of women's lives. Finally, women's work caring for their children was recognized as a job of social importance. The first sign of this recognition was a worker-protection law passed in 1900, establishing the right of married women employed in industrial jobs to take one month off work following childbirth. There was no provision for financial compensation during this period, however, which made it irrelevant to many women, since their families could not get by without their wages. A long political battle was fought over this issue, and it was not until 1931 that the first maternal insurance system was introduced in Sweden, after Swedish women had gained access to power and were able to use the political process to improve their own circumstances and those of their children.

Women gain political power

After World War I, all Swedish women were granted civil rights that put them on an equal footing with men. Unmarried Swedish women had enjoyed legal rights since 1858, but it was not until 1920 that married women gained full legal control over their property and the right to represent themselves in court. However, men were regarded as the head of the family until 1950, when both parents were given equal responsibility for and authority over their children.

In 1919, all Swedish women were given the right to vote in elections to city and county councils, as well as to be elected to those bodies. In 1921 this was expanded to include elections to the Swedish parliament. Two years later a law was passed permitting women to serve in nearly all high-level governmental positions. Resistance to women's participation was particularly strong in the church, and women were not permitted to join the clergy until 1958.

In 1927, as noted above, new educational opportunities opened up for girls as they were admitted to state-run secondary schools. At that time corporal punishment was also abolished in secondary schools.

The role of female politicians

The first elections to the Swedish parliament after the introduction of universal suffrage were held in 1921. There were only five female members at first, two Social Democrats, one Liberal, one Conservative and one, labor inspector Kerstin Hesselgren, who was elected with both Liberal and Social-Democratic votes. Kerstin Hesselgren was one of 150 members of the First Chamber, while the other women made up four out of a total of 230 in the Second Chamber.

Even before then, women had formed their own organizations within the political parties. At roughly the same time that they were granted the vote, they established nationwide women's associations. These associations played an important role in addressing current political issues and offering support to their respective parties' female members of parliament.

Throughout the years between the World War I and World War II, there were very few women in parliament, and it was not until the 1950s that women made up more than ten percent of parliament's members. The first female cabinet member, the economist Karin Kock, was not appointed until 1947. Although these women were few in number, their contributions were substantial.

Like male politicians, these women were interested in traditional political issues. However, they also added a new perspective. The first women politicians brought with them into political life specifically female areas of responsibility and experience. Issues related to the rights and needs of both women and children now took on political weight.

Kerstin Hesselgren's first parliamentary speech proposed an increase in midwives' wages. Along with the other female members of parliament, she also introduced a number of bills dealing with labor issues, notably the wages and hiring of women in state jobs. The Social Democrat Agda Östlund raised the issue of hiring conditions for cleaning women in governmental departments and offices. She also submitted a bill to improve obstetrical and newborn care and addressed the problem of domestic abuse of women.

Throughout the decades, female politicians fought tenaciously to improve the conditions affecting women and children. The importance of their efforts in bettering the position of Swedish women can hardly be overstated. During the 1970s, the number of female members of parliament rose to over twenty percent, and women regularly held important offices in government. In the late 1980s, several of the political parties sought to nominate more women, and following the 1994 elections more than 40 percent of Swedish parliamentarians were women. This is the highest percentage of women in any parliament in the world.

A recently published study shows that countries in which women gained political rights and seats in parliament early on have achieved more gender equality, as well as substantially better conditions for children, relative to countries where women were slow to gain political influence.

Since the 1930s, society has taken on more and more responsibility for children, and this has had a major impact on women's lives as well. The 1930s saw improvements in obstetrical care and the introduction of maternity allowances. Maternity and child welfare clinics were established in the 1940s, with child allowances introduced in 1948. The foundation for the present system of parental insurance was laid in 1955, when a maternity insurance plan was put into effect. During the 1970s, the number of day-care and after-school care openings rose from about 10,000 to 130,000. An additional 15,000 were added in the 1980s.

The parental insurance system initiated in 1974 established in law a revolutionary change that had taken place in the relationship between fathers and their families. Although women continued to do most of the housework as well as to take most of the parental-leave time, the change that had occurred was indeed revolutionary. The conflict between production and reproduction, which had formerly been confined to women's lives, was now relevant to men's lives as well. Now, unlike the past, children truly had two parents. It is unlikely today for a child to die because a father fails to provide proper care, as occurred in the nineteenth century and before.

The increased importance of fathers was also reflected in divorce laws. In the past, divorcing women almost always received custody of their children, but since 1983 parents have been granted shared custody. A dispute can result in custody being awarded to one of the parents—and that parent is increasingly likely to be the father.

Labor market trends

If we include part-time work, Sweden currently has Europe's highest rate of employment among women. Finnish women have the highest rate of full-time work. What trends have we seen during the twentieth century?

In the 1870s, a good 30 percent of industrial workers were women, 60 percent of them employed in the textile and clothing industries. About a third worked in food and match production, and workers in the dairy industry were almost exclusively women.

Later on, female industrial workers tended to be concentrated in certain types of businesses, particularly clothing and food manufacturing. In 1990, a total of 16 percent of industrial workers were women.

As early as the nineteenth century it was common for women to work as low-level bank clerks. With the dawn of the twentieth century, more and more women were hired as shop assistants and office secretaries. After World War II there was a dramatic increase in women's employment in the public sector—in teaching, health care, child care and social work. In 1987, more than half of all employed women in Sweden had jobs in the public sector.

At the same time, the labor market was becoming increasingly segregated. Although Swedish women today have the highest employment rate in Europe, the Swedish labor market is more segregated by gender than that of other countries.

However, in the 1990s Swedish women have made significant inroads into higher-level white-collar jobs, particularly in the public sector, although this has not been the case in industry. There has not been a corresponding influx of men into jobs dominated by women.

Trade unions

When the trade-union movement began in the late nineteenth century, there were a number of women's unions. However, before long these unions were assimilated into men's unions. Membership rates were lower among women than men, and these men's unions were primarily concerned with the interests of male workers.

The demand for equal pay for equal work by women and men did not show results until 1947, when equal pay was introduced in the public sphere. Industry still had separate pay scales for women, with the rationalization that men had to provide for their families. Not until 1960 did the Swedish Trade Union Confederation and the Employers' Confederation reach an agreement on equal pay for equivalent work.

In practice, there are still wage inequities today, and wage differentials have increased again in recent years. In 1991, women working in the public sphere were paid 85 percent of men's wages—in county jobs only 75 percent and in municipal jobs 87 percent. In the private sector, female industrial workers earned 90 percent of men's wages, while female white-collar workers in private businesses were paid only 75 percent of their male colleagues' wages.

Women's double burden: Strength or strain?

Throughout history, women have worked hard and made a substantial contribution to society. They have also carried a double burden. Historically, women have been expected to do the impossible—to be responsible for both production and reproduction, for both earning a living and caring for their households and families. As long as women lacked power, it was difficult to change this situation. As women gained power, particularly economic control over their own lives, they were able to begin changing and improving conditions for themselves, their children and their husbands.

What did this double burden mean to them, this need to achieve the impossible? Was it a weakness, or perhaps a strength? Frequently women indeed managed to do the impossible. Perhaps precisely this burden gave them a real strength, an ability to deal with and prevail in difficult situations. Might it have made them better able to handle the real world?

This would indeed appear to be the case. We know that women have always handled crises in their lives better than men, and this remains true today. When women find themselves alone, after the death of a husband or a divorce, for example, they generally do better than comparable men. Average life expectancy is approximately the same for women living alone and for women living with a partner. In contrast, married men live significantly longer than single men. As long as men were incapable of handling basic responsibilities of life—cooking dinner, running the household, doing laundry, cleaning—they were, of course, quite vulnerable when they found themselves alone. Today the average life expectancy for men in Sweden is rising rapidly. Might that be because the men who have learned the most basic tasks in life are now beginning to grow old?

Thus health in the broadest sense of the word may be closely linked with gender equality in society. The more equality is achieved, the better the life circumstances of children, women and men.

References

Artaeus I. *Kvinnorna som blev över. Ensamstående stadskvinnor under 1800-talets första hälft—fallet Västerås [Women who were left over: Single women in the city during the first half of the nineteenth century: The Västerås case]*. Uppsala: Studia Historica Upsaliensia 179, 1992.

Berggreen B. *Fra kvinnebonde til bondekvinne [From woman farmer to farmer's wife]*. Kvinnenes kulturhistorie, Vol. II. Oslo, 1985.

Bladh C. *Månglerskor. At sälja från korg och bod i Stockholm 1819–1946 [Market women. Selling from a basket and from a shop in Stockholm 1819–1946]. Stockholm, 1992.*

Damsholt N. *The Role of Icelandic Women in the Sagas and in the Production of Homespun Cloth.* The Scand. Journal of History 1984.

Carlsson S. *Fröknar, mamseller, jungfrur och pigor. Ogifta kvinnor i det svenska ståndssamhället [Young ladies, misses, maidens and maids: Unmarried women in Sweden's class society].* Uppsala: Studia Historica Upsaliensia 90, 1977.

Emanuelsson A. *Pionjärer i vitt. Professionella och fackliga strategier bland svenska sjuksköterskor och sjukvårdsbiträden, 1851–1939 [Pioneers in white: Professional and union strategies among Swedish nurses and medical assistants, 1851–1939].* Stockholm: SHSTF, 1990.

Emanuelsson A, Rendt R. *I folkhälsans tjänst. Sju decennier med den svenska distriktssköterskan [In the service of public health: Seven decades of Swedish district nurses].* Stockholm: SHSTF, 1994.

Florén A. *Genus och producentroll. Kvinnoarbete inom svensk bergshantering, exemplet Jäders bruk 1660–1840 [Gender and the role of producer: Women's work in the Swedish mining industry, illustrated by the Jäder mine, 1660–1840].* Uppsala: Opuscula Historica Upsaliensia 7, 1991.

Florin C. *Kampen om katedern. Feminiserings- och professionaliseringsprocessen inom den svenska folkskolans lärarkår 1860–1906 [Struggle for the teacher's desk: The feminization and professionalization process among Sweden's elementary school teachers 1860–1906].* Umeå: Acta Universitatis Umensis. Umeå Studies in the Humanities 82, 1987.

Henriksson H. *Kvinnor i gruvarbete. [Women in the mining industry].* Med hammare och fackla. Årsskrift för Sancte Örjans Gille 1994, pp. 111–171.

Johansson E. *Kvinnorna och lästraditionen omkring 1700. Exempel från Sverige och Tyskland [Women and the reading tradition around 1700: Examples from Sweden and Germany].* Unpublished manuscript, Umeå University, 1991.

Högberg U. *Maternal mortality in Sweden 1750–1950.* Umeå 1986.

Hörsell A. *Borgare, smeder och änkor. Ekonomi och befolkning i Eskilstuna gamla stad och fristad 1750–1850 [Citizens, blacksmiths and widows: Economics and population in Eskilstuna 1750–1850].* Uppsala: Studia Historica Upsaliensia 131, 1983.

Lenander Fällström AM. *Kvinnor i lokalhistoriskt perspektiv. Levnadsvillkor i Örebro vid 1600-talets mitt [Women from a local historical perspective: Living conditions in Örebro in the mid-seventeenth century].* In: Sawyer B, Göransson A: Manliga strukturer och kvinnliga strategier. En bok till Gunhild Kyle [Male structures and female strategies: A book for Gunhild Kyle]. Medd. från Historiska institutionen i Göteborg nr. 33. Gothenburg, 1987.

Lindegren J. *Knektänkornas land. [Soldiers' widows' land].* Ambjörnsson R, Gaunt D, Editors. Den dolda historien (Hidden history). Malmö, 1984.

Lindegren J. *Utskrivning och utsugning. Produktion och reproduction i Bygdeå [Enlistment and exploitation: Production and reproduction in Bygdeå].* Uppsala: Studia Historica Upsaliensia 117, 1980.

Lindquist (Bladh) C. *Kvinnor i tvåförsörjarfamiljen. Gifta krögerskor och månglerskor i Stockholm under första delen av 1800-talet [Women in two-earner families: Married innkeepers and market women in Stockholm during the early nineteenth century].* In: Sawyer B, Göransson A: Manliga strukturer och kvinnliga strategier. En bok till Gunhild Kyle [Male structures and female strategies: A book for Gunhild Kyle]. Medd. från Historiska institutionen i Göteborg nr. 33. Gothenburg, 1987.

Lithell UB. *Breast-feeding and Reproduction. Studies in Marital Fertility and Infant Mortality in 19th Century Finland and Sweden.* Uppsala. Studia Historica Upsaliensia 120, 1981.

Lithell UB. *Kvinnoarbete och barntillsyn i 1700- och 1800-talets Österbotten [Women's work and child care in eighteenth- and nineteenth-century Österbotten].* Uppsala: Studia Historica Upsaliensia 156, 1988.

Lundgren B. *Allmänhetens tjänare. Kvinnlighet och yrkeskultur i det svenska postverket [Public servants: Femininity and work culture in the Swedish postal system].* Carlssons 1990.

Matovic M. *Den ensammas lott. Om ensamstående kvinnor i 1800-talets Stockholm [Being alone: Single women in nineteenth-century Stockholm].* In: Sawyer B, Göransson A: Manliga strukturer och kvinnliga strategier. En bok till Gunhild Kyle [Male structures and female strategies: A book for Gunhild Kyle]. Medd. från Historiska institutionen i Göteborg nr. 33. Gothenburg, 1987.

Nyström E. *Den svenska dödsorsaksstatistikens framväxt och tidiga historia [The development of Swedish cause-of-death statistics and early history].* In: Nordenfelt L (Ed.): Hälsa. Sjukdom. Dödsorsak [Health—illness—cause of death]. Stockholm 1986.

Ohlander AS. *En utomordentlig balansakt? Kvinnliga forskarpionjärer i Norden [An extraordinary balancing act? Female pioneers in research in the Nordic countries].* Historisk tidskrift 1987:1.

Ohlander AS. *Karolina Widerström och de första kvinnliga läkarna i Sverige [Karolina Widerström and the first female physicians in Sweden].* In: I Karolina Widerströms fotspår. 100 år med kvinnliga läkare i Sverige [In Karolina Widerström's footsteps: 100 years of female physicians in Sweden]. Stockholm: Sveriges Kvinnliga Läkares Förening, 1988.

Ohlander AS. *Kvinnan—historiens huvudperson [Women: History's leading characters].* Kulturrådet 1992:1–2.

Ohlander AS. *SOU 1994:38. Kvinnor, barn och arbete i Sverige, 1850–1993 [Swedish Government Official Reports 1994:38. Women, children and work in Sweden, 1850–1993].* Report for the U.N. conference on population and development in Cairo, 1994. Stockholm: Ministry for Foreign Affairs, 1994.

Ohlander AS. *Marias döttrar. Kvinnornas Europa. [Mary's daughters: Women's Europe].* Furuhagen B (Ed.): Utsikt mot Europa [Outlook on Europe]. Utbildningsradion och Bokförlaget Bra Böcker 1991.

Qvist G. *Kvinnofrågan i Sverige 1809–1846. Studier rörande kvinnans näringsfrihet inom de borgerliga yrkena [The issue of women in Sweden 1809–1846: Studies examining women's freedom to pursue trades and crafts].* Gothenburg: Kvinnohistoriskt arkiv 2, 1960.

Sandin B. *Hemmet, gatan, fabriken eller skolan. Folkundervisning och barnuppfostran i svenska städer 1600–1850 [Home, street, factory or school: Education and childrearing in Swedish cities 1600–1850]*. Lund: Arkiv avhandlingsserie 22, 19986.

Sjöberg MT. *Dufvans fångar. Brottet, straffet och människan i 1800-talets Sverige [Dufvan's prisoners: Crime, punishment and the individual in nineteenth-century Sweden]*. Författarförlaget 1986.

Sommestad L. *Från mejerska till mejerist. En studie av mejeriyrkets maskuliniseringsprocess [From dairywoman to dairyman: A study of the masculinization of the dairy industry]*. Lund: Arkiv förlag, 1992.

Sommestad L and McMurry, S. *Farm Daughters and Industrialization: A Comparative Analysis of Dairying in New York and Sweden, 1860–1920*. Journal of Women's history 1998– Vol. 10, No.2.

Wennemo I. *Sharing the costs of children. Studies on the development of family support in the OECD countries*. Stockholm 1994.

Wieselgren G. *Den höga tröskeln. Kampen för kvinnas rätt till ämbete [The high threshold: The fight for women's right to hold office]*. Lund 1969.

Winberg C. *Fabriksfolket. Textilindustrin i Mark och arbetarrörelsens genombrott [Factory people: The textile industry in Mark and the breakthrough of the workers' movement]*. Gothenburg 1989.

Österberg E. *Bonde eller bagerska? Vanliga svenska kvinnors ekonomiska ställning under medeltiden. Några frågor och problem [Farmer or baker? The economic position of ordinary Swedish women during the Middle Ages. Some questions and issues]*. Historisk tidskrift 1980:3.

Östman AC. *Kvinnors arbete i österbottniskt jordbruk från 1880- till 1930-tal [Women's work in the farming industry in Österbotten between the 1880s and the 1930s]*. Historisk tidskrift för Finland 1994:2.

11

Women's health and changes in care for the elderly

Rolf Å. Gustafsson, Marta Szebehely

Introduction

THE SYMBOL OF HEALTH CARE in the welfare state is often a physician (male) and a nurse (female) who are curing a patient (of indeterminate sex). For the most part, however, health care involves not curing people, but providing assistance and care to frail, elderly individuals whose need for help increases as time goes by. Old people make up a very large percentage of people in need of medical and nursing care. Although most people manage to take care of themselves independently up to a relatively advanced age, those over the age of 65 account for more than three-fourths of all in-patient stays and an even larger percentage of in-home care—whether provided by the public care system or by relatives (Statistics Sweden 1993, p. 44). And, of course, those receiving help are never genderless. A majority of elderly people in need of assistance are women—in part because there are more elderly women than men, and in part because the health of elderly women is worse than that of elderly men (men die of their illnesses, while women have to live with theirs) (Statistics Sweden 1993, p. 38, Thorslund et al. 1993).

Recently major changes in the health care system have been implemented, changes that have consequences for many people's day-to-day lives and well-being:

- One affected group, of course, is those who *need medical and nursing care*—both those who receive help from the formal care systems and those who don't.

- Another affected group is those who *work in the formal (paid) care system*. However, virtually no consideration has been given to the question of how working conditions might be affected by the introduction of market-oriented systems and other organizational changes in the formal care systems.

- Even less attention has been paid to the fact that changes within the formal care system also have consequences for the *informal* care system.

All of these groups—care recipients as well as paid and unpaid caregivers—are predominately women. In this chapter we examine specifically what happens to these women, on both sides of the caring relationship, when changes are initiated in the formal system of elderly care.

245

Changes in the elderly care system

During the first two or three decades following World War II, the welfare state was widely conceived as a road to a better life for large groups of people, not least women and the elderly. During the last decade, however, there has been an ideologically-driven skepticism toward public monopolies in Sweden, as well as a more specific critique directed at the elderly care system, particularly the lack of continuity and the limited control people have over their own care. Freedom of choice has become an official watchword (Swedish National Board of Health and Welfare 1995). Both internationally and within Sweden, there has been interest in a paradigm shift in public welfare systems—from the principles of a planned economy to a market-based system of management. More drastic proposals have also been put forward. Exhortations have been heard in Sweden to "roll back the state" and "let people take care of themselves" with the help of a managed market, civil society and the family.[1] However, analyses of opinion polls show a high level of confidence among Swedes in publicly-run health and nursing care, and this has remained true over time, for both men and women (Svallfors 1994).

Financial constraints facing both Sweden as a whole and individual municipalities have contributed to a heated debate, and opinions are divided on the reasons for and extent of these economic problems (Krugman 1995). The 1980s will probably go down in history as the decade in which economists dominated the debate over the future of the welfare state (Hugemark 1994).

Of course, changes in elderly care are also affected by demographic factors. In recent years there has been much discussion of the aging explosion (Tornstam 1992). Some have spoken of a cost-driving demographic bomb; the Swedish population has the largest proportion—five percent—of people 80 years and older in the world. In Sweden, however, the most revolutionary demographic changes have already occurred: Between 1975 and 1995, the number of people over the age of 80 increased by more than 80 percent. Increases are expected to continue, but at a slower rate—by 20 percent up to the year 2015 (Government bill 1997/98:113).

However, concrete changes in the organization of and resources for elderly care are not an automatic consequence of demographic or economic developments. To a large extent, elderly care is shaped by social developments as interpreted by political parties, individual municipal and county politicians, their advisors in government service and, not least, the growing numbers of management consultants. Traditionally, politicians and government administrators have had two tools at their disposal: budgetary measures and reorganization. In Sweden, the use of these tools dates back hundreds of years.

Budget management—levying taxes to finance care and allocating these funds for specific purposes—was a method used as early as Sweden's Catholic period during the Middle Ages, when people gave their tithes to the church. In the mid-seventeenth century, there were efforts to *reorganize* the health-care structures that had been established by the medieval church. A formal division was made between the responsibility of the Crown (state) for inpatient institutional care (asylums for those suffering from infectious diseases or serious mental illness) and the role of the church/parish (later the municipality) in caring for the deserving poor (which, for a long time, primarily meant the elderly). Efforts were made to classify potential care recipients according to the likelihood that they would benefit from care. Resources were allocated to children and others who might be expected to have a chance of being cured and become "productive and loyal" citizens. The elderly and the poor were treated less generously.[2] How the lines were drawn between different budgets, how much money flowed through these channels and who was defined as a "legitimate" recipient of help had a direct effect on people's life circumstances, whether they were potential caregivers or care recipients. Cutting costs, improving efficiency and economic considerations have been important issues for the state ever since the eighteenth century.

Toward the end of the nineteenth century there was increasing interest in the *internal organization of health care.* This was triggered by the emergence of modern medical science, in turn intertwined with the rise of an urban middle class, in Sweden often in coalition with the centralized state apparatus. One effect was new ideas on treatment procedures, along with a need to strengthen the hierarchical structures in order to manage care in accordance with criteria of the medical profession. Restructuring continued into the twentieth century. In the realms of health and elderly care, some of the most important internal reorganizational efforts during the 1950s followed the pattern of "Taylorism" (i.e., an assembly-line model borrowed from industry). Later, partly as a reaction to the fragmented Taylorized care, the introduction of semi-autonomous groups—"team nursing"—followed during the 1970s.[3] Economic motives were important, but other factors played a role as well—for example, an urge to conceive the patient/care recipient in holistic terms, as well as to increase professionalism and underscore the scientific element in care management.

A central aim of elderly care since the 1950s has also been to "normalize" the lives of care recipients through deinstitutionalization. The Ädel reform, which went into effect in 1992, focuses primarily on the external organization of the care system and the boundaries between different types of care and the authorities responsible for financing them. This reform also represents a further step toward deinstitutionalization; however, we shall not go into further detail here on this organizational change.[4]

In addition, *new economic management methods* have been established within the last 5–10 years. These are based on the assumption that competition and economic incentives will foster productivity and increase the efficiency of health and nursing care. Thus three quite different management methods have been used: resource allocation/budgeting; changes in internal and external organization; and, more recently, changes in economic incentives based on neoclassical economic theories. In order to understand what is happening within elderly care—and how this may affect health and well-being—it is important to have a more detailed grasp of these methods. Accordingly, we outline below the changes that have occurred in recent years.

Changes in allocation of resources

In contrast to the costs of health care, which have declined in recent years, the total costs of elderly care (at both the county and the municipal levels) increased by 32 percent in real terms between 1984 and 1993. This increase in funds for the care of the elderly has roughly kept pace with demographic changes: Total public expenditures to care for the elderly and the handicapped (in-home and institutional care) have remained more or less constant relative to the number of individuals over the age of 80 in the population in 1984 and 1993 (Prütz & Lindgren 1994), but have declined in the last few years (Swedish National Board of Health and Welfare 1998).

Change through reorganization

In elderly care a significant first step toward deinstitutionalization occurred in 1949, when the well-known Swedish writer Ivar Lo-Johansson published a series of articles voicing scathing criticism of homes for the elderly and instead argued for home-based care. This criticism resonated with the public, and within a few years official ideology had shifted.[5] A breakthrough occurred with the government report on elderly care published in 1956, which underscored in-home care and public home-help services as the main alternative to the old system of homes for the elderly. During the 1960s, there was increasing criticism throughout the world of the inhumane consequences of institutionalization, particularly for psychiatric care. This doubtless contributed, in Sweden and elsewhere, to a general shift toward a policy of deinstitutionalization (Åman 1976, pp. 468 ff).

However, it was a long time before these ideas were put into practice. Relative to the number of elderly people in the population, institutional capacity actually continued to increase up to the early 1980s, when a substantial decline began, partly offset by an increase in sheltered housing: From 1980 to 1997 the proportion of people over the age of 80 in institutional care dropped from 24 percent to 15 percent. In the same age group, the percentage living in sheltered accommodations (service blocks) increased from 4 to 8 percent. However, the most striking trend during that period was a substantial decline in the public home-health services, which went from covering 34 percent to only 20 percent of the population aged 80 and older (Swedish Ministry of Health and Social Affairs 1999, p. 40). This drastic decline in home-based services is peculiar to Sweden. Today the home-help services in the other Scandinavian countries reach a share of the elderly population that is two to three times as high as in Sweden (Swedish National Board of Health and Welfare 1998; see also Szebehely 1998a).

This reflects two priorities:

- *Who is to receive help.* A general principle has been to concentrate both public home-help services and institutional care on the most needy (reducing the number of people covered).

- *Certain kinds of assistance.* Priority has been given to the kinds of help deemed most essential—personal nursing care rather than help with household chores—which affects the degree of assistance. This means that even those who still receive home-help services often find that the help they receive is limited to fewer of the tasks necessary for keeping the household functioning.

Note that the principle and practical consequences of setting priorities for care recipients and types of help are of critical importance. Giving priority to certain people and services inevitably means reduced priority for others.

Change through a new system of economic management

Today, the new systems of economic management that have been put in place in elderly care are marked by an almost impenetrable jungle of different measures. Similar systems have been introduced for health care as well (see Gustafsson (ed.) 1994). The most important organizational changes follow:

- *Profit centers.* This refers to a distinct organizational unit that has been assigned responsibility for personnel, finances and results. Decision-making tasks and responsibilities that used to be handled in a more centralized manner "higher up" in the administrative structure have been delegated to these units to facilitate adapting the organization and resources to a given situation. When profit centers were first established within the health care system in the mid-1980s, one goal was to increase staff participation in decision making (Borgert 1992 and Dahlström & Ramström 1990). As time went by, however, the focus shifted to breaking down activities into small units so that higher levels of management might better identify the role of individual working sites or teams in production and resource use.

In the health care system, the attempt is to establish a direct connection between units' utilization of resources and their performance (the profit centers receive payment for each treatment episode in accordance with a predetermined rate of compensation). However, this system has not been as common in elderly care, probably because it is even more difficult to develop a fair and well-functioning system of performance-based remuneration in that arena than it is in somatic health care.

In the fields of care for elderly and disabled individuals, approximately half of all municipalities had introduced profit centers by 1993 (Swedish National Board of Health and Welfare 1994a, pp. 19–20).

- *Purchaser-provider model.* Basically, the goal is to split the responsibilities between those in political and management positions who formulate and contract out a given service, on the one hand, and those performing the actual care work, on the other. By establishing a clear relationship between those two parties—frequently in the form of a contract or agreement—the aim is in part to clarify the objective, volume, goal fulfillment, etc., and in part to encourage or necessitate competition between various providers. The idea is that competition will help increase productivity and efficiency—which, to put it mildly, has triggered considerable scientific and political debate.[6]

In elderly care, a good 10 percent of municipalities had introduced some form of purchaser-provider model by 1993. A little more than half of these municipalities applied a purchaser-provider model in which the political leadership, in the form of a committee responsible for contracts (production board etc.), is part of the process (Swedish National Board of Health and Welfare 1994a, pp. 15–16). In other cases, there are internal divisions within the administrative structure, which usually means that officials responsible for evaluating the needs of elderly persons are considered the purchaser, while those actually managing home-help services are defined as the providers.[7]

Both purchaser-provider models and profit centers help provide the organizational framework for the third component of the new system of economic management in the sphere of elderly care: contracting out and "privatization."[8]

- *Competitive tendering and "privatization"* may be the most controversial elements of recent changes. While competitive tendering has long been used in other activities carried out by the Swedish municipalities, such as street cleaning and garbage collection, the idea of instituting a similar system in the realm of health and nursing care has drawn particular attention.

- Advocates have often argued that individual *freedom of choice* would be expanded this way. Both consumers and producers should be able to choose among various alternatives to the state and municipal monopolies. Furthermore, it is argued that competition would have a positive effect on quality and costs. ". . . All experience has shown that increased competition improves quality and reduces costs. Thus it is important to have more alternatives—independent entrepreneurs, employee cooperatives, consumer cooperatives, etc." (Swedish Ministry for Health and Social Affairs 1994, p. 12. See also Swedish Government Official Reports 1991:104).

Critics have expressed concern about privatization, worrying that the profit motive might become a factor in health care if private business entered the managed market system based on the idea of competitive tendering. Moreover, it might be the first step toward a situation in which health care financing, as in other markets, is increasingly the responsibility of the individual (Dahlgren 1994). This could possibly trigger a process by which citizenship is transformed into "consumership" in local government (Montin & Elander 1995). The contract system also requires that municipalities be capable of making the proper decisions on contracting services and following up on the performance of profit-driven providers. Offering choices requires consumer access to information, and presumes that people have both the desire and the energy to take advantage of that information (Swedish National Board of Health and Welfare 1995). All of these matters are the subject of considerable debate.

For the time being, however, the concept of privatization should be placed in quotation marks. Current law expressly states that responsibility for carrying out official duties (assessment of need, following up on the quality of care, and setting fees) may not be assigned to a private enterprise. Furthermore, under the contract system, services continue to be financed through tax revenues, although the organization and implementation of care services are carried out on a private basis.[9]

It is important to delineate which aspects of the actual, day-to-day work of providing social care services are contracted out:[10]

In the sphere of home-help services, the most common arrangement has been to contract out *specific services* (meals-on-wheels, cleaning, shopping, security systems, etc.). This has the disadvantage of reducing personnel continuity and making it more difficult for service providers to view their clients in holistic terms. By 1993, one in four municipalities had experimented with this type of contract system in some aspect of its home-help services. More recent figures are not yet available, but most probably this trend has continued.

The next most common area where contracts are used involves special living arrangements (service blocks, homes for the elderly, nursing homes, group homes). In 1993, a good 20 percent of Sweden's municipalities had contracted out some of these services.

A less common situation is when one or more *home-help service districts are contracted out entirely.* In 1993, this was the case in about 5 percent of the municipalities.

All of the above figures refer to the share of municipalities that have tried some kind of contracting arrangement in their care for the elderly, and thus they provide an indication of the interest that exists in such arrangements. How widespread different forms of contracting out services are among the Swedish municipalities remains unclear. Communities that have experimented with contractual arrangements tend to be large and medium-sized cities with Liberal and Conservative governments (The Expert Group on Public Finance 1995, pp. 55–57). It should also be noted that the role of non-profit organizations (foundations or cooperatives) has declined in favor of business arrangements aimed at financial profit.[11] Finally, we note that privatization in the field of elderly care remains limited, although it is increasing: In 1997, private providers accounted for about 10 percent of institutional care for the elderly and about 4 percent of home-help services—in both cases a two-fold increase in the number of care recipients since 1993 (Swedish National Board of Health and Welfare 1998).

- *Customer-choice system/vouchers.* This feature of the new economic management systems, finally, is the one most reminiscent of a market in the traditional sense. The local-authority social worker assesses an individual's need and determines the type and amount of assistance to be granted, which is "translated" into a voucher amount. The voucher can then be used to pay those providers—privately or publicly run—that are accredited by the municipality. The care recipient, or "customer," can choose freely among the alternatives and "shop around" much as in a traditional market.

The system has been tried out in four Liberal/Conservative suburban communities in the Stockholm area, i.e., in about 1 percent of the country's municipalities (1993). However, only 10 percent, at most, of aid recipients in these communities have chosen to participate in the voucher system (Swedish National Board of Health and Welfare 1995, p. 34). This system has given rise to intense debate, not least because aid recipients may end up supplementing the vouchers with money out of their own pockets. This runs counter to the equality principle to which municipal services are legally required to adhere, since access to elderly care is not supposed to depend on an individual's financial resources.[12]

Toward marketization and informalization of care

In the preceding section, we have offered an overview of recent changes in Swedish elderly care. Taken together, trends in *resource allocation,* internal and external *reorganization* and the new *economic management system* have changed the boundaries between different care systems and led to a shift toward both more market-oriented care and more informal care.

About 4 percent of elderly care has been turned over to the market in the literal sense: Social care services that used to be publicly provided have now been contracted out to private enterprise. The percentages are small, but changes have been occurring rapidly in recent years. The aim is to introduce competition into the care system, which is also expected to have an impact on the elderly care services that remain publicly provided (Swedish National Board of Health and Welfare 1995, p. 30 and Ström 1994). However, there are further implications of a marketization of the care system: Organizational models imported from the production industry have long been used in public care services. Jobs are fragmented, the pace is accelerated, the time for providing help declines to the minimum time required for carrying out only those tasks that can be measured.[13] A new language is evolving, and there are changes in the criteria used by politicians and superiors to evaluate performance. This, in turn, affects employees' motivation and behavior. It is by no means clear how these things will affect relationships, among care workers as well as between them and the people they are helping. These changes in the way work is organized mean changes both for paid workers (the overwhelming majority of whom are women) and for care recipients.

The *informalization* of the care system means that a decreasing proportion of elderly people benefit from the resources of the formal care sector: In 1980, 62 percent of the oldest individuals (80 years old and above) received either home-help services or institutional care, while in 1997 the corresponding share was only 43 percent (Swedish Ministry of Health and Social Affairs 1999).

There are no corresponding official statistics on informal, unpaid care, since it is significantly more difficult to measure the efforts made by family caregivers such as spouses and children, or by close friends. Not until recently were these efforts examined more closely in Scandinavian research (Johansson 1991, Lingsom 1997). However, those studies that have been done indicate an increase in care by family members during the 1980s. According to a Swedish study, the share of elderly people in need of practical assistance who received public home-help services decreased, while there was an increase in the percentage receiving care from their families. These changes are especially true for women; for elderly men, there was no change in the percentage receiving home-help services or help from family caregivers during the 1980s (Szebehely 1993).[14]

According to a Norwegian study, both women and men provide informal care to persons outside their own households, but women are responsible for a larger proportion of such help. Men and to a greater extent women increased their caregiving activities during the 1980s: In 1980, 11 percent of men and 15 percent of women provided informal help to persons outside their own households. In 1990, the corresponding percentages were 24 and 32, respectively (Lingsom 1993, p. 311). Women were responsible for two-thirds of the informal help provided in 1980, measured in hours spent, compared with three-fourths of such help in 1990. A reasonable explanation is that "the slow pace of efforts to expand public in-home and institutional care services relative to population trends in the 1980s has led to an increased need for private care" (Lingsom 1993, p. 314). The study indicates that it is mainly women who take on such responsibilities, no matter how much they work outside the home.

All of this points to a shift in the line between the formal and the informal care sectors—a change we refer to as a process of informalization.[15] The informalization of care affects women in particular—as both care recipients and caregivers.

Consequences for the elderly, families and paid caregivers

Seen in terms of day-to-day implications, the movement toward more informal and market-oriented elderly care has consequences for at least three groups: *those who need help, their families and paid care workers.* Moreover, these changes not only have a direct effect on these groups, but also affect the relationships among them.

In the following sections we focus in turn on those who need help, their families and paid caregivers. Since we are also interested in the relationships among these groups, the sections will overlap to some degree.

Elderly individuals who need help

As we have noted above, fewer elderly people received help from the formal sector in the 1980s—whether in the form of institutional care or home-help services. Deinstitutionalization has meant that today more people who are in need of substantial help are living at home. Home-help services have assigned priority to this group at the expense of other groups. For the most needy, the shift in the boundary between the formal and informal care systems has meant that these individuals receive help either exclusively from the formal system, or from both the formal and the informal sectors. Less-needy elderly people receive only informal help or they manage on their own.

A close look at the data shows that it is primarily *single women with a moderate need for assistance as well as married couples who end up outside the formal system of elderly care.* Single men, in contrast, are given priority. Thus elderly women have been more affected than elderly men by the concentration of in-home care resources, since they are more frequently expected to take care of their own needs or to rely completely on help from their families. However, even those women who continue to receive home-help services are more likely than men to find that their level of assistance has been reduced. Unlike elderly men, these women increasingly perceive the help they receive as inadequate (Szebehely 1993).

This is true despite the fact that elderly women are in greater need of formal care services than men are. Men's needs in their old age are largely taken care of by their wives. Women tend to be dependent on either the formal sector or their children. This is partly because women's health is worse than men's, and partly because there are substantially more elderly women living alone (a result, in turn, of the fact that women live longer and that women frequently marry older men). Approximately 70 percent of elderly men die before their wives do, while only 25 percent of elderly women precede their husbands in death (Lundin & Sundström 1994).

Demands to limit home-help services have required officials to "examine more closely than before what relatives might be able to contribute."[16] The formal care system has increased its requirements that families of the elderly provide help. Relatives have increased their contributions mainly in two ways:

First, as supplementary assistance to elderly people who are still receiving help from the formal sector, but at an increasingly inadequate level. This kind of help has primarily increased among elderly persons living alone who are in great need of help (Szebehely 1993, p. 12).

Second, as a replacement for assistance to elderly people who no longer have priority in the formal elderly care system, i.e., those who receive help only from the informal sector. This includes both single elderly people (mainly women) who receive help from their children and other family members and elderly married couples in which, to an increasing extent, one spouse is dependent for help on the other (Sundström 1994, p. 33, Szebehely 1998b).

These changes can be summarized as follows:

- As a result of prioritization and concentration, fewer elderly people are receiving help exclusively from the formal sector.

- More elderly people—primarily women—are receiving help from their families along with assistance from the formal care system.

- More elderly people—primarily women and married couples—are receiving help only from their families. Here there are significant gender differences, with women at a disadvantage: When single elderly people receive help from their families, the caregiver is frequently a woman. When elderly couples care for each other, it is usually the woman who is taking care of her older husband.

We do not know whether the concentration of publicly-financed services provided by the formal elderly care system is offset by an expansion of informal care, i.e., whether relatives fill the entire gap left when resources of the formal care system are concentrated on fewer elderly individuals, or whether more older people now find themselves without any help at all.

We know, however, that *elderly individuals prefer help from the formal sector* to assistance from their families. This is true particularly for elderly women, probably because they know what it "costs" to help and support someone in need.[17] Those who criticize the welfare state sometimes argue that a well-developed system of formal care poses a threat to intergenerational solidarity. This argument is not new; as early as the beginning of the nineteenth century, British authorities worried that the introduction of the Poor Laws would damage the social fabric (Daatland 1990). However, there is no evidence to support the idea that intergenerational contact would improve if families had more responsibility for the care of the needy. Today, elderly people have at least as close contact with their relatives as they had in the 1950s, when formal care for the elderly was much less well established (Sundström 1983). There is no reason to believe that these relationships would be improved if relatives had caregiving responsibilities in addition to maintaining their social contacts. On the contrary, good relationships are fostered when both the decision to *offer* informal assistance and the decision to accept such help are made freely. The opposite case has been called "compulsory altruism" (Land & Rose 1985, p. 93). The disadvantages for both parties when relatives are coerced into caring for the elderly are obvious.[18] Thus the reduced level of formal assistance probably constitutes a burden on the well-being of needy elderly women. If and when people are forced to ask their families for help, this is quite likely to have an adverse effect on their relationships.

Thus far, our discussion has focused on the quantitative shifts between the formal and the informal sectors. In addition, however, changes *within* the formal care system have consequences for care recipients. Studies of various aspects of the quality of elderly care all show that one of the most important things for the elderly is to have as few people as possible involved in their care, i.e., to have a *high degree of personnel continuity*.[19] The current movement toward a market system of elderly care, however, poses a threat to continuity. When portions of home-help services are contracted out (such as cleaning and grocery shopping) while municipalities retain responsibility for other services, more people are inevitably involved on a day-to-day basis. A report by the Swedish National Board of Health and Welfare discusses the consequences of the changes between 1989 and 1992 for home-help recipients in Stockholm:

> The quality of care has declined. Often elderly people are no longer receiving help with food preparation at home, and they are not able to go out shopping as often as before; cleaning is done less and less frequently, perhaps once a month, and personal contact is replaced by equipment like security systems (Swedish National Board of Health and Welfare 1994c, p. 32).

Care workers express concerns about health consequences for the elderly when they are increasingly unlikely to receive approval for help with their grocery shopping. These workers often see elderly women carrying heavy grocery bags and wonder how they manage to cope (ibid., p. 25). Twenty-nine percent of those receiving help regard it as inadequate:

> The most common problems are that retired people are forced to do things they really cannot handle, they are forced to burden other people, and this leads to anxiety and insecurity (ibid., p. 26).

Families of the elderly

We have established that changes in elderly care have led to an increase in assistance from the family, both as a supplement to formal care and as a replacement. To understand better the consequences of this increase in the role of families, we need to distinguish among different groups of relatives. Indeed, the relationship between an individual needing help and his or her relatives differs a great deal depending on whether it is a spousal relationship or one between a parent and adult children or other close kin. In Sweden, most family care is provided by a spouse.

· *Elderly spouses.* Elderly spouses receive only a limited amount of help from the formal care system and other relatives. This means that older couples are often forced to rely on each other. The promise of for better or for worse is taken very seriously. Only 5 percent of retirees living with a partner received home-help services in 1990, compared with 28 percent of retired people living alone (Szebehely 1993, p. 16). Even when people require a great deal of physical assistance or are suffering from dementia, it is not unusual for their spouses to receive no formal help (Grafström 1994, Szebehely 1998b).

It is mainly women who are affected by the lower priority given to married couples by the formal care system. The gender-neutral term spouse often really means a woman who is responsible for providing care. Given demographic factors and traditional marriage patterns, we frequently find that when elderly couples are afflicted with poor health, it is the woman who ends up caring for an older, ailing husband. So with fewer elderly spouses receiving formal care, elderly women generally have more responsibility for taking care of their elderly husbands. In addition, however, there appears to be a gender gap in the treatment of elderly spouses by the formal care system: Elderly men caring for their wives receive more formal assistance than do elderly women in a similar situation.[20]

In other words, elderly wives often bear a great deal of responsibility for caregiving. What this increasing burden means for women's own health is not entirely clear, but a Danish study suggests that the responsibility of caring for a spouse may put the caregiver's health at risk. According to this study, elderly women who are married experience worse health than single women in the same age group. The reverse is true for men (Due 1991). This suggests that elderly women's responsibility for their husbands' health constitutes a risk to their own well-being.[21]

- *Other relatives.* Aside from spouses, adult children (including daughters-in-law) are the most important group of family caregivers for the elderly. It is not uncommon for both daughters and sons to help their parents, but more daughters are involved, and their help is more extensive.[22]

Daughters' contributions should be seen in the context of the high employment rate of Swedish women, even in the age groups (i.e., approximately 50–65 years of age) of women whose parents are beginning to require assistance. Compared with other countries, there is an exceptionally high percentage of women working outside the home in this age range (Vogel 1997, p. 38).

Today, there is heightened interest in Sweden in the situation faced by relatives who are caring for elderly individuals (Government bill 1997/98:113).[23] Yet there are few (if any) Swedish studies of the health consequences of combining gainful employment with increased responsibility for caring for elderly relatives. We do know, however, that early retirement and long-term work absences increased among older women (but not among older men) toward the end of the 1980s (Diderichsen et al. 1993). This may well indicate a link between the increase in poor health among older female workers and the increasing informalization of the elderly care system.

Overall, we know little about the extent to which caregiving responsibilities pose a risk to the health of elderly spouses and gainfully employed daughters. Studies should be conducted to determine how the relationships between elderly people and their families are affected when relatives are required to provide help, although the elderly themselves would prefer help from the formal sector. Moreover, research should address the question of the relationships between the families of care recipients and paid care workers. Although an increasing number of the elderly are receiving help from both the formal and the informal sector, there is rarely a forum for contact between care providers from both systems, which probably places strain on both parties.

Women as paid caregivers

In all, about 250,000 persons are employed in the elderly care system (i.e., home-help services/home health care and municipal institutions). More than 90 percent of them are women (Swedish National Association of Local Authorities 1999, p. 79).

People who work in caregiving occupations are at risk. Municipal home helpers and nursing assistants find themselves in the two women's occupations with the highest incidence of stress injuries. People providing home-help services run a risk of such injuries that is five times as high as that of the average worker, a rate exceeded only by firefighters. Unlike most other occupations, municipal home helpers experienced an increase in stress injuries in 1990 (Arbetsmiljö-fonden informerar [Information from the Foundation for the Workplace] 1992, No. 6). Home helpers had substantially more back and shoulder problems than forestry workers or automobile mechanics (Thulin 1987). In addition, psychosocial problems related to work are more common among home helpers than other groups, and work absenteeism and employee turnover are substantially above average (Aronsson et al. 1994).

Practical nurses in the care system are also at risk. More than any other group, they encountered increased stress on the job during the 1980s. While the psychological demands of their jobs increased, practical nurses were not given more decision latitude to deal with those new demands (Szulkin & Thålin 1994, p. 106). Although all of this is well known, authorities seeking to establish a new, market-oriented management system have failed to analyze possible consequences of such systems for the working environment (Gustafsson (Ed.) 1994).

Cutbacks, whether actual or planned, also mean that the employment situation of paid care workers is less secure. An increasing percentage of workers are hired on a temporary basis (Swedish National Association of Local Authorities 1999, p. 30).

The changes that are taking place in the care system—reallocation of funds, organizational changes and the introduction of new market-oriented management systems —and the increased demands and stepped-up pace that are likely to follow pose a threat not only to the work environment. *Such changes also affect the character and scope of social interactions between the elderly and their caregivers.* Within the sphere of home-help services, we have seen that the encounter between care workers and care recipients, which has traditionally been a positive one, is at risk of becoming unsatisfactory for both parties (Eliasson-Lappalainen & Motevasel 1996).

Care for the elderly rarely involves the hope that individuals will regain their health and independence, and this has certain consequences for the relationships among care personnel, care recipients and families. Kari Wærness (1984) distinguishes between "resultless" caregiving and care efforts aimed at achieving a cure or recovery. Caregivers interacting with elderly people in frail health generally have no other measure of their job performance than the subjective well-being and trust of the person for whom they are caring. If the elderly are not content with the assistance they receive (owing to a lack of time or organizational arrangements that are not suited to their needs), care workers cannot find consolation in the prospect of future recovery. Work satisfaction in a care system that, by its very nature, does not show results in terms of recovery or improved health is directly and negatively affected by dissatisfaction on the part of the elderly themselves.

Accordingly, good working conditions in this kind of relational and interactive work involve not only those factors that have been shown to promote good health among production workers (e.g., a variety of tasks, appropriately challenging work, control of the work process, etc.). *Good working conditions in the caregiving sector also mean being able to provide adequate care.*[24]

As we have already pointed out, the current trend toward a market-oriented system of home-help services brings with it a decline in the continuity of relationships between care workers and care recipients, which in turn means that the elderly are likely to be less satisfied with their care. We also know that elderly women who receive home-help services increasingly perceive those services as inadequate. This is probably a consequence both of organizational changes and of the lower priority assigned to household chores by the home-help service system. This increased dissatisfaction not only puts a strain on care recipients and their families, who may end up filling in the gaps, but affects the working environment of care workers as well, and thus also their well-being and health.

Does the responsibility women bear for others' health pose a risk to their own well-being?

Anna Bexell, a physician specializing in social medicine, has raised the question of whether women's responsibility for others' health puts their own well-being at risk (Bexell 1985). Our findings indicate that the answer, unfortunately, is yes.

It is important to bear in mind that on the whole the reduction in the total number of elderly people receiving help from the formal sector has so far occurred without a drastic drop in the total financial resources allocated for elderly care. Yet, as we have also pointed out, there have been clear negative consequences that have primarily affected women. Now that there are indications of the beginning of a real decline in financial resources, it is even more important to follow these developments closely. One important lesson is that few, if any, changes have been gender-neutral. Elderly care is not simply a matter of "cost containment," "efficiency," "new systems of management," "incentives," etc. Elderly care involves day-to-day relationships between human beings of flesh and blood—men and women, fathers and mothers, sons and daughters, people with plans and hopes. Abstract and genderless concepts could be misleading, even destructive, in social contexts like the care of elderly and frail human beings.

Frequently, women are doubly affected by cuts and structural changes in the formal care system. They experience both an increase in their workload on the job and a heavier burden as caregivers in the informal system. It is not unusual for female care workers to assume their role as mothers when they come home, and then, in the evenings or on their days off, to take on traditional responsibilities as daughters caring for aging parents. Eventually they, too, become grandmothers who may find themselves forced to ask their own daughters for help.

It is perhaps harsh, but unfortunately increasingly true, to conclude that working-class women often take care of both middle-class elderly people for low wages and their own elderly relatives for no compensation at all.[25]

The trend in elderly care toward "informalization" and "marketization" leads to a *shift in care services*. This shift not only means a decline in paid caregiving services, but also affects the very character, content and terms of care.

Examining who takes care of whom and how the system is organized helps us to understand important and fundamental social conditions. The changes that are taking place within the formal care system affect more than just those individuals who remain within the system; they also mean that some people are forcibly removed from the system. New relationships also need to be established between the formal and the informal care systems.

The reduction in public care services has most probably led to both increased amounts of care work performed by other caregivers (within the informal as well as the market-based care system) and unmet care needs among elderly people. As the historian Lena Sommestad (1994, p. 628) has noted, the reproductive and caregiving responsibilities of society cannot be streamlined or eliminated in the interest of cost cutting. A certain amount of care work is necessary and thus will have to be either reorganized or neglected.

Notes

1 An enormous body of literature on the international and Swedish debate on the welfare state has emerged in recent years. The following selection is a personal one, and these works have shaped the content and design of this chapter: Antman 1994, Krugman 1995, Glennerster & Le Grand 1995, Glennerster & Midgley 1991, Whitehead et al. 1997.

2 See also Gustafsson 1989.

3 See also Gardell & Gustafsson 1979 on health care and Eliasson (ed.) 1992 on home-help services.

4 With the Ädel reform in 1992, the municipalities became the primary authority responsible for elderly care, except for medical rehabilitation. The aim of this change was, first of all, to increase the efficiency of resource utilization. Among other things, by making municipalities responsible for paying for elderly patients whose immediate medical treatment has been completed, an incentive has been

created for transferring such elderly patients from the relatively more expensive acute-care system into municipal nursing homes or homes for the elderly, or offering them in-home care. With this reform, some 55,000–65,000 employees and one-fifth of the county councils' expenditures on health and nursing care were transferred from the county to the municipal level.

5 See Edebalk 1990 and Szebehely 1995, Chapter 2.

6 According to Swedish Government Official Reports 1991:104, ". . . it is the presence of competition—rather than who is carrying out production—that offers the opportunity to reduce costs and increase efficiency." This view has been criticized; for an overview, see also Gustafsson 1996, Glennerster & Le Grand 1995 and Jonsson 1993.

7 Without going into detail on the extensive debate regarding the various manifestations of the purchaser-provider model in the sphere of health and nursing care—and its actual or presumed effects—we should note here that relevant analysis has so far been limited in both scope and focus (Gustafsson 1995). However, a number of studies of the concept are beginning to appear; see Swedish National Board of Health and Welfare 1994b on elderly care. The English-speaking debate is quite similar to the debate in Sweden. There, too, analyses have been few; see, however, Robinson & Le Grand (Eds.) 1994.

8 As early as 1991, it was explicitly stated in the state report on competition (Swedish Government Official Reports 1991:104) that the purchaser-provider model can be viewed as a step on the road to total privatization.

9 See also Swedish National Board of Health and Welfare 1994a, p. 28 and The Expert Group on Public Finance 1995, pp. 26–27.

10 The following information is based on Swedish National Board of Health and Welfare 1994a, p. 29.

11 Stock companies made up 50 percent in 1994, according to the Expert Group on Public Finance 1995, p. 53.

12 See also Swedish National Board of Health and Welfare 1994a, p. 24, Swedish National Board of Health and Welfare 1995, pp. 34–38 and von Otter & Tengvald 1992.

13 For home services, see Swedish National Board of Health and Welfare 1994c, Szebehely 1995 and Eliasson-Lappalainen & Motevasel 1996.

14 See also Sundström 1994, p. 33 for an analysis of developments between 1988/89 and 1994. The author finds relatively minor changes, but sums up the trend by noting: "Overall, the pattern may indicate that families are doing more and the state somewhat less."

15 See also Barker & Mitteness (1990), who use the term "informalization" to refer to the fact that a reduction in the length of hospital stays has led to increased responsibility for care being placed on loved ones. Another term for the shift from paid to unpaid work is "work transfer" (Glazer 1993). Changes in the distribution of work between the family and the formal sector are referred to in the English-language literature as "shifting boundaries of public and private" (Showstack Sassoon 1987).

16 Stockholm Social Service Department 1989. In addition, the Swedish National Board of Health and Welfare (1994c, p. 29) has noted an increase in municipalities' demand for family participation.

17 See Daatland 1990, Andersson 1994. Svallfors 1994, p. 45, shows that between 1986 and 1992 the percentage of people who thought that relatives were best suited for providing assistance to the elderly dropped from 11 to 5 percent.

18 See, for example, Wærness 1990, Odén 1992, Andersson 1994 and Szebehely 1994.

19 See Swedish National Board of Health and Welfare 1994d for an overview.

20 Sundström 1994, Szebehely 1998a. A smaller (and declining) percentage of all relatives providing care are paid. The large majority of such individuals are women, but male relatives who are paid for their care services generally receive more help from the formal care system than women in the same situation (Mossberg 1996).

21 Another indication that caregiving responsibilities constitute a risk to the health of elderly women is that many relatives who are paid to provide care services (most of whom are women) have developed their own physical problems as a result (Mossberg 1996).

22 Daughters do more of the urgent tasks (nursing care, laundry, grocery shopping, meal preparation), while sons do more things that can be planned in advance, such as repairs, larger-scale shopping, help with taxes (Lingsom 1987, p. 48, Sundström 1994, p. 34).

23 See also Johansson 1991, Grafström 1994, Mossberg 1994. There has long been a wealth of international research on "caregiver burdens" and "caregiver stress," see Braithwaite 1992, among others. In light of the large number of empirical studies, one prominent figure in the research tradition exclaimed: "Do we need another 'stress and caregiving' study?" (Zarit 1989, p. 147). English-language research on caregiving from a women's studies perspective has also shown interest in women's unpaid caregiving services. Examples of studies dealing with the consequences of caring for elderly relatives for women's lives and well-being include Ungerson 1987, Lewis & Meredith 1988 and Abel 1990.

24 See also Astvik & Aronsson 1994, p. 101 on home-help services: "Research on and discussion of good working conditions have usually overlooked the fact that relationships with the people for whom work is performed—care recipients, clients— can be an important aspect of a positive evaluation of working conditions."

25 The decline in the number of home-help recipients has primarily affected the elderly with little education, while highly educated elderly people continue to receive help. In-home care priorities have benefited middle-class elderly individuals, probably because they have more resources to make their voices heard (Szebehely 1993 and Sundström 1994).

References

Abel EK. Family care and the frail elderly. In: Abel EK, Nelson M (Eds.): *Circles of Care. Work and Identity in Women's Lives*. State University of New York Press, 1990.

Åman A. *Om den offentliga vården. Byggnader och verksamheter vid svenska vårdinstitutioner under 1800- och 1900-talen [The public care system. Swedish care institutions during the nineteenth and twentieth centuries: The buildings and the activities].* Liber Förlag och Arkitektmuseum, 1976.

Andersson L. *Äldre och äldreomsorg i Norden och Europa [The elderly and elderly care in the Nordic countries and Europe].* Socialstyrelsen [Swedish National Board of Health and Welfare], Ädelutvärderingen 1994:2.

Antman P. *Vägen till systemskiftet—den offentliga sektorn i politiken 1970–1992 [The road to the paradigm shift: Public sector policy 1970–1992].* In: Gustafsson RÅ (Ed.), 1994.

Arbetsmiljöfonden informerar [Information from the Swedish Work Environment Fund] 1992, No. 6.

Aronsson G et al. *Vårdbiträde i öppen hemtjänst och vid servicehus. [Home-care workers in open home-care services and at service-houses].* Arbetsmiljöinstitutet [National Institute of Occupational Health], Arbete och hälsa 1994:32.

Astvik V, Aronsson G. Det goda arbetet i hemtjänsten [Good jobs in home care]. In: Aronsson G et al. (Eds.), 1994.

Barker J, Mitteness L. Invisible Caregivers in the Spotlight: Non-Kin Caregivers of Frail Older Adults. In: Gubrium J, Sankar A (Eds.): *The Home Care Experience. Ethnography and Policy.* Newbury Park: Sage, 1990.

Bexell A. Stort ansvar—liten makt [Heavy responsibility—little power]. *Socialmedicinsk tidskrift* 1985;8–9:353–358.

Borgert L. *Organiserandet som mode—perspektiv på hälso- och sjukvården [Management as fashion—a perspective on health care].* Nerenius & Santérus förlag, 1992.

Braithwaite V. Caregiving Burden. *Research on Aging* 1992;14:1:3–27.

Daatland SO. What are families for? On family solidarity and preference for help. *Ageing and Society* 1990;10:1:1–15.

Dahlgren G. *Framtidens sjukvårdsmarknader—Vinnare och förlorare [Health-care markets of the future: Winners and losers].* Natur och Kultur, 1994.

Dahlström A, Ramström D. *Att leda och styra hälso- och sjukvård—en utvärdering av hälso- och sjukvårdens politiska ledningsorganisation inom Stockholm läns landsting [Directing and managing health care: An evaluation of the political system of Stockholm's county council].* IKE 1990:23. University of Stockholm, Department of Business Economics.

Diderichsen F, Kindlund H, Vogel J. Kvinnans sjukfrånvaro [Women's work absences]. *Läkartidningen* 1993;90:4:289–292.

Due P. Enlige, gamle kvinder: Et proletariat med et stærkt socialt netværk [Old women living alone: A proletariat with a strong social network]. In: Helset A (Ed.): *Gamle kvinner i Norden—deres liv i tekst og tall [Elderly women in the Nordic countries: Their lives in words and statistics].* Report 6/1991, Norsk gerontologisk institutt, Oslo.

Edebalk PG. *Hemmaboendeideologins genombrott—åldringsvård och socialpolitik 1945–1965 [The ideological shift toward "aging in place": Elderly care and social policy 1945–1965].* Meddelanden från Socialhögskolan 1990:4, University of Lund.

Eliasson R (Ed.). *Egenheter och allmänheter. En antologi om omsorg och omsorgens villkor* [*Peculiarities and generalities: On carework and the conditions of caregiving*]. Lund: Arkiv förlag, 1992.

Eliasson-Lappalainen R, Motevasel I. Ethics of care and social policy, *Scandinavian Journal of Social Welfare* 1996;6:189–196.

Expert Group on Public Finance. *Vad blev det av de enskilda alternativen? En kartläggning av verksamheten inom skolan, vården och omsorgen* [*What happened to the private alternatives in schools, health care and elderly care*]. Loord-Gynne U, Mann CO: Rapport till expertgruppen för studier av offentlig ekonomi (ESO) Finansdepartementet Ds 1995:25.

Gardell B, Gustafsson RÅ. *Sjukvård på löpande band* [*Assembly-line medical care*]. Stockholm: Prisma, 1979.

Glazer N. *Women's Paid and Unpaid Labor. The Work Transfer in Health Care and Retailing.* Philadelphia: Temple University Press, 1993.

Glennerster H, Midgley J (Eds.). *The radical right and the welfare state.* Harvester Wheatsheaf, 1991.

Glennerster H, LeGrand J. The development of quasi-markets in welfare provision in the United Kingdom. *International Journal of Health Services* 1995;25:2.

Government bill 1997/98:113. *Nationell handlingsplan för äldrepolitiken* [*National plan for a policy on aging*].

Grafström M. *The experience of burden in the care of elderly persons with dementia.* Stockholm: Karolinska Institute, 1994.

Gustafsson RÅ (Ed.). *Köp och sälj, var god svälj? Vårdens nya ekonomistyrningssystem i ett arbetsmiljöperspektiv* [*Buy and sell? The new purchaser-provider systems and the work environment in health care*]. Arbetsmiljöfonden, 1994.

Gustafsson RÅ. Origins of Authority: The Organization of Medical Care in Sweden. *International Journal of Health Service* 1989;19.

Gustafsson RÅ. Valfrihet och konkurrens inom den offentliga sektorn—en kritisk analys [Freedom of choice and competition within the public sector: A critical analysis]. *Sociologisk Forskning* No. 3, 1995.

Gustafsson RÅ. Freedom of choice and competition in the public sector—a conceptual analysis. In: Iliffe S, Deppe HU (Eds.): *Health Care in Europe: Competition or Solidarity?* Proceedings of the 9th Conference of the International Association for the Study of Health Policy. Frankfurt-Bockenheim: Verlag für Akademische Schriften 1996.

Hugemark A. *Den fångslande marknaden. Ekonomiska experter om välfärdsstaten* [*The captivating market: Economic experts on the welfare state*]. Lund: Arkiv Förlag, 1994.

Johansson L. *Caring for the Next of Kin. On Informal Care for Elderly in Sweden.* University of Uppsala, 1991.

Jonsson E. *Konkurrens inom sjukvården. Vad säger forskningen om effekterna?* [*Competition in health care: What does research tell us about its effects?*] SPRI, 1993.

Krugman P. *Peddling prosperity : economic sense and nonsense in the age of diminished expectations.* London : W.W. Norton, 1995.

Land H, Rose H. Compulsory altruism for some or an altruistic society for all. In: Bean P, Ferris J, Whynes DK (Eds.): *In Defence of Welfare*. London: Tavistock, 1985.

Lewis J, Meredith B. Daughters caring for mothers: The experience of caring and its implications for professional helpers. *Ageing and Society* 1988;8:1–21.

Lingsom S. *I eget hjem med andres hjelp [Staying at home with the help of others]*. Report 3/1987, Institutt for sosialforskning, Oslo.

Lingsom S. Fra studentopprør til eldreomsorg [From student rebellion to elderly care]. *Tidskrift for samfunnsforskning* 1993;34:297–317.

Lingsom S. *The Substitution Issue. Care policies and their Consequences for Family Care*. NOVA-Report 6/1997, Norwegian Social Research, Oslo.

Lundin L, Sundström G. Det riskabla åldrandet [Dangerous aging]. *Välfärdsbulletinen* 1994;2:7–9.

Montin S, Elander I. Citizenship, Consumerism and Local Government in Sweden. *Scandinavian Political Studies*. 1995; 18:25–51.

Mossberg AB. "Jag tar en dag i sänder." Om anställda ålderspensionerade anhörigvårdare ["I take one day at a time." Retired people employed as caregivers for their relatives]. In: Eliasson R (Ed.): *Omsorgens skiftningar [Nuances of care]*. Lund: Studentlitteratur, 1996.

Mossberg AB. Anhörigvårdare—informella vårdare i ett formellt vårdsystem [Family members employed as caregivers: Informal care in a formal care system]. *Socialvetenskaplig tidskrift* 1994;2–3:177–192.

Odén B. Bilden av anhörigvård förr är romantisk och genomfalsk [The picture we have of how people used to care for their relatives is romantic and utterly fictitious]. *Social Forskning*, 1992;2.

Prütz C, Lindgren B. *Produktions-, kostnads- och produktivitetsförändringar inom äldre- och handikappomsorgen 1984–1993 [Changes in production, costs and productivity in the system of care for elderly and disabled persons 1984–1993]*. Socialstyrelsen, Ädelutvärderingen 1994:15.

Robinson R, LeGrand J (Eds.). *Evaluating the NHS reforms*. Kings Fund Institute, 1994.

Showstack Sassoon A (Ed.). *Women and the State, the shifting boundaries of public and private*. London: Hutchinson, 1987.

Sommestad L. Privat eller offentlig välfärd? Ett genusperspektiv på välfärdsstatens historiska formering [Private or public welfare? A gender perspective on the historical development of the welfare state]. *Historisk Tidskrift* 1994;4:601–629.

Statistics Sweden. *Pensionärer 1980–1989 [Retired persons 1980–1989]*. Levnadsförhållanden rapport 81. *Stockholm: SCB, 1993*.

Stockholm Social Service Department. *Tjänsteutlåtande [Official report] 11/23/1989*.

Ström P. Hur påverkas de gamla och personalen av hemtjänstens privatisering? [How are the elderly and care personnel affected by the privatization of home care services?]. In: Gustafsson (Ed.), 1994.

Sundström G. *Caring for the Aged in Welfare Society*. Socialhögskolan, University of Stockholm, 1983.

Sundström G. *Hemtjänst före och efter Ädel [Home care before and after the Ädel reform]*. Socialstyrelsen, Ädelutvärderingen 1994:17.

Svallfors S. Svenskarna och välfärdsstaten [The Swedes and the welfare state]. *Häften för kritiska studier* 1994;2–3:39–52.

Swedish Government Official Reports 1991:104. *Konkurrensen inom den kommunala sektorn [Competition in the municipal sector]*.

Swedish Ministry of Health and Social Affairs. *Valfrihetsrevolutionen i praktiken [The freedom-of-choice revolution in practice]*. Ds 1994:50.

Swedish Ministry of Health and Social Affairs. *Välfärdsfakta Social 1999. [Facts on welfare 1999]*.

Swedish National Association of Local Authorities. *Vår framtid. Äldres vård och omsorg inför 2000-talet. Slutrapport [Our future: Care of the elderly in the twenty-first century. Final report]* 1999.

Swedish National Board of Health and Welfare (1994a). *Alternativa styr- och driftsformer i äldreomsorgen. En kartläggning [Alternative forms of governing and management in the care of the elderly and disabled : A survey]*. SoS report 1994:24.

Swedish National Board of Health and Welfare (1994b). *Konsekvenser av beställar-utförarmodellen inom äldre- och handikappomsorgen [Consequences of the purchaser-provider model in the care of the elderly and disabled]*. Socialstyrelsen, 1994.

Swedish National Board of Health and Welfare (1994c). *Äldreomsorg i nedskärningstider [Elderly care in a time of cutbacks]*. Main report. SocialstyrelsenSocialstyrelsen, 1994.

Swedish National Board of Health and Welfare (1994d). *Utvärdering av kvalitet [Quality evaluation]*. SoS report 1994:13.

Swedish National Board of Health and Welfare (1995). *Alternativa styr- och driftsformer i äldreomsorgen—Valfrihet [Alternative forms of governing and management in the care of the elderly and disabled: Freedom of choice]*. SoS report 1995:11.

Swedish National Board of Health and Welfare (1998). *Äldreuppdraget. Årsrapport 1998 [Report on elder care in Sweden 1998]*. Stockholm: Socialstyrelsen 1998

Szebehely M. *Hemtjänst eller anhörigvård? Förändringar under 1980-talet [Home-help services or informal care? Changes in the 1980s]*. Stockholm: Socialstyrelsen, 1993.

Szebehely M. Ger minskad offentlig omsorg varmare relationer? [Does a reduction in public care services lead to better relationships?] *Socialvetenskaplig tidskrift* 1994;4:326–346.

Szebehely M. *Vardagens organisering. Om vårdbiträden och gamla i hemtjänsten [The organization of everyday life—on home helpers and elderly people in Sweden]*. Lund: Arkiv förlag, 1995.

Szebehely M. *Hjälp i hemmet i nedskärningstid—hemtjänstens och anhörigas insatser för gamla kvinnor och män. [Practical assistance at home in times of cut-backs: Home-help services and family help for older women and men]*. Stockholm: Swedish Association of Local Authorities, 1998a.

Szebehely M. Changing divisions of carework. Caring for children and frail elderly people in Sweden. In: Lewis J (Ed.): *Gender, Social Care and Welfare State Restructuring in Europe*. Aldershot: Ashgate, 1998b.

Szulkin R, Tåhlin M. Arbetets utveckling [The development of work]. In: Fritzell J, Lundberg O (Eds.): *Vardagens villkor [Conditions of everyday life]*. Brombergs, 1994.

Thorslund M, Lundberg O, Parker M. Klass och ohälsa bland de allra äldsta [Class and ill health among the oldest old]. *Läkartidningen* 1993;60:41:3547–3553.

Thulin AB. *Arbetsförhållanden inom hemtjänsten [Working conditions in home care]*. Report No. 80, Stockholms socialförvaltning [Stockholm Social Service Department], 1987.

Tornstam L. Den demografiska bomben och de nya kraven på den informella omsorgen—framtidshot eller myt? [The demographic bomb and new demands placed on informal care: Future threat or myth?]. *Aldring & Eldre*, 1992;2:22–28.

Ungerson C. *Policy is Personal: Sex, Gender and Informal Care*. London: Tavistock, 1987.

Vogel J. *Living conditions and inequality in the European Union 1997*. Eurostat Working Paper. European Commission, 1997.

Von Otter C, Tengvald K. Vouchers: A revolution in social welfare? *Economic and Industrial Democracy*, 1992;13.

Wærness K. The Rationality of Caring. *Economic and Industrial Democracy* 1984;5:185–211.

Wærness K. *Informal and formal care in old age: What is wrong with the new ideology in Scandinavia today?* In: Ungerson C (Ed.): Gender and Caring. New York: Harvester Wheatsheaf, 1990.

Whitehead M, Gustafsson RÅ, Diderichsen F. Why is Sweden rethinking its NHS-style reforms? *British Medical Journal* 1997; 315.

Zarit SH. Do we need another "Stress and caregiving" study? *The Gerontologist* 1989;29:2:147–148.

12

The future of gender inequalities in health

Annika Härenstam, Gunnar Aronsson, Anne Hammarström

Introduction

THE PURPOSE OF THIS CHAPTER is to discuss social changes likely to occur in the future, particularly in the spheres of working and private life, as they relate to health trends among women and men. The impact of changes in society on people's living conditions may affect the health of women and men in similar or different ways. Our comments on what the future may bring should be viewed as a basis for discussion rather than as predictions.

This chapter is based on two assumptions regarding health and the spheres of employment and private life. First, it is beneficial to the health of both women and men to be actively involved in both working and private life. This is a normative statement, but it is also supported by empirical data. While a balance between different aspects of life is desirable, it is, in itself, insufficient. Stress can be too great—which is our second assumption. Further on we shall offer empirical support for these assumptions, followed by discussion. We focus particularly on two life phases: youth, when people are establishing themselves in the adult world and beginning their careers, and the period in which people are combining work with parental responsibilities. Finally, we outline several possible scenarios in which social changes could have a positive or negative effect on the health of various groups of women and men.

An important starting point in evaluating and assessing trends in society and working life is to examine how various changes affect the balance between men's and women's involvement and opportunities in both working life and the private arena. Our discussion and conclusions are based on certain assumptions and causal arguments. In order to assess overall health trends, it is important to take into account complex and dynamic interactions; for example, changes for the worse in one area may be offset by improvements elsewhere. Health risks may decline for one group but increase for another. Conditions outside of working hours affect how people deal with the stresses of their jobs, just as the effects of working conditions extend into hours spent off work. There are a number of potential conflicts between paid employment and private life, which is why we need to take a "twenty-four hour perspective" (Salomon & Grimsmo 1994). The fact that there are more working parents with small children exacerbates the conflict between the stresses of work and private life. Complicating matters is the fact that although there is a generally positive association between paid employment and health, this does not apply to all individuals. Certain people may find that paid employment has a more negative effect on their health than unemployment or early retirement.

Social and working conditions

A high level of economic growth appears to have a more favorable effect on working conditions and the job environment than low growth. This applies particularly to physical job stress, hiring conditions and opportunities for decision-making on the job. However, high economic growth can also lead to increased time constraints and greater psychological demands at work, which, in turn, may result in further tension between work and family roles (Salomon & Grimsmo 1994).

High demand for workers puts employees in a stronger negotiating position with respect to a number of matters directly or indirectly associated with health. High rates of economic growth make it easier to maintain society's systems of economic, social and medical security. When the individual has to assume more of the economic costs, his or her contact with these systems is more likely to be delayed, which presumably has negative health consequences. Cutbacks in the social security system would probably be felt most strongly by low-wage earners, i.e., blue-collar workers, particularly women.

The 1990s saw the emergence of a phenomenon that is likely to have signicant health consequences: unemployment has remained at a rather high level despite strong economic growth within most industries. Even if the prognosis for Sweden's economy is largely hopeful, most experts are pessimistic about reducing the unemployment rate, which is currently high in historical terms. Internationally, Sweden's economy has become increasingly dependent on other countries, most recently because of Sweden's entry into the European Union, several of whose member states have long had mass unemployment. Fighting inflation may become an overarching goal, taking precedence over full employment.

Employment has been shown to be of great significance to one's health. The link between working conditions and health varies substantially from one type of work to another, with certain occupations closely associated with an increased risk of poor health. Furthermore, working conditions vary over the life course, as people move from one position to another. Women's and men's job situations are characterized by gender segregation (Jonung 1997; Gonäs, Plantenga & Rubery 1999): horizontal segregation means that women and men work in different occupations and have different employers, while vertical segregation means that women and men have different opportunities when it comes to advancement and mobility, control of their own work and flexibility in their jobs and careers. Owing to these types of segregation, women and men are exposed to different risks on the job, which, in turn, affect their health in different ways (Lagerlöf 1993, Kilbom, Messing, Bildt Thorbjörnsson 1999). Accordingly, structural changes in the labor market can be expected to affect both the degree and the type of health problems people encounter. Health differences between women and men stem, for example, from the fact that women and men are recruited for different jobs and responsibilities. They also reflect the degree to which the respective interests of women and men are taken into consideration in the face of structural changes, business shutdowns and personnel cuts.

Gender segregation offers a point of departure for further discussion of work-related health issues that will affect women and men in the future. It may be appropriate here to consider both quantitative and qualitative changes occurring in the labor market, the former being changes in the number of people working in a particular field, the latter involving changes in employees' working conditions as new technologies and organizational innovations are introduced. The most negative development, in terms of public health, is that more employees are working in fields with poor working conditions.

It is beyond the scope of this chapter to detail every type of industry. Instead, we concentrate on three major sectors: the public sector, industry, and the private service sector, each of which has different features and is currently undergoing certain changes.

A not unlikely scenario is that the national economy is splitting into two parts, with strong growth and profitability in high-tech, export-oriented businesses but personnel and financial cuts in publicly financed areas (such as health and nursing care). It does not appear to work as well as it did in the past to transfer profits from the first sector to shore up welfare services. The private service sector, which is closely linked with both the industrial and the public sector, is expected to show some employment growth. It is becoming more difficult to make a clear distinction between services and goods. Since goods increasingly involve services, such a distinction no longer applies to the modern working world (Aronsson & Sjögren 1994).

The public sector: Downsizing and structural change

The public sector has undergone substantial and continuing downsizing and structural changes during the 1990s. Following several decades of strong growth, employment has stagnated or even declined in the fields of health care and public administration.

From a perspective of gender, class and health, changes occurring in the realms of health and nursing care are of particular interest, since the current cutbacks involve a sector that is highly gender-segregated and employs a disproportionate number of women. Changes in the public sector affect a large number of women whose training has prepared them for today's public-sector jobs. Women have a particular stake in what happens in the spheres of child and elderly care, since their role in those areas goes beyond paid employment. Cutbacks may well mean that women who are now providing care for pay will find themselves performing the same services without compensation. Cutbacks in this sector, leading to a lower level of investment in elderly care, may also put increased pressure on women who work outside the home.

Bengt Furåker (1993) discusses alternatives for women in the labor market at a time of substantial cuts in the public sector. He sees three main options:

1. *Creating new jobs in the private sector responsible for the same kinds of work currently carried out as part of the public sector—particularly teaching, nursing care and social work.* It is difficult to economize on welfare services, whether offered on a private or public basis. Making services less expensive will very likely mean a decline in quality or fewer jobs, or both.

2. *Creating new job opportunities in other areas of the private sector, such as retail trade, hotels and restaurants.* A decrease in public expenditures and lower taxes might be expected to lead to an increase in private consumption, and in turn to the expansion of certain types of businesses. For at least some of these businesses—retail enterprises, banks and insurance companies—the situation is more likely to be reversed, with a decline in employment and economic difficulties probably continuing over the long term.

3. *Women entering male-dominated occupations.* In an economic slump with low demand for labor, anyone who has a job will be anxious to keep it. It is unlikely that women from the public sector will be able to compete with men and enter existing male-dominated occupations. A shortage of workers, however, would change the situation.

Furåker concludes that it is very difficult in the short term to create new jobs for women forced out of the public sector. Restructuring takes time, and many people, particularly older individuals, will find themselves outside the labor market as this process is taking place. If new jobs are created later on, they will, to a large extent, be filled by workers other than those who were let go. Furåker underscores the importance of age and education. Several studies of structural change in the public sector indicate that educational level is a decisive factor. Highly educated women seem to do relatively well, while older women in low- or middle-level jobs have the worst prospects of ever returning to the labor market. Early retirement is frequently the solution for such women (Gonäs & Spånt 1997; Marklund 2001). However, new regulations governing early retirement benefits may mean that these women will find themselves dependent on public assistance.

Assuming that the quantitative and qualitative changes outlined above occur, the end result will be fewer employees and more stress on those who manage to keep their jobs. Job quality would likely deteriorate, as fewer people would find themselves responsible for an equal or greater amount of work. This would primarily affect the large numbers of women working in the care sector, where it is unlikely that technical developments or new technologies would be able to reduce job stress to any substantial degree. From a health standpoint, such a situation would benefit neither caregivers nor care recipients.

Production industries

Basic industries and the production industry are in the midst of major techno-logical and organizational changes that have dramatically increased productivity and efficiency (Aronsson & Sjögren 1994). There is a long-term, stable trend toward a reduction in the number of workers involved in raw material extraction (forestry, agriculture and mining). The percentage of workers employed in pro-duction jobs has been declining since the early 1960s. There was a sharp decrease in employment at the beginning of the 1990s, followed by some recovery begin-ning in 1995. Over the long term, however, it is expected that employment will continue to decline. More and more goods are being produced by multinational corporations, and reduced trade barriers and free movement of capital have enabled businesses to move their production easily from one country to another. This results in uncertainty for workers and requires them to be able to adapt to change and job insecurity.

The production industry encompasses a wide range of activities, with a vari-ety of different ways in which production is organized. The industry is over-whelmingly male-dominated, with women constituting only about one-sixth of the labor force. The production industry is characterized by considerable ill health, a high rate of illness-related absences, high mortality risks, injuries and work disabilities/early retirement. Injuries from stress and overwork are common in all production-related industries. In addition, there is a disproportionate inci-dence of coronary infarctions, skin problems, hearing damage, etc. However, the number of accidents on the job and work-related illnesses has been steadily declining in the production industry since the late 1980s. A study has shown that of the 27,000 oldest members (over 60) of the Swedish Metalworkers Union, a striking number have left their jobs to take early retirement. Only 5 percent of the union members over the age of 60, most of whom are men, work full-time.[1]

Women who work in production have a higher frequency of ailments of the muscles and joints than men. Although these jobs had been regarded as tempo-rary, many women have found themselves staying in such repetitive, fixed jobs with little opportunity for influence or control, for lack of alternatives. Women in production jobs are among the most vulnerable women in the labor force in terms of health. Many jobs in this sector have begun to require more training than in the past. However, in this process of upgrading skills, new forms of stratifica-tion are created, as those women who regard their work in the production sector as temporary stay in the worst jobs (Swedish Foundation for Working Life 1995).

New technologies and innovative organizational models involving more var-ied work tasks are reducing the rate of physical injury. The use of robots is help-ing to lower the rate of injuries resulting from heavy, noisy and dirty industrial environments, since workers are physically removed from the most dangerous environments. Within the electronics industry and the field of micro-assembly, however, where women make up a large proportion of workers, it is still difficult to replace human labor with robots.

The new organizational concepts include the "just-in-time" inventory method, overtime as the norm, and high expectations of loyalty and teamwork. This increases the risk of physical strain, stress and error. During the economic slump of the early 1990s, many businesses undertook harsh personnel and organizational cutbacks. These measures, combined with overtime work to meet the needs of the given economic situation, appear to be the solution preferred by businesses in the ideological vanguard. Following on the heels of computerization, it is likely that shift work will also become more common. This is largely because round-the-clock production with limited employee participation has become more feasible, and because investment costs have risen, spurring efforts to increase the level of resource utilization. Overtime work and shift jobs often make it difficult to combine jobs with responsibilities for children and home, which has a negative effect particularly on women.

Based on employment prognoses and the percentage of workers in problematic job environments, a Norwegian study, "Arbeidsliv mot år 2010" [Working life up to the year 2010], calculates the distribution of work-related stress factors (Salomon & Grimsmo 1994). The prognosis is for improvements in fields involving industrial production. Fewer people will be exposed to physically and ergonomically stressful conditions, noise, vibration or chemicals. Similar conclusions are reached by the authors of a Dutch study (Steering Committee on Future Health Scenarios 1994).

There is the danger that structural change toward high-tech production will result not in a positive working environment for all, but instead in further polarization of high- and low-level jobs. High-tech industry employs a large percentage of highly qualified and trained personnel in the product-development phase. The manufacture of high-tech products frequently involves a complicated division of labor and repetitive kinds of work. In those industries with the best employment record, a large proportion of more sophisticated tasks tend to be performed by white-collar workers, while manual workers carry out largely routine jobs. However, there is a very conscious attempt in some quarters to broaden the scope of tasks performed by manual workers and eliminate the stark boundary between the work of technicians/engineers and other employees.

Reducing the amount of mass production, increasing variation and adapting products to customers' needs all require a more highly skilled work force. From a health perspective, this should be beneficial to both men and women, but particularly women, who are overrepresented in mass production jobs. However, the need for higher qualifications may lead businesses to seek new employees with advanced technical training, which women are less likely to have.

We do not anticipate much change in the number of employed persons. While the physical work environment is likely to improve in many respects, over the medium term many workers will continue to carry out repetitive jobs that pose the risk of stress and overuse injuries. There is a disproportionate number of women in such jobs.

Factors such as streamlined organization, "just-in-time" production methods, managing customer orders and adapting to customers' needs increase time pressures and businesses' need for flexible work hours and overtime work. This heightens the tension between the demands of the job and private life, and may result in fewer women working in the industrial sector, either because women are forced out of such jobs or because fewer women are hired. There are trends that point in this direction. For men, these factors may make it difficult for them to play an active role in both their jobs and the private sphere, even if they wish to do so, since job demands take priority.

The private service sector

Private services are a growth industry, although to some extent this growth is deceptive, since the services performed by private service companies show up more clearly in statistics than the same services did when performed by other businesses or government authorities as part of a larger whole. It is difficult to assess just how working conditions and health risks are affected when service responsibilities are taken out of a business and contracted out to specialized, for-hire service providers, and little research has been devoted to this question. The accessibility of services is a very strong competitive argument for service providers. As society moves toward more businesses in the service sector and increased service production, the demand for flexibility in working hours and job tasks is likely to increase. It is clearly impossible to store services; they need to be rendered when the demand arises.

Private service production involves a large proportion of "atypical" jobs, with irregular work hours, temporary hiring, non-standardized contracts and part-time work. Computer technology makes possible sophisticated scheduling and a wide variety of working hours. This offers both risks and opportunities for employees and the work environment. For example, computerized accounting systems in commercial businesses can precisely record the level of transactions at different times of the day or over an extended period. Demand patterns can then be used to determine minimum staffing requirements. This may result in eliminating low-stress periods and thus reduce or eliminate altogether the opportunity for workers to relax. There are also examples of quite sophisticated computer-generated scheduling systems where individual preferences can be taken into account.[2]

While technological innovations are leading to a decrease in manual labor during the extraction and production stages, this is less apparent in the areas of transportation, retail trade and the hotel and restaurant businesses. It is probably most difficult to use technology in these fields to address the traditional problems of the working environment and the issues of work-related accidents and illnesses. In contrast to industrial workers, employees in these areas cannot be replaced in high-risk jobs by robots or other technological means. In trade and transportation, as well as in the hotel and restaurant businesses, risks related to manual labor and heavy lifting are still common, with the ensuing problems of excess strain and a variety of injuries. In addition, it is not possible to make the same kinds of changes in the working environment as one might in an industrial setting, and problems that industry would address are ignored. For example, certain types of restaurants inevitably involve evening and night hours, a high level of noise, smoke and crowding, as well as different spatial levels and situations in which employees have difficulty moving about. These kinds of businesses are segregated by gender, both horizontally and vertically. Men predominate in transportation work, while women occupy most of the low-level positions in sales, hotels and restaurants.

In terms of the future, it is interesting to look at the trends in modern information-related businesses with decentralized and less hierarchical organizational structures. Computer and consulting companies are one familiar example, both of which are growth industries that will play a central role in the future. Two Swedish doctoral dissertations focus on working conditions and gender relations in such businesses (Blomqvist 1994, Roman 1994). It appears that equal treatment is the rule, rather than the gender discrimination often found in more traditional businesses. This holds true both for hiring and for the distribution of responsibilities within these companies. Gender-integrated workplaces are seen to be more advantageous than gender-segregated workplaces. Traditionally "female" characteristics like the ability to communicate with clients and personnel have proved to be commercially beneficial. The women in these studies were also focused on both their jobs and their families. The quality of their jobs is high. However, equal treatment also seemed to mean that "women were expected to adapt to 'male' working conditions, and no heed was paid to gender differences in life circumstances" (Roman 1994). Neither working nor career conditions were designed to meet the needs of employees with responsibilities for their children and families.

Future working conditions in the private service sector and the ensuing health consequences for women and men are hard to assess in terms of quantitative and qualitative change. It is likely that the number of job opportunities will increase, and that this sector will include both stressful jobs with little opportunity to adapt one's work hours and duties to one's own needs and jobs that can evolve and offer flexibility.

Some general conclusions on trends in working life, as they relate to gender and health

To sum up: In structural terms, i.e., when we look at where jobs are available and where they are being eliminated, women may be most vulnerable, particularly to economic cutbacks in the public sphere and exclusion from industrial jobs, where the increased importance of technical skills also frequently prevents women from being hired. Within the private service sector, the picture is mixed. We find poor working environments with little hope of change, but also a trend toward favorable working conditions. Women may be better equipped than men to make their way into the expanding knowledge-intensive branches of the service sector. They have more unrealized human capital, with experience that makes them well suited to the job world of the future. This applies particularly to jobs in which the decision-making process is conducted not by sluggish hierarchies, but through compromise, negotiation and adaptation, and by maintaining internal and external relationships.

Family and work

So far, we have presented various scenarios for changes in society and working life, i.e., the sphere of life that involves gainful employment. What about the private sphere, and what effect does combining private life and employment have on health? What we term the private sphere includes the efforts people make to ensure the functioning of home, family and social relationships. It also involves volunteer work of a social nature, such as coaching young people in a sport or volunteering in one's neighborhood or in a day-care cooperative run by parents.

Work in the private sphere is, by definition, unpaid, and whether or not it is done has consequences for other people. American researchers have defined work in terms of eight categories, two of which are paid (House & Kahn 1984; Kahn 1991). The other six categories are housework, child care, household maintenance, volunteer work in organizations, helping relatives and friends, and helping people with chronic or acute problems. Estimates indicate that unpaid work is nearly as extensive as paid work in Sweden. Women perform substantially more unpaid work than men, particularly housework (Björnberg 1998; Gonäs & Spånt 1997; Härenstam et al. 2000). Men are more involved than women in volunteer work for organizations, most commonly athletic clubs (Jeppson Grassman 1993; Wijkström 1994). A comparison over the course of people's lives shows that particularly for women, the level of unpaid work is at least as high after retirement as before (Jeppson Grassman 1993).

The division of labor between women and men is very clear, but it has shifted over time, depending largely on where women's contributions have been needed (Wikander 1992). The labor market is gender-segregated, both vertically and horizontally. This division of paid and unpaid work, sometimes referred to as the gender contract, is now being strongly called into question by many women, but also to some degree by men, mainly in connection with custody disputes in divorce situations. A substantial rise in women's employment rates and a gradual increase in men's work as caregivers and their childcare responsibilities have called into question the traditional norms governing who is expected to do what in society.

Much of what is termed the welfare society is based on women's work in low-paying jobs and on decades of strong economic growth. Like the gender contract,[3] the social contract, which regulates the paid work performed by society and unpaid contributions by families, neighborhoods and organizations, is also in a state of crisis (Åström & Hirdman 1992). The public sector is shrinking, and more and more tasks are now being transferred from the world of employment back to the private arena. Dependence on the family as a social and economic safety net is again increasing.

The unfavorable trend in women's health during the 1980s may be rooted in an increased discrepancy between society's values and women's opportunities. Although women today have as much education as men and have grown up with the ideal of gender equality, women continue to have more limited control over their life circumstances, as a result of such factors as less representation in decision-making bodies, lower earnings, smaller pensions and fewer capital assets. Men's predominance in working and social life has meant that men have usually been the ones to identify and define problems, determine solutions and decide how resources are to be used. Combined with a high overall level of job stress, increased frustration with limited opportunities can lead to higher rates of illness among women (cf. Johannisson's analysis of the transition to an industrialized society, Chapter 4).

Health consequences of combining work and family

Our basic assumption is that health improves for both women and men if they can participate in both spheres, with a moderate level of stress and sufficient opportunity for influence and personal development. We focus here particularly on the life stage in which people are combining parenthood with gainful employment. Reconciling the two spheres during this stage produces the most conflict and results in high levels of stress for the individual. How women and men combine their work and their private lives is largely determined by socio-cultural factors. Thus studies from other countries and cultures of the health consequences of reconciling work and family cannot be directly applied to conditions in Sweden.

As Ohlander (Chapter 10) points out, women have always done most of the unpaid work involved in running their households and taking care of children, and they have frequently had jobs as well to help support their families. What is really new, in historical terms, is that men are beginning to participate in housework and child care (Ohlander 1993).

There are numerous hypotheses regarding women's work in both spheres and how it relates to their health.[4] We shall summarize two of the most common ones, the expansion hypothesis and the stress hypothesis, although these have been tested primarily in countries other than Sweden, particularly the United States.

According to the *expansion hypothesis,* people who have many roles[5] or responsibilities in their lives do better than those with only a few. A person with several different positions can use positive conditions in one sphere to offset occasional stress in other areas (Gove & Zeiss 1987; Thoits 1983). Experience and competence in the world of work and in home and family life seem to produce a higher level of social integration and a greater capacity to deal with different situations, thus giving the individual more control over his or her life situation (Barnett et al. 1994; Lennon & Rosenfield 1992). Increased self-confidence and economic independence outweigh the additional stress that comes from the responsibilities of several positions (Barnett & Baruch 1987; Pugliesi 1995).

Second, there is the *stress hypothesis.* Here the focus is on human limitations. Having a number of responsibilities in life means increased stress, more conflict and, in turn, increased risk to health. The primary roles assigned to people—for men, productive work and the responsibility to support a family; for women, reproductive work at home and within the family—are so demanding that any additional responsibility increases the risk of negative health effects (Coser 1974; Goode 1960; Slater 1963). The stress hypothesis as it was originally formulated may appear outdated, but similar biologically-based hypotheses continue to be offered as an explanation of poor health among women. Some researchers suggest that trying to "tamper with nature" may increase the risk of poor health or result in other negative consequences.[6] Particularly in the media and in popular science literature, a great deal of attention is given to the differences between women's and men's biological constitutions. This type of literature explains such phenomena as aggressive, outgoing and dominating behavior among men and relating, submissive and sensitive behavior among women in terms of natural hormonal differences between the sexes.[7]

Most studies of women support the expansion hypothesis over the stress hypothesis, but empirical studies lend some credence to both. Chapter 9 shows that women who work outside the home live longer than housewives do, and this cannot be explained in terms of selection mechanisms (Vågerö & Lahelma 1996). A number of population studies indicate that work circumstances are more closely linked to women's health than family circumstances (Kindlund 1993; Szulkin & Thålin 1994). Other studies point to a negative effect of women's twofold responsibilities (Bird & Fremont 1991; Frankenhaeuser et al. 1989; Hall 1992; Rosenfield 1989). If total stress is too great, the risk of negative health effects increases (Lundberg et al. 1994). Much points to the conclusion that a combination of both hypotheses is required to understand the links between work and health, i.e., that having several responsibilities in life is good for one's health, provided that one's overall stress level is not excessive.

Gender research is beginning to focus more attention on the importance of men's actions and activities for their own health and women's health. However, the health consequences for men of combining gainful employment and work in the private sphere remain largely unexplored. There are few studies, for example, of the health consequences of how men divide their time between gainful employment, on the one hand, and housework and caregiving activities at home, on the other—even though the quality of their private lives appears to be at least as important to men's health as conditions on the job (Barnett et al. 1987; 1992; Pugliesi 1995). Since most men are actively involved in only *one* sphere, they are worse off than women, according to the expansion hypothesis. If men were to expand their work and responsibilities to include the private sphere, this might lead to a change in social roles and behavior, improved well-being and perhaps also longer lives.[8] Moreover, it would also benefit women's health, since it would reduce the overall burden on them.

The importance of being able to adjust one's stress level

A high level of demands and stress over which one has no control is associated with a high risk of poor health. Influence over one's work situation has been shown in numerous studies to be a very significant factor in people's health.[9] Somewhat less attention has been given to the question of people's influence over their lives as a whole (Lindbladh 1993; Syme 1989; Wallston 1987; Östergren et al. 1995). Women and men who are involved in both spheres of life are able to adjust their stress level, partly by dividing up housework, and partly because they can better adjust the demands of work to accommodate the private sphere.

The interface between gainful employment and the private sphere highlights the opportunities that exist for keeping total stress at a manageable level. Research on living arrangements has examined how people combine work and family (Jakobsen & Karlsson 1993). The traditional worker's lifestyle is based on the idea that paid work, the sphere of necessity, provides the means for shaping one's free time, the sphere of one's free choice. Here the line is clear between the time that belongs to one's working life and one's leisure time.

Work organization and new company cultures demand commitment, flexibility and overtime work. The boundary between work and leisure time is breaking down, even for manual workers (Jakobsen & Karlsson 1993; Wiklund & Härenstam 1995). This can affect health in both positive and negative ways. Central considerations in combining the two spheres will include both the amount of paid work and the allocation of work hours (Puranen 1995).

Influence over one's work hours has been shown to be of great importance to health, particularly for women. Women, but not men, who do a great deal of overtime work have an increased risk of cardiovascular disease (Theorell & Härenstam 2000) and elevated levels of adrenaline (Lundberg & Palm 1989). Many men today have the advantage of being able to arrange their time in accordance with the demands of their jobs. According to a Swedish survey, 63 percent of men but only 54 percent of women felt that they had some control over the allocation of their work hours (Statistics Sweden 2000). It has also been shown that women do most of the regular work at home that needs to be done at a certain time, while men take on more of the responsibilities that can be put off until later (Rydenstam 1992).

In different life stages, opportunities vary to achieve a balance between the two spheres at a manageable stress level. Since people are entering the work force later, the first years of employment may well coincide with marriage and starting a family. The conflict between work and family has become a more and more common problem for men, too, particularly white-collar workers (Nilsson 1992). How well these spheres are balanced during this period can also affect both men and women in later years. Too much stress over a limited number of years can wear people out and contribute to illnesses that may not show up until later in life. Similarly, too little stress, as in the case of unemployed young people with few responsibilities in the private sphere, is also associated with the risk of poor health.

What factors influence how work and responsibility are distributed between women and men?

Gender differences in the amount of time spent on paid and unpaid work have declined in Sweden, although there are still large differences in the case of housework. Women have become just as involved in the job world as men. The situation with respect to housework is less clear, and differs somewhat depending on such things as whether one looks just at people working full-time or at the overall population (Lundberg et al. 1994, Rydenstam 1992). A study of changes in life circumstances in Sweden between 1981 and 1991 shows that men were generally doing more of the housework than before,[10] but this did not apply to all men. Housework done by younger men increased more than among older men (Nermo 1994). Time-use studies also show that no one works as much—in terms of both paid work alone and total paid and unpaid work—as fathers of small children (Rydenstam 1992). But the percentage of men who stay home with their children continues to be very low.

Men and women who defy traditional gender roles in one sphere are more inclined to do so in the other sphere as well (Bejerot & Härenstam 1995). Highly educated men who have children at home and work in female-dominated occupations take on a larger share of unpaid responsibilities than do men in other kinds of jobs (Bejerot & Härenstam 1995). Highly educated women working in male-dominated occupations are less likely to have children than other women.

When these women do have children, they are more likely to share responsibility for housework with their husbands (ibid.). There are a number of possible explanations for this: It may be, of course, that women and men choose their occupations because they want to focus on their spouse and children. There may also be a socialization and learning process that goes on at work and at home in which men and women influence each other. The gender-segregated labor market may thus work against a balance between the two spheres.

There is a link between women's social position (e.g., level of education, income and job status) and the extent to which their husbands participate in housework and child care (Roman 1992; Bejerot & Härenstam 1995; Nermo 1994; Statistics Sweden 1994).[11] The amount of housework done by men whose female partners hold a low-level blue-collar job has not increased as much as it has for other men (Nermo 1994). In addition, the working conditions of many women in blue-collar jobs worsened in the 1980s (Szulkin & Thålin 1994). Not only have female blue-collar workers seen a disproportionate increase in their total workload, then, but many of them have also experienced a decline in the conditions they find on the job.

Highly educated women have more opportunities to find jobs with good working conditions (Nermo 1994). However, they may have to contend with unacceptable stress, particularly women in high-level positions. Up to now health trends have not been as favorable for these women as one might expect, given their social position (see Chapter 9). This may reflect the fact that women are not as able to unwind after work as men in similar jobs (Frankenhaeuser 1989). A high-level position alone does not relieve them of the responsibility of housework. Men with careers frequently have a wife to take care of things and support them at home, while women in high-level positions bear such responsibilities themselves (Jakobsen & Karlsson 1993; Bejerot & Härenstam 1995; Billing 1991).

The most common family model in Sweden still assigns to women primary responsibility for home and children, even though there are two earners in most families with children (Björnberg 1995). The increase in women's employment does not appear to have brought about a decrease in the time women spend caring for ill relatives or ensuring that the emotional and physical needs of their husbands and children are met (Moen et al. 1994). Both men's and women's job stress spills over into their family life. Women seem to be more likely to adjust the work they do at home to offset the effects their partners' stress may have on the family (Bolger et al. 1989).

A study of highly educated employed women and men (Bejerot & Härenstam 1995) examined the links between health and various ways of dividing up responsibility for earning a living and caring for home and family. It was most favorable to the health of both women and men when husband and wife shared equally in breadwinning and household responsibilities. Men in a traditional family situation, who bore primary responsibility for earning a living and whose wives did most of the housework, reported a lower level of well-being than other men. The situation of single mothers was no worse than that of doubly-burdened women, i.e., those who held jobs that were at least as demanding as those of their husbands as well as primary responsibility for home and children. The quality of their jobs was of great importance to single mothers and to both men and women who worked outside the home as well as at home. It is reasonable to assume that when people have substantial responsibilities in the private sphere, the stress they encounter at work is critical to their health.[12]

Paid and unpaid work in the future

How will people reconcile work and home responsibilities in the future? Is it only a historical anomaly that most women work outside the home and men are involved in home and family responsibilities? Will more people be volunteering to help others? How will paid and unpaid work affect future health? These things depend on such factors as the extent to which caregiving will be an unpaid job, who will take on that responsibility, which people will find themselves in either positive or stressful job environments or perhaps unemployed, and whether men will take on more responsibilities in the private sphere. These issues involve both structural and individual factors.

Surveys of young people's attitudes suggest that unpaid work will become more common among men, and that women will insist on meaningful work and equal pay (Swedish Government Official Reports 1994). The majority of young Swedish women and men believe that both partners should help provide for the family, work full-time and share home and family responsibilities equally (ibid.). People generally feel that when there are children under the age of seven, both women and men should work part-time and share responsibility for housework (Statistics Sweden 1994). Compared with the 1960s, men are more family-oriented and more favorably disposed toward women working outside the home (Nilsson 1992). The meaning of fatherhood has changed, from being mainly a matter of earning a living to being involved on a daily basis (Åström 1990). However, there are clear differences between attitudes on home responsibilities and reality (Edlund et al. 1990; Nilsson 1992). For instance, older fathers take more days of parental leave. The lowest level of gender equality was found for the youngest couples (Bejerot & Härenstam 1995; Statistics Sweden 1994).

Total work time is at an all-time high for families in which both parents are employed.[13] Stress on the family is growing, and it is increasingly important for people to be able to adjust their work hours to their life situations. Which people will have sufficient power and self-confidence to make their desires and needs known? They will have to negotiate mainly with their employers, but also with colleagues, for example in questions of overtime work. Employees' autonomy will depend on their jobs, the sector in which they are employed, how much they earn and how secure their jobs are. Everyone in a family is affected by the work hours of both husband and wife. Job demands that are better attuned to a given life situation will improve the quality of the private sphere, which, in turn, is beneficial to the health and well-being of women, men and children.

Structural conditions are crucial for achieving a balance between spheres and an appropriate degree of work stress. Changes in the job world help determine how many and which people will find employment, who will get a job that offers room for advancement and who will find a job that leaves sufficient time and energy for the private sphere. Family, social and distribution policies provide the framework in which women and men can divide their time, both between themselves and between the two spheres of their lives. Changes occurring at the societal level that affect matters like the parental leave system, sick leave and unemployment benefits are in danger of fostering inequality, particularly between different groups of women and between women and men.

An increase in class differences in health appears to have a more negative effect on women's health than men's. This, according to the British sociologist Ann Oakley (1994), is because when class differences increase, poverty spreads more rapidly among women and children than men. In addition, more and more women are in a position of having to support their families on inadequate material resources, which takes a toll on them personally. At present, the gap is widening between different groups in Sweden. Many immigrants, long-term unemployed workers and single parents find themselves in a vulnerable position (Swedish Trade Union Confederation 1995). Women in blue-collar jobs are frequently under a great deal of stress and have only limited control over their situations, both at work and in the private sphere, compared with other women and men (Hall 1991; 1992; Härenstam et al. 2000; Westberg 1998)). If class and gender differences observed in Great Britain hold for Sweden as well, this means worse health for large numbers of women, particularly those in blue-collar jobs.

The future is brighter for highly educated women and men. Women with advanced training in a field that is also in demand outside the public sector are likely to be sought-after in the job market and well able to compete for good positions. If present trends continue, their husbands will be taking on more and more responsibility for unpaid work at home.

Today's young people: Tomorrow's adults

Youth is the time of life when young women and men are socialized into adult life. It is a period filled with change, in which young people try out various options so that later on they will be able to establish their own families and careers. During this time the groundwork is laid for their adult lives, first through their educational choices and then through their choice of an occupation and a spouse. While it is possible to go back for additional training later on, this frequently involves substantial hurdles, not least financial ones. The young adult years seem to be growing more and more stressful and demanding, with the requirements of the labor market increasing and a high rate of unemployment apparently a permanent feature of our society. This makes it more difficult to bring the private sphere and the demands of one's job into equilibrium.

The future health of young men and women depends to a large extent on gendered power imbalances. These power imbalances mean that men have more influence and power than women do, and thus a better basis for achieving good health (see Chapter 1). However, we show in this chapter that power structures represent an obstacle to improving not only women's, but also men's health.

Young people's health and their health-related habits

A pattern emerges at an early age, with girls having more physical and psychological symptoms, while boys have a higher rate of accidents and mortality (Hammarström 1996; Children's Ombudsman 1995). This pattern is magnified in adulthood. The trend is toward an increase in poor health due to psychological and psychosocial factors, particularly among girls (Children's Ombudsman 1995). Boys have a higher mortality rate than girls, but it is declining more rapidly than the mortality rate of girls (Swedish National Board of Health and Welfare 1991), primarily because of a longstanding public-health effort to prevent accidents.

Young people's health habits lay the groundwork for their future health. There are substantial gender differences in these habits that appear to affect people's health, some immediately, others not until ten or twenty years later. Teenage boys have worse health habits than girls in a number of respects. They brush their teeth less often, consume more alcohol, have worse sleeping and eating habits and are more careless with contraception (Hammarström 1996). On the other hand, girls exercise less than boys and smoke more cigarettes, although Swedish boys' use of snuff balances out the gender difference in tobacco consumption (ibid.). These habits shed light on how gender is constructed within any given society. The construction of the dominant form of masculinity means, among other things, an achievement orientation, risk-taking and a focus on proving themselves. As Connell points out, patriarchy has emotional and physical costs for males, often associated with the stress and violence needed to maintain hierarchies (Connell 1996). The construction of the dominant form of femininity, on the other hand, tends to be based on taking responsibility and on a relational orientation (described in more detail below), which have a more beneficial effect on health. Compared with males, females are, for example, less likely to take risks, and more likely to use bicycle helmets, seatbelts and other safety equipment (Hammarström 1992).

Early on, health and health habits are already unevenly distributed in the population, depending primarily on gender, age, socioeconomic status and ethnic background. Those with the worst health status are young women from socially disadvantaged environments who find themselves unemployed at an early age (Hammarström 1996). It is important to address the conditions affecting these teenage girls, particularly in view of their relatively high rates of alcohol consumption, cigarette use and sexual risk-taking, coupled with poor psychological and physical health and pessimism about the future. A common denominator for many of these girls is a lack of self-confidence and control at school, in their leisure time and in their relationships with boys.

Eating disorders constitute a serious threat to the health and well-being of young women. Studies indicate that as early as sixth grade, girls are restricting their food intake in hopes of losing weight. Anorexia nervosa and bulimia have attracted increasing attention in recent years. The number of diagnosed cases of anorexia has risen markedly over the past two decades (Szmukler 1985, Swedish National Board of Health and Welfare 1991). It is uncertain to what extent this reflects an increase in incidence or an increase in diagnosed cases. However, it appears clear that the incidence of bulimia has indeed risen. There is a widespread misconception that eating disorders are most likely to develop in high socioeconomic groups. A literature review shows no scientific foundation for this belief (Gard & Freeman 1997). On the contrary, increasing evidence suggests that the opposite may be true with respect to bulimia nervosa.

One of the most serious and at the same time one of the least visible public health problems today is the violence, oppression and exploitation that girls, and to a lesser degree boys, are exposed to, mostly at the hands of their fathers, stepfathers and other men they know well. Fear, shame and depression prevent most victims from telling others about such abuse, especially when the perpetrator is a relative (Gillander-Gådin & Hammarström 2000). Accordingly, there is a substantial problem that is not reflected in the statistics we have available. A Swedish study has estimated that seven percent of all women and one percent of all men have been exposed to sexual abuse before they reach the age of 18 (Rönnström 1986). More and more psychological, somatic and social problems turn out to be related to sexualized violence in childhood. Experiences of sexual abuse can, among children and youth, manifest themselves as anxiety, depression, difficulty in making contacts, drug abuse, suicide attempts, eating disorders and headaches (Martins 1989).

Gender relations

In order to understand the origin of gendered health differences, it is important to shed light on unequal power structures in the relationships between girls and boys as well as between women and men.

A study of children in the elementary grades shows gender differences with respect to how children take responsibility and their degree of relational orientation (Gillander-Gådin & Hammarström 2000). Among 11- to 12-year-old children, a gendered pattern emerges, with girls performing more domestic tasks than boys, such as cleaning and washing dishes. The study also showed gendered expectations with respect to domestic duties in adulthood. One in five boys expects to do less housework than his partner, while eight in ten assume that they will share responsibility equally with their partners. Virtually none of the boys expects to do most of the housework. In contrast, 28 percent of the girls assume that they will do most of the domestic work, while 70 percent expect to do an equal share and only two percent anticipate doing less than their partners.

This suggests that there will be continued inequality in the distribution of household responsibilities, even if more young people today than in the past share such responsibilities. This conclusion is backed up by the youth surveys conducted by the Institute for Future Studies (Andersson et al. 1993). The three areas to which young people give highest priority are the family and social relationships, work or school and personal health. Young women attach highest priority to the family, while work is most important to young men. The same study notes that women still choose courses of study that involve social interaction, while men focus on technical subjects. This reinforces gender segregation in the labor market.

Gender-oriented classroom research has shown how gender is constructed at school (Spender 1980; Mahony 1983; Käller 1990; Thorne 1993). While boys are taught to develop a strong sense of self-confidence and encouraged to dominate, girls are brought up to wait, to expect to be interrupted and to accept the fact that boys dominate. Girls are expected to take responsibility for maintaining harmony in the classroom, which gives them less opportunity than boys to develop self-confidence and assertiveness, as well as less influence and control at school. The low level of influence girls have, combined with the responsibility and demands placed upon them, is associated with an increased risk of both psychological and physical illness, even at a young age (Hammarström et al. 1988). Boys, on the other hand, are permitted to dominate, to avoid responsibility and to disparage girls. This leads to obvious health risks for them as well as for girls. Dominance and a lack of a sense of responsibility are important factors in injuries and violence at school, where boys cause at least four out of five injuries to both girls and boys (Hammarström & Janlert 1994). Other boys end up very low in the hierarchy, or find themselves excluded entirely, which leads to a clear increase in their risk not only of injuries, but also of stress and psychological difficulties.

In recent years, more and more attention has been paid to the conditions affecting girls at school. Some schools have initiated classroom training to counteract the dominance of boys and to reinforce girls' self-confidence. The idea of changing boys' behavior provokes strong objections in some quarters (Sinkkonen 1992; Kryger 1993). The objections are based on an interpretation of boys' (and girls') behavior from a prevailing biological model.[14] If this view were to predominate in shaping people's expectations and behaviors, there is a clear risk that sex and gender stereotypes might persist or perhaps worsen, which could in turn lead to negative health effects.

Statistics show that youth violence has increased in recent years. Assault is by far the most common violent crime. The number of assaults committed by boys, primarily between the ages of 15 and 17, more than doubled over the ten-year period from 1984 to 1994 (Olsson 1995). Assaults occur both during and after school hours. Studies show that one in four injuries occurring during school hours is caused by other pupils, mainly boys (Hammarström & Janlert 1994). Girls are particularly vulnerable to violence perpetrated by boys at school; their risk of being injured at school is about three times as high as their risk of injury outside of school (ibid.). For boys the risk is twice as great. Injuries with more serious medical consequences, like injuries to the head region, are more common in school than outside of school.

There are some indications that violence may continue to increase as the unemployment rate increases. An ecological study conducted in the United States and covering the period from 1947 to 1976 shows that an increase of one percent in youth unemployment led to an increase of between 6 and 20 percent in violent crimes, including sexualized violence,[15] such as rape and prostitution (Brenner 1980). The mortality rate among nonwhite young men was estimated to increase by between 4 and 7 percent, as a result of murder, motor-vehicle accidents and suicide.

The consequences of youth unemployment

What will the future bring for the generation of young people who are hard-hit by the effects of unemployment today? Unemployment immediately upon completing basic schooling is linked to a high risk of later unemployment, particularly for young men (Hammarström & Janlert 1999). This is true despite the major efforts that have been made to reduce youth unemployment. The health consequences of youth unemployment have been widely documented, in terms not only of physical and psychological health, but also of poor health habits and social consequences such as financial problems, lower work motivation and increased passivity (Winefield 1995, Hammarström 1994). Research has shown that exposure effects are greater than selection effects, that is, poor health among the unemployed can be more readily ascribed to unemployment per se than to the personal characteristics of the unemployed. There are clear gender differences, with a much higher increase in alcohol consumption and sexual risk-taking among young men, while unemployed young women smoke more and experience more somatic symptoms (Hammarström 1996). Thus, the future is not particularly bright for today's unemployed youth, at least for those with the most limited job prospects.

The unemployment rate increased dramatically in Sweden in the early 1990s. From a level of 4 percent in 1990, the youth unemployment rate quadrupled among women and increased seven-fold among men by 1993, after which it remained stable for a few years at about 20 percent. Since 1997 the rate has been declining. Many young people who experience unemployment come from families where at least one parent is unemployed. Consequently, in areas of Britain with high levels of unemployment we are seeing a third generation of unemployed people, with all the problems of isolation and pessimism about the future one might expect (Roberts 1997). This may be in store for Sweden, too, unless the unemployment rate declines. Mass unemployment can lead to a number of other negative consequences for jobless workers. In Sweden, unemployment benefits were cut when unemployment became a widespread phenomenon. A loss of financial resources increases the risk of poor health. Furthermore, it is considerably more difficult for people who are unemployed during a recession to return to work when the economic climate improves. When many people are looking for work, it is easier for employers to rule out job seekers who are not in perfect health, which leads to a more stringent selection process in hiring workers. Even minor health problems, such as mild allergies or less serious psychological difficulties, may make it hard for people to return to work. A society appears to be emerging in which two-thirds of the population are well-off, while one-third find themselves excluded from jobs, prosperity and good health.

Work is crucial to young people's identity development and socialization (Hammarström 1996; Ovesen 1978), since it offers them an environment in which they can experience a sense of self-worth and personal development. If young people are deprived of the opportunity for work, they may be forced to choose other, more negative frames of reference to create their own identity, which may leave a lasting mark on their health. The effects of unemployment may have different consequences for women's and men's future health. Long-term unemployed men describe how unemployment makes them lethargic and passive. They have stopped struggling and live one day at a time, without thought of the future. The construction of the dominant form of masculinity among these working class, long-term unemployed young men is built up around compensating for not having a waged work, through e.g. out-acting behaviour in driving, fighting, etc., resulting in increased risk for high alcohol consumption, sexual risk taking and an overall more anti-social performance (Hammarström 1996).

The femininity of long-term unemployed young women tends to be constructed around a traditional female model, based on motherhood, marriage and domestic duties. Therefore, some of these young women end up on the fringes of society as well, just as unemployed men do, but for other reasons. A study performed during a period of economic prosperity shows that nearly half of these long-term unemployed young women have children by the age of 21, and they frequently end up bearing sole responsibility for their children (Hammarström 1996). They are forced to cope with this difficult task on extremely limited financial resources. They choose their jobs based on whether or not those jobs can be combined with family responsibilities, which drastically reduces these women's advancement in the job world.

In the above-mentioned Swedish study, the risk of future unemployment was much higher for the long-term unemployed young men than for the long-term unemployed young women, a remarkable finding in view of the fact that the young men were more integrated into the labor market (Hammarström & Janlert 1999). The women seem to have more strategies for ending their period of unemployment, for example by migrating, pursuing further education or taking any available job. Their higher rate of activity may be related to how femininity is developed from responsibility-taking and a relational orientation; they suffer not only from their own situation, but also from the problems they cause their children, husband/boyfriend and parents. Compared with men, women are more sensitive to the needs of others and thus more willing to break vicious circles (ibid.).

Relational orientation

The fact that these women seem to handle unemployment better than men does not point to any major inherent differences between men and women. In our society, women most frequently take on most of the responsibility for relational tasks in the family and society at large. This fact does not reflect female characteristics or genes, but is rather a result of gendered differences in power and influence in society. An ability to relate to others does not develop in a social vacuum, unaffected by the hierarchical conditions that surround women in their daily lives. Instead, it appears that the ability to relate to others is characteristic of people in a socially subordinate position (Miller 1976), who develop a heightened sensitivity to the demands and wishes—both spoken and unspoken—of those in a position of dominance. Subordination also means that women become responsible for the "relational work" within the family, in the workplace and in society as a whole. These tasks are often regarded as low-status work by men with power and have therefore been assigned to women, who have lower status. It fits well into this power imbalance that femininity in our society is largely constructed from a relational orientation. Women often seek to remain in fairly constant and close contact with people in their immediate environment, and they find this to be beneficial to their health (Surrey 1991; Miller 1991).

An orientation toward relationships can be assumed to have major effects on health, both positive and negative. For example, in contrast to men, women often reduce their alcohol consumption when they have children, which shows that taking responsibility can have positive consequences, at least in the short term (Hammarström 1996). Positive effects are also associated with the beneficial aspects of having a social network of friends with whom one can discuss problems, and with an ability to share worries and concerns in close reciprocal relationships (Östergren 1991). Over the longer term, however, it is unclear what women's acceptance of responsibility and their relational orientation mean for their health and life circumstances.

Although international research clearly shows that social support has positive health effects, less attention has been paid to the gendered effects of such support. A Swedish study of people between the ages of 65 and 74 shows that among persons with a high degree of social support, women have higher mortality from coronary heart disease than men (Orth-Gomer & Johnson 1987). The gender difference might be explained by the gendered nature of social support; while for men it is a beneficial factor that leads to improved health, for women it also means that there are more demands on them to perform the supporting tasks. Thus, social support means extra work for women and increases their risk of burnout. It is usually women who need to arrange their lives to combine reproductive work at home with gainful employment.

Gender-oriented research has shown that boys and men would have much to gain if they, too, were better able to relate to others (Askew & Ross 1988; Bergman 1991). They would likely be better able to handle crises in their lives if they increased their social competence and had better support networks. The family would also benefit if men assumed more responsibility at home.

How will young women and men respond to changes in the future? As Sweden moves from an industrialized to a post-materialistic society, according to the Institute for Future Studies, there is a clear dichotomy between those born in the 1970s who are leading the way and their peers who would prefer to avoid change. Women with an academic education who come from highly educated backgrounds are among the leaders, while men with practical training tend to resist change. Women often attach more importance to internationalism, flexibility, independent organization and creativity than to productivity, and they value equality, particularly with respect to gender and ethnic background (Anderson et al. 1993). A government report entitled "Young people's welfare and values" (Swedish Government Official Reports 1994), however, reaches quite different conclusions from similar data. According to this report, it is young men who are behind the trend toward change, since they are more market-oriented than women are. Young men are more likely to attach importance to good pay, a secure job and career opportunities (Swedish Government Official Reports 1994). Nearly one-third of young men regard the industrialized society as the ideal, compared with about one in ten women. The report sees women's more collective orientation in their attitude toward the welfare state as reactionary in its effects. Clearly, then, assessments of what is progressive, and perhaps what is desirable, will differ, depending on one's own value system.

General conclusions and some speculation

Change can be viewed from a gender perspective at both the individual and the societal level. There is reason to believe that women will be more vulnerable than men to the effects of societal and labor-market changes. Finding work will be more difficult, and unpaid work is likely to increase. Poorly educated women in occupations involving manual labor will be particularly affected. Women with more education, however, will be well equipped to deal with changes in society and working life by virtue of as-yet untapped skills. Many women today have more education than required by their jobs. In general, women's experience combining family and paid work and bearing responsibility for their children has enhanced their social skills and made them more flexible in dealing with changes in work demands.

The effects of structural changes seem to be more positive for men. Men's training is more likely to correspond to the needs of the labor market. At the individual level, however, the picture for men is less positive. Since men are used to concentrating on one sphere, many of them are not as well equipped to deal with the changes we are witnessing. Men have less experience than women with social relationships, and they appear to have a harder time dealing with unemployment.

Accordingly, it is likely that women will have an easier time meeting the demands of the knowledge society for flexibility, an ability to work with others and the skill of relating and communicating in network organizations. Social integration and self-confidence gained in a variety of life spheres are mediating factors between working conditions and health (Moen et al. 1989). Women's health would benefit if their experience and interests could be put to greater use in working life.

Both women and men need time and financial resources if they are to be involved in the private sphere. There is much to indicate that workplaces in which there is a more equal distribution of men and women doing similar jobs enhance people's consciousness of gender equality. Reducing gender segregation at work and changing how gainful employment is distributed at different stages of life and among different population groups should benefit the health of both women and men. Table 12.1 outlines possible health consequences of different ways of combining gainful employment and unpaid work in the private sphere

Table 12.1. Different ways of combining employment and private life, and how they affect health

Employment	Unpaid work in the private sphere		
	Primary responsibility	Shared responsibility	Little responsibility
Stressful	1. Major risk to health	2.	3. Risk to health
Good	4.	5. Best health	6.
None	7. Risk to health	8.	9. Major risk to health

The table presumes that the association between an individual's life situation and his or her health is the same for women and men. This assumption is supported by recent empirical studies, carried out at a time when the ideals of democracy and equality are generally accepted, as well as by published historical analyses. Since women's life circumstances differ from those of men (most women are found in groups 1 and 4 and most men in groups 3 and 6), it is important to focus on gender-specific measures to improve health.

It is almost exclusively women who have both a stressful job and primary responsibility for their home and children (group 1). In this not uncommon situation, women are involved in both spheres, but their total stress level is too high. If the trend begun in the 1980s continues—with an increased percentage of women under a great deal of stress—many women may find their health deteriorating (Szulkin & Thålin 1994).

It is usually men whose activities are restricted to one sphere (groups 3 and 6). We know very little about what this means for men's health. However, men who are involved in both spheres seem to do better than those who focus only on work (Barnett et al. 1992, Bejerot & Härenstam 1995). It would benefit the health of both women and men if male involvement in the private sphere began when boys were still in school and continued in a job world that provided more parental leave and offered shorter work hours for employees with small children.

Overtime requirements at work limit the amount of time people can spend with their families. The parents of small children are under particular pressure in a labor market with intense competition for jobs. Furthermore, many families with young children are under a great deal of economic pressure and in need of additional income. Even when men are willing to do more of the work at home, financial considerations may force them to concentrate on their jobs. The other side of the coin is that men who do more of the unpaid work in the private sphere find a better balance between the two life spheres, which can help to improve both women's and men's health. Less support from society means greater dependence on family members, both socially and economically. It is likely to be women, particularly in low-income families with substantial needs to be met, who will end up assuming responsibility for most of the family's unpaid work, while they also work outside the home wherever possible to maintain the family's standard of living.

Unemployment creates an imbalance for both women and men (groups 7, 8 and 9 in Table 12.1) and has major health implications for young people as well as adults (Public Health Group 1992). When an individual also has little responsibility in the private sphere (group 9), as is often true of unemployed young people, the result is understimulation and a lack of social integration, leading to negative health consequences. Unless unemployment is reduced, more women and men will find their health at risk.

If unemployment remains at its current high level or rises further, societal factors will have a significant impact on health trends. Large numbers of women are at risk of unemployment and a decline in their quality of life when the public sector downsizes and other sectors fail to pick up the slack. There is a great deal of pressure on those who are able to keep their jobs as well as those who are let go.

Women's future health will depend on what jobs are available, as well as how they are treated within the medical system when they seek help for problems related to their life circumstances. It is very tempting to seek a *medical* diagnosis for the symptoms people develop, even when they are only a natural reaction to problems in their lives. Excessive reliance on the biological models may lead to labeling women as sick when their problems are really the result of a difficult situation in their lives, such as an excessively high stress level, relationship problems or financial concerns. Unnecessary gender differences in health may develop when medical theory and practice focus on the biological and disregard the sociocultural differences that exist between the sexes. More insight into women's illnesses should be accompanied by more insight into women's life circumstances, as well as further information on methods and conditions for preventive and rehabilitative measures geared to women's needs.

How women and men act and react in response to social changes is a function of the ideals communicated to them. School, the mass media and the culture play an important role, especially for young people. Particularly in commercials, young women seem more and more to be presented as thin, passive children with erotic appeal or as submissive "victims," while young men are shown as muscular, active, dominating and aggressive. A gap between the ideals presented in the media and a young person's perception of his or her own circumstances can undermine self-esteem. Such individual-level factors obviously affect people's identity development and health.

Many other factors will also affect women's and men's health in the future. We have not mentioned such environmental factors as air and water pollution, nor the increased incidence of allergens. These factors are of obvious significance for public health, and they may affect women's and men's health in different ways.

A rise in the share of elderly people in the population, coupled with fewer resources for elderly care, may result in more people suffering from significant health problems than ever. Since women will probably take on the bulk of responsibility for care that is no longer provided by the public sector, women's health will be at particular risk.[16] How immigrants are integrated into Swedish society will affect their health, too. There is cause for concern in this context that women from an immigrant background will be especially vulnerable, with a further increase in illnesses of the musculoskeletal system and mental-health problems as possible consequences. Children who have escaped war and torture to come to Sweden, as well as children growing up in disadvantaged, segregated areas, will be future risk groups, particularly in terms of mental health.

Offsetting these disheartening prospects are increased knowledge of the causes of women's and men's ill health and the determination to put that knowledge to work through practical medical care and preventive public health efforts. Also significant are a heightened health consciousness among the population, increased interest among young people in an ecologically sound society and in post-materialistic values that attach more importance to quality of life than to material goods. Such attitudinal shifts affect what happens at the structural and political level, which in turn may have a long-term positive effect on health.

In this chapter we have dealt primarily with changes in working life and the private sphere. The distribution of work and power between women and men (the gender contract) and between the public and the private sector (the social contract) form the context for individuals' life circumstances.

If changes were to occur in both the social and the gender contract, class differences in health might take precedence over gender differences. If the social contract continues to change, with responsibilities transferred from the public to the private sector and increasing numbers of women unwilling to put up with subordination to men and demanding equal pay and power (changed gender contract), the political and economic system might consider facilitating the purchase of household services. The lives of well-educated and well-paid women would then become more similar to those of men, resulting in reduced stress and improved health. It is doubtful that low-income women and men would have the resources to purchase help with household and family responsibilities, even with tax subsidies. Thus women with little education could well experience an increase in overall stress, resulting in worse health.

Trends in both women's and men's health would benefit if the responsibilities transferred from the public to the private sector (changed social contract) were shared by men much more than they are today (changed gender contract). However, there would have to be a substantial increase in men's contributions in order to equalize the gender differences that already exist, as well as to offset the greater burden resulting from a changed social contract. To keep men's total stress at a manageable level, major changes would be required on the job to enable men to invest more time in their homes and families. A movement in this direction, however, appears unlikely.

A third vision of the future, and the most positive scenario, is one in which the burden of work on the job and at home is distributed more evenly between women and men in all social classes and at all life stages. That, too, would presuppose a change in the social and gender contracts as well as a decrease in unemployment. Such changes at both the societal and the individual level could be expected to lead to an improvement in women's and men's health.

We see a danger that changes in society and working life may result in health consequences that differ depending on an individual's class, gender and ethnicity. A change in the social contract would affect everyone, but particularly people dependent on society's support. Accordingly, class, gender and ethnic differences in health are likely to increase. The well educated, particularly those in technical fields, most frequently men, will have the easiest time finding jobs. Unemployment is likely to increase among the poorly educated as well as those trained for work in the public sector, primarily women.

A common family scenario today, in which the husband works full-time in the private sector and the wife works part-time in the public sector, may become less common. Instead, we may see an increase in the number of one-earner families, with more women financially dependent on their husbands, increased financial stress and worse health for both men and women. This may lead to a society marked by a larger gap between one- and two-earner families and heightened class differences between women. In the past, class differences in women's health have not been as great as among men.

Economic and social vulnerability limits opportunities for changing the relationships between women and men by restricting individuals' choices and ability to negotiate. Many women and men are constrained by necessity and unable to alter their life circumstances. A changed gender contract, then, is likely to have disparate effects on different social classes, particularly if society's role in caregiving responsibilities decreases and the high rate of unemployment continues. Class differences would increase, both in life circumstances and health, and gender differences in health would decrease, but only among the well-educated. We can only hope that we are mistaken in these more pessimistic prognoses for the future.

Notes

1 Study summarized in the article "Extrem utslagning av äldre industriarbetare" [Elimination of older industrial workers from the job world] published in Svenska Dagbladet, December 30, 1993.

2 See article entitled "Jobb när det passar dig bäst" [Work when it's most convenient] from Dagens Nyheter 1994–04–24, which describes the use of this type of system by Karolinska Hospital's orthopedic department.

3 For a discussion of views on the gender division of labor and the concepts "gender system" and "gender contract," see the anthology "Kontrakt i kris" [Contract in crisis] by Gertrud Åström and Yvonne Hirdman (Eds.) and SOU 1990: 44, Chapter 3, Genussystemet [Gender system].

4 See, for example, Søgaard 1994.

5 The role concept is analyzed from a historical and theoretical perspective in Chapter 1, p. 2.

6 See for example Kerstin Uvnäs-Moberg (1988): "Kvinnligt och manligt. En skapelsesaga i nytt biologiskt perspektiv" [Female and male: A creation story from a new biological perspective]. Läkartidningen, 10:814–818.

7 See for example Hon och han, födda olika [Male and female: Born different] by Rigmor Robert and Kerstin Uvnäs-Moberg, Brombergs, Stockholm 1994 and Sedan du fött [After you have given birth] by Maria Borelius, Stockholm 1994.

8 See Chapter 10.

9 For a summary, see Karasek & Theorell 1990.

10 See also an article by Ann Marie Berggren entitled "Ökad tryck på kvinnor i hårdnad arbetsmarknad" [Increased pressure on women in a difficult job market"] in

Svenska Dagbladet, December 3, 1995, and Lars Jalmert: "Den svenske mannen" [The Swedish man], 1984. Approximately 30 percent of men report that they share housework and home and family responsibilities, 20 percent leave these things to their wives, and about 50 percent say that they would like to share such responsibilities, but it is not feasible.

11 The concepts of "power," "status," "relative number" and "opportunities" have been developed for studying in structural terms what factors affect women's position in the job world (Moss Kanter 1977). These concepts have also been used in studies to determine what affects women's negotiating position with respect to housework (Bejerot & Härenstam 1995; Björnberg 1992; Roman 1992).

12 See also Diderichsen et al. 1993, Björnberg 1992.

13 See also the article "Fri tid åt alla" [Free time for all] by Christer Sanne, appearing in Dagens Nyheter, October 7, 1995, and Sanne C 1995.

14 See for example Robert & Uvnäs-Moberg 1994.

15 Sexualized violence refers both to individual incidents of violence against women (physical, psychological) and to structural violence against women (pornography, prostitution, etc.).

16 See Chapter 11.

References

Andersson Å, Fürth T, Holmberg I. *70-talister—om värderingar förr, nu och i framtiden [The 70s generation: Values systems past, present and future].* Stockholm: Natur och Kultur, 1993. (Available in Swedish only).

Aronsson G, Sjögren A. *Samhällsomvandling och arbetsliv. Omvärldsanalys inför 2000-talet [Social change and working life: A pre-millennial analysis].* Fakta från Arbetsmiljöinstitutet, 1994. (Available in Swedish only).

Askew S, Ross C. *Boys don't cry.* Milton Keynes, 1988.

Åstrom G, Hirdman Y. *Kontrakt i kris. Om kvinnors plats i välfärdsstaten [Contract in crisis: Women's role in the welfare state].* Stockholm: Carlsson Bokförlag, 1992. (Available in Swedish only).

Åström L. *Fäder och söner. Bland svenska män i tre generationer [Fathers and sons: Three generations of Swedish men].* Stockholm: Carlssons Förlag, 1990. (Available in Swedish only).

Barnett R, Baruch G. *Social roles, gender and psychological distress.* In: Barnett R, Biener L, Baruch G (Eds.): Gender and Stress. New York: Free Press, 1987; 122–143.

Barnett R, Brennan R, Marshall N. *Gender and the relationship between parent role, quality and psychological distress.* Journal of Family Issues, 1994; 15:229–252.

Barnett R, Marshall N, Pleck J. *Men's Multiple Roles and their Relationship to Men's Psychological Distress.* Journal of Marriage and the Family, 1992; 54:358–367.

Bejerot E, Härenstam A. *Att förena arbete och familj [Combining work and family].* In: Westlander et al.: På väg mot det goda arbetet [On the way toward good working conditions], Solna: Arbetslivsinstitutet, 1995:123–147. (Available in Swedish only).

Bergman JS. *Men's psychological development: A relational perspective.* Stone Center, Wesley College: Work in Progress, 1991.

Billing Dye Y. *Køn, karriere, familie [Gender, career, family].* Copenhagen: Jurist- og Økonomforbundet, 1991.

Bird C, Fremont A. *Gender, Time Use, and Health.* Journal of Health and Social Behavior, 1991; 32:114–129.

Björnberg U. *Family Orientation Among Men—Fatherhood and Partnership in a Comparative Context.* In: Drew E, Emerek R, and Mahon E, *Families, Labour Markets and Gender Roles.* A Report on a European Research Workshop, Dublin, 7-9 September 1994. European Foundation for the Improvement of Living and Working Conditions. Luxembourg, Office for Official Publications of the European Communities, ref. nr. EF/95/12/EN, 1995.

Björnberg U. *Well-being among Swedish employed mothers with preschool children.* In: Orth-Gomér K, Chesney M, Wenger N (Eds): *Women, Stress and Heart Disease.* London: Lawrence Erlbaum Associates, Publishers, 1998;133-149.

Blomqvist M. *Könshierarkier i gungning. Kvinnor i kunskapsföretag [Gender hierarchies in flux: Women in knowledge industries].* University of Uppsala: Department of Sociology, 1994. (English summary).

Bolger N, Delongis A, Kessler R, Wethington E. *The contagion of stress across multiple roles.* Journal of Marriage and the Family, 1989; 51:175–183.

Borelius M. *Sedan du fött [After you have given birth].* Stockholm: Fischer, 1994. (Available in Swedish only).

Brenner MH. *Estimating the social costs of youth unemployment problems 1947–1976. The Vice President's task force on youth unemployment.* Waltham: Brandeis University, Center for Public Service, 1980.

Children's Ombudsman [Barnombudsmannen]: *Upp till 18 — fakta om barn och ungdom [Up to 18: Facts about children and youth].* Stockholm: SCB, 1995. (Available in Swedish only).

Connell RW. *Teaching the boys: New research on masculinity, and gender strategies for schools.* Teachers College Record 1996; 98:207–35.

Coser L. *Greedy institutions.* New York: Free Press, 1974.

Diderichsen F, Kindlund H, Vogel J. *Kvinnans sjukfrånvaro. Arbetsmiljön orsak till kraftig ökning [Women's work absences: The work environment as a cause of a substantial increase].* Läkartidningen, 1993; 90:289–292. (English summary).

Edlund C, Ahltorp B, Andersson G, Kleppestø S. *Karriärer i kläm. Om chefen, familjen och företaget [Careers caught in the middle: Boss, family and business].* Stockholm: Nordstedts förlag, 1990. (Available in Swedish only).

Frankenhaeuser M, Lundberg U, Fredrikson BM, Toumisto M, Myrsten AL. *Stress on and off the job as related to sex and occupational status in white-collar workers.* Journal of Organizational Behavior, 1989; 10:321–346.

Furåker B. *Vad händer med kvinnornas jobb när den offentliga sektorn bantas? [What happens to women's jobs when the public sector downsizes?]* In: Kvinnors arbetsmarknad. 1990-talet—återtågets tionde? Arbetsmarknadsdepartement [Ministry of Labor]. Stockholm: Allmänna förlaget, Ds 1993:8. (Available in Swedish only).

Gard MC, Freeman CP. *The dismantling of a myth: A review of eating disorders and socioeconomic status.* Int J Eat Disord 1996 Jul;20(1):1–12.

Gillander-Gådin K, Hammarström A. *School-related health—a cross-sectional study among young boys and girls.* Int. J. Health Serv. 2000;30(4):797–820.

Gillander-Gådin K, Hammarström A. *Betydelsen av att synliggöra unga flickors hälsa och livsvillkor ur ett könsteoretiskt perspektiv [The importance of visualizing the health and life circumstances of young girls from a gender perspective].* Socialmedicinsk tidskrift 1999;75(1–2):53–56. (Available in Swedish only).

Goode WA. *Theory of Strain.* American Sociological Review, 1960;25:483-496.

Gonäs L, Plantenga J & Rubery J (Eds.). *Den könsuppdelade arbetsmarknaden—ett europeiskt perspektiv. Kunskapsöversikt [The gender-segregated labor market—a European perspective. A review of what we know].* Arbetslivsinstitutet, 1999. (Available in Swedish only).

Gonäs L, Spånt A (1997). *Trends and Prospects for Women's Employment in the 1990s.* Arbete och Hälsa, [Work and Health], 1997;4. National Institute for Working Life, Stockholm, Sweden.

Gove WR, Zeiss C. *Multiple roles and happiness.* In: Crosby F (Ed.): Spouse, parent and worker: On gender and multiple roles. New Haven: Yale University Press, 1987.

Hall E. *Gender, Work Control and Stress: A Theoretical Discussion and an Empirical Test.* In: Johnson J, Johansson G (Eds.): The Psychosocial Work Environment: Work Organization, Democratization and Health. New York: Baywood Publishing Company, Inc., 1991:89–107.

Hall E. *Double exposure: The combined impact of the home and work environment in psychosomatic strain in Swedish women and men.* International Journal of Health Services, 1992;20:239–260.

Hammarström A. *Skaderegistreringen i Gällivare sjukvårdsdistrikt [Registry of injuries in the Gällivare health care district].* Report from Socialmedicinska forskningsenheten [Research unit for social medicine] in Luleå 1992 (Available in Swedish only).

Hammarström A. *Health consequences of youth unemployment—review from a gender perspective.* Soc Sci Med 1994;38:699–709.

Hammarström A, Hovelius B. *Kvinnors hälsa ur ett könsteoretiskt perspektiv [Women's health from a gender-theory perspective].* Nordisk Medicin 1994;109:288–291. (English summary).

Hammarström A, Janlert U, Theorell T. *Youth Unemployment and Ill-Health: Results from a 2-Year Follow-Up Study.* Soc. Sci. Med, 1988;26(10):1025–1033.

Hammarström A, Janlert U. *Epidemiology of School Injuries in the Northern Part of Sweden.* Scand J Soc Med 1994;22(2):120–126.

Hammarström A, Janlert U. *Do early unemployment and health status among young men and women affect their possibility of later employment?* Scand J Public Health [2000;28(1):10–15].

Hammarström A. *Arbetslöshet och ohälsa—om ungdomars livsvillkor [Unemployment and ill health: Young people's life circumstances].* Studentlitteratur 1996. (Available in Swedish only).

Härenstam A, Westberg H, Karlqvist L, Leijon O, Rydbeck A, Waldenström K, Wiklund P, Nise G, Jansson C. *Hur kan könsskillnader i arbets—och livsvillkor förstås? Metodologiska och strategiska aspekter samt sammanfattning av MOA-projektets resultat ur ett könsperspektiv.* Arbete och Hälsa, 2000;15. [Work and Health], (English summary).

House JS, Kahn RL. *Productivity, stress and health in middle and late life.* Proposal to the National Institute on Aging, 1984.

Jakobsen L, Karlsson JC. *Arbete och kärlek. En utveckling av livsformanalys [Work and love: Developing lifestyle analysis].* Lund: Arkiv, 1993. (Available in Swedish only).

Jalmert L. *Den svenske mannen [The Swedish man].* Tidens Förlag, Stockholm 1984. (Available in Swedish only).

Jeppson Grassman E. *Frivilliga insatser i Sverige—en befolkningsstudie [Volunteer work in Sweden: A population study].* In: Socialdepartementet: Frivilligt socialt arbete. Stockholm: Statens offentliga utredningar, 1993:82. (Available in Swedish only).

Jonung C. *Yrkessegregeringen mellan kvinnor och män [Occupational segregation of men and women].* In: Persson I & Wadensjö E (Eds.). Glastak och glasväggar? Den könssegregerade arbetsmarknaden [Glass ceiling or glass walls? The gender-segregated labor market]. SOU 1997:137, Fritzes, Stockholm. (Available in Swedish only).

Kahn RL. *Work and everyday life.* In: Enander A, Gustavsson BO, Karlsson JC, Starrin B (Eds.). Work and Welfare. Papers from the Second Karlstad Symposium on Work. Research Report 91:7, University of Karlstad, 1991.

Käller KL. *Fostran till andrarang [Bringing them up to be second-rate].* Uppsala: Acta universitatis Upsalienses, 1990 [Uppsala studies in education 34]. (English summary).

Karasek R, Theorell T. *Healthy Work—Stress, Productivity, and the Reconstruction of Working Life.* New York: Basic Books Inc., Publishers, 1990.

Kilbom Å, Messing K, Bildt Thorbjörnsson C (Eds.). *Women's health at work.* Swedish National Institute for Working Life, 1999.

Kindlund H. *Kvinnoroll och sjukfrånvaro [The female role and work absences].* In: Vogel J, Kindlund H, Diderichsen F (Eds.). Arbetsförhållanden, ohälsa och sjukfrånvaro 1975–1989. (Report 78:135–148). Stockholm: Statistiska Centralbyrån 1993. (Available in Swedish only).

Kryger N. *Om pojkars svårigheter att anpassa sig till skolan [Boy's difficulties adjusting to school].* In: Visst är vi olika, Stockholm: Utbildningsdepartementet, 1993;15–17. (Available in Swedish only).

Lagerlöf E. *Women, Work and Health.* National Report Sweden. Ministry of Health and Social Affairs, Regeringskansliets tryckeri, Ds 1993:83.

Lennon MC, Rosenfield S. *Women and Mental Health: The Interaction of Job and Family Conditions.* Journal of Health and Social Behavior, 1992;33:316–327.

Lindbladh E. *Fallgropar vid mätning av kontroll [Pitfalls in measuring control].* Socialmedicinsk tidskrift, 1993;5:252–256. (Available in Swedish only).

Lundberg U, Palm K. *Workload and catecholamine excretion in parents of preschool children.* Work and Stress, 1989;3:255–260.

Lundberg U, Mårdberg B, Frankenhaeuser M. *The total workload of male and female white collar workers as related to occupational level, age, number of children.* Scandinavian Journal of Psychology 1994;35:315–327.

Mahony P. *Schools for the boys?* London: Hutchinson, 1985.

Marklund S. (ed). *Working Life and Health in Sweden.* National Institute for Working Life, Stockholm, 2001.

Martens PL. *Sexualbrott mot barn [Sexual crimes against children].* Stockholm: Allmänna Förlaget, 1989. (Available in Swedish only).

Miller JB. *Toward a New Psychology of Women.* Boston: Beacon Press, 1976.

Miller JB. *Development of Women's Sense of Health.* In: Jordan J et al.: Women's Growth in Connection. New York: Guilford Press 1991;11–26.

Moen PH, Dempster-McClain D, Williams R. *Social integration and longevity: An event history analysis of women's roles and resilience.* American Sociological Review 1989;54:635–647.

Moen PH, Robinson J, Fields V. *Women's work and caregiving roles: A life course approach.* Journal of Gerontology: Social Sciences, 1994;49:176–186.

Moss Kanter R. *Men and women of the corporation.* New York: Basic Books Inc., Publishers, 1977.

Nermo M. *Den ofullbordade jämställdheten [Incomplete equality].* In: Fritzell J, Lundberg O (Eds.): Vardagens villkor. Stockholm: Brombergs, 1994. (Available in Swedish only).

Nilsson A. *Den nye mannen—finns han redan? [The new man: Does he exist yet?]* In: Acker et al. Kvinnors och mäns liv och arbete. Stockholm: SNS Förlag, 1992. (Available in Swedish only).

Oakley A. *Who cares for health? Social relations, gender and public health.* Journal of Epidemiology and Community Health, 1994;48:427–434.

Ohlander A. *Den historiska konflikten mellan produktion och reproduktion [The historical conflict between production and reproduction].* In: Modernt familjeliv och familjeseparationer. En antologi från ett forskarseminarium [Modern family life and family separations: An anthology from a research seminar]. Socialvetenskapliga forskningsrådet. Kommittén för FN:s familjeår, Socialdepartementet. Stockholm 1993. (Available in Swedish only).

Olsson M. *Ungdomar och våldsbrott [Young people and violent crime].* Apropå 1995;2–3,22–27. (Available in Swedish only).

Orth-Gomer K, Johnson J. *Social network interaction and mortality—a six-year follow-up study of a random sample of the Swedish population.* Journal of Chronic Diseases 1987;40:949–957.

Östergren, PO. *Psychosocial resources and health—with special reference to social network, social support and cardiovascular disease.* Malmö: Dept of Social Medicine 1991 (academic thesis).

Östergren PO, Lindbladh E, Isacsson SO, Odeberg H, Svensson SE. *Social Network, Social Support and the Concept of Control—A Qualitative Study Concerning the Validity of Certain Stressor Measures Used in Quantitative Social Epidemiology.* Scand J Soc Med, 1995;23:95–102.

Ovesen E. *Arbetslöshetens psykiska följdverkningar* [*The psychological consequences of unemployment*]. Stockholm: Raben & Sjögren, 1978. (Available in Swedish only).

Public Health Group [Folkhälsogruppen]: *Arbetslöshet som folkhälsoproblem* [*Unemployment as a public-health problem*]. Stockholm, 1992:17. (Available in Swedish only).

Pugliesi K. *Work and wellbeing: Gender differences in the psychological consequences of employment.* Journal of Health and Social Behavior, 1995;36:57–71.

Puranen B. *Finns en konflikt mellan arbetstid, hälsa och välfärd?* [*Is there a conflict between working hours, health and welfare?*] Socialmedicinsk tidsskrift, 1995;2–3:74–86. (Available in Swedish only).

Robert R, Uvnäs-Moberg K. *Hon och Han. Födda Olika* [*Male and female: Born different*]. Stockholm: Bromberg, 1994. (Available in Swedish only).

Roberts K. *Is there an emerging British "underclass"?* In: MacDonald R (Ed.). Youth, the "underclass" and social exclusion. London: Routledge, 1997.

Roman, C. *Yrkesliv och Familjeliv. En studie av kvinnor i arbetslivet* [*Working life and family life: A study of women in working life*]. Uppsala: Sociologiska Institutionen, 1992. (Available in Swedish only).

Roman C. *Lika på olika villkor. Könssegregering i kunskapsföretaget* [*Equal under unequal conditions: Gender segregation in the knowledge industry*]. Stockholm/Stehag: Symposium Graduale, 1994 (academic thesis). (English summary).

Rosenfield S. *The Effects of Women's Employment: Personal Control and Sex Differences in Mental Health.* Journal of Health and Social Behavior, 1989;30:77–91.

Rydenstam K. *I tid och otid. En undersökning om kvinnors och mäns tidsanvändning 1990/1991* [*At all times and seasons: A study of women's and men's time use 1990/1991*]. Levnadsförhållanden [Living conditions] Report No. 79. Stockholm: Statistiska Centralbyrån, 1992. (Available in Swedish only).

Rönnström A. *Den smärtsamma verkligheten* [*The painful reality*]. Stockholm: Rädda Barnen, 1986. (Available in Swedish only).

Salomon R, Grimsmo A. *Arbeidsliv mot år 2010* [*Working life up to the year 2010*]. Notat 4/94. Oslo: Arbeidsforskningsinstituttet, 1994. (Available in Norwegian only).

Sanne C. *Arbetets tid* [*Working time*]. Paper No. 15. Nordiska Institutet för samhällsplanering. Stockholm: Carlssons bokförlag, 1995. (Available in Swedish only).

Sinkkonen J. *Till små pojkars försvar* [*In defense of young boys*]. Helsingborg: Forum, 1992. (Available in Swedish only).

Slater P. *On social regression.* American Sociological Review, 1963;28:339–364.

Søgaard A. *Är det verkligen sunt att jobba?* [*Is it really healthy to work?*] In: Schei B, Botten G, Sundby J (Eds.): Kvinnomedicin [Women's medicine]. Falköping: Bonnier Utbildning, 1994. (Available in Swedish only).

Spender D. *Learning to Lose, Sexism and Education.* The Women's Press, 1980.

Statistics Sweden [SCB]: *The Work Environment 1999.* Stockholm: Statistiska centralbyrån 2000. (English summary).

Statistics Sweden [SCB]: *Att klara av arbete–barn–familj [Dealing with work–children–family].* Demografiska rapporter. 1994:1. Stockholm: Statistiska Centralbyrån 1994. (Available in Swedish only).

Steering Committee on Future Health Scenarios: *Work and Health—risk groups and trends.* Dordrecht: Kluwer Academic Publishers, 1994.

Surrey J. *The "Self-in-relation": A Theory of Women's Development.* In: Jordan J et al.: Women's Growth in Connection. New York: Guilford Press, 1991;51–66.

Swedish Foundation for Working Life [Arbetslivsfonden]: *Arbete i utveckling—på kvinnors vis [Work in transition: Women's way].* Final report of the ALFA Q program, Arbetslivsfonden, 1995. (Available in Swedish only).

Swedish Government Official Reports [SOU]: Maktutredningen [Report on power], Chapter 3, Genussystemet [Gender system]. Stockholm: Statens offentliga utredningar, 1990:44. (Available in Swedish only).

Swedish Government Official Reports [SOU]: *Ungdomars välfärd och värderingar [Young people's welfare and value systems].* Stockholm: Statens offentliga utredningar, 1994:73. (Available in Swedish only).

Swedish National Board of Health and Welfare [Socialstyrelsen]: *Folkhälsorapport 1991 [Public Health Report 1991].* SoS-rapport 1991:11. Stockholm, 1991. (Available in Swedish only).

Swedish Trade Union Confederation [LO]: *Klass och kön 1995 [Class and gender 1995].* Stockholm: Landsorganisationen i Sverige, 1995.

Syme L. *Control and health—a personal perspective.* Steptoe A, Apples A (Eds.): Stress, Personal Control and Health. Chichester: John Wiley & Sons, 1989.

Szmukler GI. *The Epidemiology of Anorexia Nervosa and Bulemia.* J Psychiat Res 1985;19(2/3):143–153.

Szulkin R, Tåhlin M. *Arbetets utveckling [The development of work].* In: Fritzell J, Lundberg O (Eds.): Vardagens villkor [The conditions of everyday life]. Stockholm: Brombergs, 1994. (Available in Swedish only).

Theorell T, Härenstam A. *Influence of Gender on Cardiovascular Disease.* In *Handbook of Gender, Culture and Health.* Eisler R M and Hersen M (Eds). Lawrence Erlbaum Associates, Inc, Publishers. 2000:161-177.

Thoits P. *Multiple identities and psychological well-being.* American Sociological Review, 1983;48:174–187.

Thorne B. *Gender play. Girls and boys in school.* Buckingham: Open University Press, 1993.

Uvnäs-Moberg K. *Kvinnligt och manligt. En skapelsesaga i nytt biologiskt perspektiv [Female and male: A creation story from a new biological perspective].* Läkartidningen 1988;10:814–818. (Available in Swedish only).

Vågerö D, Lahelma E. *Women, work and mortality: An Analysis of the relation between female labor force participation and female mortality rates.* In: Orth-Gomér K, Chesney M, Wenger NK (Eds.): Women, stress and heart disease. Mahwah, N.J.: Erlbaum, 1998.

Wallston KA, Wallston BS, Smith S, Dobbins CJ. *Perceived control and health.* Current Psychological Research and Reviews, 1987;6:5–25.

Verbrugge LM. *Women's social roles and health.* In: Berman P, Ramey E (Eds.): Women: A developmental perspective (Publication No. 82–2298). Washington DC: U.S. Government Printing Office, 1982.

Westberg H. *Different worlds.* In Kilbom Å, Messing K, Bildt Thorbjörnsson (eds). *Women's Health at Work.* National Institute for Working Life, Solna, 1998; 27-57.

Wijkström F. *Det organiserade ideella arbetet i Sverige [Organized non-profit work in Sweden].* EFI Research Report. Stockholm School of Economics, 1994. (Available in Swedish only).

Wikander U. *Delat arbete, delad makt: om kvinnors underordning i och genom arbetet [Shared work, shared power: Women's subordination at and through work].* A historical essay. In: Åström G, Hirdman Y. Kontrakt i kris [Contract in crisis]. Stockholm: Carlssons Bokförlag, 1992. (Available in Swedish only).

Wiklund P, Härenstam A. *Eremitkräftan utan skal. Om arbetsförhållanden av betydelse vid organisationsförändring. En kvalitativ studie [Hermit crab without a shell: Working conditions relevant to organizational change. A qualitative study].* Report from the MOA project. Yrkesmedicinska enheten NVSO, Report 1995:9. Stockholm 1995. (Available in Swedish only).

Winefield AH. *Unemployment: its psychological costs.* In: Cooper CL, Robertson IT (Eds.). International Review of Industrial and Organizational Psychology. New York: John Wiley & Sons Ltd., 1995:169–212.

List of Authors

GUNNAR ARONSSON is a Professor of Psychology, specializing in work organization and health, at the Swedish National Institute for Working Life. His research deals primarily with people's control and influence over their working conditions and labor market situation. He has focused in his studies on the working conditions of academics, as well as work in sawmills, local traffic, offices, schools, and social services offered to people in their homes.

MARIA DANIELSSON is a physician with special training in social medicine at the Karolinska Institute, Department of Public Health, Division of Social Medicine. Her recent research is in social epidemiology with main focus on issues related to gender.

FINN DIDERICHSEN is a Professor in social epidemiology and health policy research at the Karolinska Institute, Department of Public Health Sciences, Division of Social Medicine. His research and development work deals mainly with the mechanisms of social aetiology and social inequalities in health as well as the development of epidemiological tools for health policy and planning.

ROLF Å GUSTAFSSON is a Professor of Medical Sociology and has carried out both action-oriented research and historical analysis of work environments and the organization of nursing care. Most recently his interest has focused on the welfare state's new system of economic management. He is currently a researcher at the Swedish National Institute for Working Life.

ANNE HAMMARSTRÖM is a Professor of Public Health, focusing on gender research at the Department of Public Health and Clinical Medicine at Umeå University. She is also a specialist medical doctor in social medicine, working part of her time as a general practitioner. Her overall research program addresses gender and feminism in the new public health, with special focus on reducing gender inequities in health. More specifically her research deals with gender theoretical issues, gender bias in medical research, gender constructions of diseases as well as the gendered health consequences of sexualised violence, unemployment, waged work, school environment and domestic work.

ÖRJAN HEMSTRÖM is a Doctor in sociology, specializing in medical sociology, in the Centre for Health Equity Studies (CHESS) at Stockholm University and at the Swedish National Institute for Working Life. In his thesis he examined particularly the social causes of the gender gap in mortality. His other research is in the area of general social epidemiology such as socioeconomic health differences and alcohol epidemiology.

TORE HÄLLSTRÖM is a Professor of Psychiatry who specializes in social psychiatry at the Karolinska Institute. He is also head of the Psychiatric Research and Development Unit, Huddinge University Hospital as well as the Resource Centre on Eating Disorders, Stockholm County Council. His research focuses largely on women's mental health.

ANNIKA HÄRENSTAM, PhD., is a senior researcher in work psychology at the Swedish National Institute for Working Life. She has conducted research into work organization, stress and health, and is head of the project "Modern working and living conditions of men and women," an interdisciplinary project aimed at developing population studies methods.

KARIN JOHANNISSON is a Professor of History of Ideas and Science at Uppsala University, specializing in History of Medicine. Her publications include *Medicinens öga (Medicine's eye)*, 1990; *Den mörka kontinenten (The dark continent)*, 1994, *Kroppens tunna skal (Body under the skin)*, 1997, and *Nostalgia: History of a diagnosis*, 2001. She is currently working on a history of physical examination.

ÅSA KILBOM is a physician and Professor of Work Physiology at the Swedish National Institute for Working Life. Her research deals with physical work capacity in the context of the demands of working life as well as with the short- and long-term effects of various occupations on illnesses of the locomotor system.

KAREN LEANDER is a *Juris doctor* from the United States. She is employed at the Center for Safety Promotion, Stockholm County Council, and is associated with Karolinska Institute, Department of Public Health Sciences, Division of Social Medicine. Her fields include the study of violence and violence prevention and she serves as an external lecturer at Stockholm University, Department of Criminology.

GUDRUN LINDBERG is a Bachelor of Arts and co-ordinator at the Centre for Epidemiology, Swedish National Board of Health and Welfare. She has been project director for four National Public Health Reports and was formerly in charge of the health component of Statistics Sweden's studies of living conditions (ULF).

ANN-SOFIE OHLANDER is a Professor of History at Örebro University. She has conducted research on Swedish emigration to the United States, the history of women and children, and the history of mental health, including a study of suicide in Sweden from the Middle Ages to the Twentieth Century.

KAJSA SUNDSTRÖM, Professor, MD. PhD, specialist in obstetrics and gynecology. She has been coordinator of Swedish national programs on family planning, abortion, antenatal care and parenthood education, and affiliated to the Karolinska Institute, Department of Public Health Science, Division of International Health, IHCAR. Her research and writing is on women's reproductive health and living conditions.

MARTA SZEBEHELY is an Associate Professor at the Department of Social Work in Stockholm. Her research focuses on care for the elderly in Scandinavia, with particular attention given to changes occurring in home-based care, from the perspectives of care recipients and providers.

TÖRES THEORELL is a Professor of Psychosocial Environmental Medicine at the Karolinska Institute and Director of the Swedish National Institute for Psychosocial Factors and Health. He is a specialist in internal medicine and has conducted research into psychosocial stress and its links to cardiovascular disease, psychosomatic illnesses and physiological responses.

EVA VINGÅRD is an occupational physician and associate professor at the Karolinska Institute in Sweden Her research deals primarily with the risk and health factors for musculoskeletal disorders in men and women, particularly arthrosis and low back pain, and work and health in the public sector.

PIROSKA ÖSTLIN, PhD, is a medical sociologist at the Karolinska Institute, Department of Public Health Sciences, Division of Social Medicine. Her research concerns primarily methodological problems in studies of labor epidemiology, as well as the significance of job environment for women's and men's health.

Index